Pediatric Oncology

Arthur Zimmermann • Giorgio Perilongo
(Editors)

Marcio Malogolowkin • Dietrich von Schweinitz
(Co-Editors)

Pediatric Liver Tumors

Springer

Editors
Arthur Zimmermann
Institute of Pathology of the University
Murtenstrasse 31
3010 Berne
Switzerland
zimmerma@patho.unibe.ch

Giorgio Perilongo
Pediatric Hematology Oncology Division
Pediatric Department
University of Padova
Via Giustiniani 3
35128 Padova
Italy
giorgio.perilongo@unipd.it

Co-Editors
Marcio Malogolowkin
Children's Hospital Los Angeles
Division of Hematology-Oncology
4650 Sunset Blvd., MS #54
Los Angeles CA 90027
USA
mmalogolowkin@chla.usc.edu

Dietrich von Schweinitz
Kinderchirurgische Klinik im
Dr. von Haunerschen Kinderspital
Universität München
Lindwurmstrasse 4
80337 München
Germany
dietrich.schweinitz@med.uni-muenchen.de

ISBN 978-3-642-14503-2 e-ISBN 978-3-642-14504-9
DOI 10.1007/978-3-642-14504-9
Springer Heidelberg Dordrecht London New York

Library of Congress Control Number: 2010938858

Cover design: eStudioCalamar, Figueres/Berlin

Printed on acid-free paper

Springer is part of Springer Science+Business Media (www.springer.com)

Foreword

Even though malignant liver tumors are rare in children, they have attracted interest and best effort, not only of pediatric oncologists and surgeons, but also tumor biologists and geneticists. The result is a significant improvement in our understanding of these tumors, patient's outcome especially those with hepatoblastoma (HB). New developments in diagnostic imaging, tumor biology, pathology, surgical, and orthotopic liver transplant (OLXT) techniques and chemotherapy have contributed to the continued improvement in the survival of children with HB.

The beneficial effect of post-operative adjuvant chemotherapy in patients with completely resected HB and hepatocellular carcinoma (HCC) was first documented by Evans in early 1990. However, the same chemotherapeutic regime failed to improve survival for patients whose tumors were either unresectable or incompletely resected. For many years, complete surgical resection of the tumor was the only treatment modality that could offer children with hepatic malignancy a reasonable opportunity for cure.

The success of doxorubicin (DOX) and cisplatin (CDDP) as the most effective agents in the therapy of HB lead to the North American (Children Oncology Group) and the International Society of Pediatric Oncology (SIOP) collaborative groups to the design and implementation of chemotherapy regimens combining these two agents. Results of these studies established the combination chemotherapy of CDDP/DOX as the most successful therapy in inducing surgical resectability in children with HB, thus making long-term survival an obtainable goal for patients with unresectable tumors. However, the timing of the primary surgery has varied among different groups. The North American and German studies systematically use surgical resection at diagnosis as determined by surgeons (primary surgery). The SIOP studies on the other hand, mandate preoperative chemotherapy. The beneficial effect of the different surgical timing became, for some time, an issue of discrepancy among investigators. Comparison of the data generated by these studies was difficult due to the difference in staging criteria among these groups.

The SIOP group uses the pretreatment extent of tumor grouping system (PRETEXT) based on the extent of the primary tumor as determined by imaging information. The North American and German groups employ a grouping system based upon the outcome of the up-front surgical intervention. To this date, results of the data generated from different studies have not been conclusive with respect to the significance of the timing of the hepatic resection since outcomes have not been significantly different. However, they have reaffirmed that complete resection of the primary tumor continues to be the primary goal in clinical management of pediatric liver tumors.

A recent analysis of pretreatment prognostic factors in the outcome of children with HB seems to indicate that both the COG and PRETEXT grouping system are both good predictive indicators of long term survival. PRETEXT may be used to identify patients who may be amenable to up-front surgical resection and may achieve long-term survival with less intensive chemotherapy since less chemotherapy-related toxicity.

The current COG study evaluates both grouping systems. Considering that most children with HB are younger than two years old, it is of utmost importance to eliminate or reduce the risks of long term chemotherapy-related toxicities without jeopardizing the results of the past. Results of the recently published SIOPEL III documented that PRETEXT standard risk patients achieved with CDDP monotherapy similar rates of complete resectability and survival compared to CDDP/DOXO, thus eliminating the potential cardiotoxicity of the anthracycline.

The significant improvement in survival of children with surgically resectable HB, achieved using CDDP-based chemotherapy unfortunately has not been observed in patients considered at high risk for failure. Among high risk patients are children with persistently unresectable disease, metastatic disease at diagnosis, recurrent disease, slowly declining alphafetoprotein (AFP) or less than 100 ng/mL at diagnosis, and small cell undifferentiated (SCU) histological subtype. In order to improve the outcomes of this group of patients novel therapeutic approaches are required.

High-dose chemotherapy has been used in an effort to improve long-term disease-free survival, but results so far have been disappointing. Irinotecan, a topoisomerase I inhibitor, has been shown in limited studies to have some activity against HB. Its role should be defined in the near future, especially when combined with CDDP/DOXO.

A more recent treatment modality, consisting of hepatic arterial chemoembolization, may be helpful in facilitating tumor resectability in a select group of patients. However, experience with this treatment modality is limited in children. Another potential treatment strategy is orthotopic liver transplant (OLXT). Recent series published by various pediatric liver transplant programs documented that children with unresectable non-metastatic HB transplant, had a similar survival rate as those who achieve complete resectability by conventional surgical procedures. A multinational registry (PLUTO) has been implemented to determine the feasibility and efficacy of OLTX in a large population of children with non-resectable HB.

The significant improvement in disease outcome observed in the last two decades in children with HB unfortunately has not been shared by those with (HCC). Even when these children with HCC have consistently been treated according to HB therapeutic trials, results have so far been extremely disappointing. This confirms the dissimilarity of these two epithelial malignancies of the liver. Surgery for these patients has seldom been complete, and chemotherapy with CDDP/DOXO has not produced the same results as seen with HB.

While adult HCC is associated with etiological factors that lead to liver cirrhosis such as viral hepatitis and alcohol consumption, the same is not observed in children with HCC. While a variety of genetic changes have been identified in adult HCC which may offer the opportunity for the development of novel therapeutic approaches, further evaluation of these changes in pediatric HCC is needed. Similarly, the importance of angiogenesis in the development of HCC should continue to be explored in the quest for effective therapeutic modalities. At the present time, complete tumor resection by standard surgical procedure, or OLXT, constitutes the only therapeutic alternative associated with long-term survival for these patients.

Given the rarity of childhood malignant liver tumors, international collaboration is needed in an effort to identify new treatment strategies, to establish the role of OLXT and development of novel therapeutic approach for patients at high risk of failure (metastatic, SCU, and low AFP patients at diagnosis). The implementation of an international childhood hepatic tumor data base is of utmost importance. It will allow for the identification of prognostic factors independent of the initial therapeutic approach, and the creation of a registry that can be used in the development of future studies.

Jorge A. Ortega

Contents

Contributors

Gianni Bisogno Hematology Oncology Division, Department of Pediatrics, Clinica di Oncoematologia, Via Giustiniani 3, I-35100 Padova, Italy
gianni.bisogno@unipd.it

Jillian M. Birch Cancer Research UK Paediatric and Familial Cancer Research Group, The Medical School, Stopford Building, Room 1.900, University of Manchester, Oxford Road, M13 9PT Manchester, United Kingdom
jillian.birch@manchester.ac.uk

Penelope Brock Department Paediatric Oncology, Great Ormond Street Hospital, NHS Trust and Institute of Child Health, Great Ormond Street, London WC1N 3JH, United Kingdom
brockp@gosh.nhs.uk

Laurence Brugières Dépt. de Pédiatrie, Service d' Oncologie Pédiatrique, Institut Gustave Roussy, 11, Rue Camille Desmoulins, 94805 Villejuif, France
brugiere@igr.fr

Piotr Czauderna Department of Surgery and Urology for Children and Adolescents, Medical University of Gdansk, Ul. Nowe Ogrody 1-6, 80-803 Gdansk, Poland
pczaud@gumed.edu.pl

Michael Grotzer Head of Pediatric Neuro-Oncology, University Children's Hospital, Steinwiesstrasse 75, 8032 Zurich, Switzerland
michael.grotzer@kispi.uzh.ch

Roland Kappler Kinderchirurgische Klinik, Dr. von Haunersches Kinderspital, Ludwig-Maximilians-Universität München, Lindwurmstrasse 2a, 80337 München, Germany
roland.kappler@med.uni-muenchen.de

Gill Levitt Department Paediatric Oncology, Great Ormond Street Hospital, NHS Trust and Institute of Child Health, Great Ormond Street, London WC1N 3JH, United Kingdom
levitg@gosh.nhs.uk

Dolores Lopez-Terrada Molecular Oncology Laboratory,
Department of Pathology, Baylor College of Medicine, Texas Children's Hospital,
1 Baylor Plaza, Suite 286A, Houston, Texas 77030, USA
Dhterrad@texaschildrens.org

Rudolf Maibach IBCSG Coordinating Center, Effingerstrasse 40,
CH-3008 Berne, Switzerland
rudolf.maibach@ibcsg.org

Marcio Malogolowkin Division of Hematology-Oncology,
Children's Hospital Los Angeles, 4650 Sunset Blvd., MS #54, Los Angeles,
CA 90027, USA
mmalogolowkin@chla.usc.edu

Rebecka L. Meyers Primary Children's Medical Center, University of Utah,
100 N. Mario Cappechi Drive, Suite 2600, Salt Lake City, UT Utah 84113, USA
rebecka.meyers@hsc.utah.edu

Bruce Morland Birmingham Children's Hospital, Steelhouse Lane,
Birmingham B4 6NH, United Kingdom
bruce.morland@bch.nhs.uk

Jean-Bernard Otte Department of Paediatric Surgery, Cliniques Universitaires
Saint-Luc, Av. Hippocrate 10, 1200, Brussels, Belgium
otte@chex.ucl.ac.be

Giorgio Perilongo Pediatric Department, University of Padua, Padua, Italy
Department of Pediatrics "Salus Pueri", University-Hospital of Padua, Italy,
Via Giustiniani 3, 35128 Padua, Italy
giorgio.perilongo@unipd.it

Jack Plaschkes Dalmazirain 22, 3005 Berne, Switzerland
jack.plaschkes@bluewin.ch

Derek J. Roebuck Department of Radiology, Great Ormond Street Hospital,
NHS Trust Institute of Child Health, Great Ormond Street, London WC1N 3JH,
United Kingdom
roebud@gosh.nhs.uk

Dietrich von Schweinitz Kinderchirurgische Klinik im Dr. von Haunerschen
Kinderspital, Universität München, Lindwurmstrasse 4,
80337 München, Germany
dietrich.schweinitz@med.uni-muenchen.de

Tarek Shalaby Pediatric Neuro-Oncology, University Children's Hospital,
Steinweisstrasse 75, 8032 Zurich, Switzerland

Arthur Zimmermann Institute of Pathology of the University,
Murtenstrasse 31, 3010 Berne, Switzerland
zimmerma@patho.unibe.ch

Jozsef Zsiros Département de Pédiatrie, Service d'Oncologie Pédiatrique, Institut
Gustave Roussy, 11 Rue Camille Demoulins, 94805 Villejuif, France

Introduction

1

Primary childhood liver tumors are indeed quite rare neoplasms; their estimate incidence worldwide is of about less than one case per million children aged less than 14 years. In these last three decades, a great amount of basic and clinical research on these tumors, notably hepatoblastoma, have been conducted. Because of all this, solid hallmarks regarding the modern clinical and histopathologic diagnostic approach to these neoplasms, the definition of their risk profile and their management have been elaborated. Concurrently, a significant progress in the prognosis of those children affected by hepatoblastoma has been achieved. Furthermore, the most recent basic researches have opened convincing ways along which the ultimate mechanisms sustaining their growth, which, for hepatoblastoma, have to be referred to derangements of the molecular genetic processes regulating normal hepatic organogenesis can be understood. If all this stands true for hepatoblastoma, it does not apply to childhood hepatocellular carcinoma. Some progress has been made in gaining knowledge of it, particularly in the direction of distinguishing this tumor from the much more common adult counterpart; however, much more should be understood about its etiopathogenesis and definitely much more should be done to develop effective therapies. If at the present standard of care we can convincingly affirm that more than 70% of the children affected by hepatoblastoma are expected to be cured, this is true for only less than 30% of those affected by hepatocellular carcinoma.

The quantity and more importantly the quality of the data produced in all these years have made it possible to conceive the idea of "making the point" on where we are in understanding the genesis of these neoplasms and on what we know regarding their management. We believe that it is the first time that a comprehensive view of the information available regarding childhood liver tumors is provided. In summary, in the last few decades relevant basic and clinical science regarding these quite rare childhood tumors has been produced and this justifies the effort of summarizing it in a book.

Furthermore, also for childhood liver tumors, probably the end of an era has to be marked. This was the period during which conventional diagnostic and therapeutic approaches have given the most they could to define the risk profile of young patients affected by these diseases and to cure them. This implies that it is realistic to hypothesize that further significant progress will be achieved only through a better understanding of the genetic bases of their growth and progression and by developing biologically driven innovative therapies.

The progress in the knowledge of these neoplasms has been made possible only thanks to large scale cooperation that has seen institutions throughout the world working together and sharing precious data. The large panel of clinical and basic scientists intervening in writing this book is the concrete sign of this cooperation which, as stated earlier, has been the conditio sine qua non for obtaining the progress we are claiming.

The Editors

A. Zimmermann et al. (eds.), *Pediatric Liver Tumors*, Pediatric Oncology,
DOI: 10.1007/978-3-642-14504-9_1, © Springer-Verlag Berlin Heidelberg 2011

Historical Background

Jack Plaschkes

2

Contents

J. Plaschkes
Dalmazirain 22, CH-3005 Berne, Switzerland
e-mail: jack.plaschkes@bluewin.ch

2.1 Introduction

Liver Tumors in children encompass a wide spectrum of entities ranging from benign to semimalignant to malignant (see Chaps. 8 and 14).

Each entity would tend to have its own historical (especially treatment related) perspective and thus make an overview unnecessarily complicated.

So in this chapter, we intend to focus mainly on the two clearly defined malignant tumors. Hepatoblastoma is the most common and relevant in childhood. The other, namely hepatocellular carcinoma has many similarities to the adult variety, though, not in all aspects (especially not the same etiology).

The most dramatic improvement in outcome has occurred in hepatoblastoma since the introduction and use of chemotherapy in the late 1970s. Thus, one can think of and divide the history of progress into three distinct eras.

1. The "dark ages" pre systematic surgery – from the "beginning" to the 1940s
2. The "industrial revolution" in surgery and their pioneers – 1940s to 1970s, predominantly adult surgeons
3. The "enlightenment" – introduction of chemotherapy and collaboration of specialties – from the 1970s onward.

Neither the terms used nor the dates need to be taken too literally or strictly as the cut offs are not necessarily so sharp.

We shall try to follow this outline throughout and add some thoughts about the future.

Naturally, the last period is of the most topical interest and actually having lived through and taken part in it, could be biased, but is the most detailed and hopefully informative one.

A. Zimmermann et al. (eds.), *Pediatric Liver Tumors*, Pediatric Oncology,
DOI: 10.1007/978-3-642-14504-9_2, © Springer-Verlag Berlin Heidelberg 2011

In Hepatocellular Carcinoma, the improvements have been mainly due to better and safer surgical techniques based on more accurate anatomical knowledge but far less spectacular (Czauderna et al. 2002). The pioneers in all these fields clearly need to be mentioned in a historical review.

The same applies to a much better and still ongoing refinement of the pathology and the authors of early texts devoted entirely to pediatric tumors deserve the same attention.

Equal merit also goes to the development of national and international cooperative and multidisciplinary groups. (see Sect. 2.8) Collaboration is the key word to the successful management of liver tumors in children.

2.2 The Dark Ages

In this protracted period over many centuries, children were hardly considered to be part of society with little attention being given to their plight and especially their diseases. It is therefore not surprising that it is hard to find any reference of their role in medical literature, even in the extensive, early, mostly encyclopedic German literature of the late eighteenth century. Tumors of any organ including liver were recorded as curiosities due to all sorts of mystical or religious causes with corresponding treatments, e.g., exorcism, counteracting bad vapors. Surgery was the realm of barber surgeons who performed dramatic "primitive live" surgery often as a spectacle for curious onlookers.

The advent of printing made it possible to publish extensive illustrated treatises on these curious procedures. (see Sect. 2.3)

An exception to these aberrations is possibly the somewhat more rational approach of some of the early medieval Arab thinkers and also Maimonides (1,135–1,204).

A light in this period was to come from the early "foundling" hospitals and their enlightened benefactors, later to become the first children's hospitals. (see Sect. 2.4)

2.3 Advent of Printing

Histoire de la Médicine et du Livre Médical (1978) Paule Dumaitre, Editions Pygmalion, Olivier Perrin.

2.4 Early Children's Hospital

Some selected ones are:

The Great Ormond Street Hospital for Sick Children founded in 1852 by Dr. Charles West, associated with the Peter Pan Foundation and the Coram Trust

Hôpital des Enfants Malades Paris 1802

Anna Kinderpital Vienna 1850

Kinderspital Bern 1862

Pediatric ward in Charité Hospital Berlin 1829

Bambino Gésu Rome 1869

The Children's Hospital of Philadelphia founded in 1855

The Chicago Hospital for Women and Children 1865

The Boston Children's Hospital 1869

New York Babies and Children's Hospital 1887

Alder Hey Children's Hospital Liverpool 1914.

Kings College Hospital London 1913 has a special hepatology unit and transplant center for children.

None, because of their early founding times, initially specialized in the treatment of liver tumors in children, but it is worthwhile mentioning that later on, many of them developed such services or units that were often associated with distinguished pioneering personalities in relevant specialties (often pediatric surgery or pathology). In order to avoid repetition, these are mentioned under other appropriate headings.

Rare hospitals treating only cancer, e.g., Sloan Kettering Memorial Hospital, New York 1884 (founded as the New York Cancer Hospital), The Royal Marsden Hospital London 1851(founded as The Cancer Hopital) with a Pediatric Branch in Sutton 1962, Institute Gustav-Roussy 1913 (as a development of the Hospice Paul Brousse Paris), and the A.C. Camargo Cancer Hospital Sao Paolo 1934 (as a development from the Antonio Prudente Foundation) did and do have special units for pediatric oncology and surgery.

St Jude's Childrens Hospital 1962 (initially funded by the Danny Thomas Lebanese Foundation) is the only one known to me as treating solely children with cancer.

Incidentally, Odile Schweisguth, the founding mother of SIOP started a 16 bed pediatric oncology service in 1952 in Paris (Coppes-Zantinga et al. 2000; Schaison and Sommelet 1995).

It goes without saying that this cannot be an exhaustive list, but hopefully a balanced, though personal, selection between various countries and personalities.

2.5 Pioneer Pathologists and/or Their Textbooks

One of the first of modern pathologists to devote himself to write a monograph on children's tumors was Willis (1962).

He clearly made the distinction between the embryonal type and carcinoma. Interestingly enough, he mentions the occasional difficulty in making a distinction between the two showing the insight and predating the recently described "transitional type" (Prokurat et al. 2002). Other pioneers are E. Potter (Wiedermann 1994) and J. Keeling (Keeling 1960). Both concentrated on the pathology of the fetus and newborn in their texts, but the latter's particular interest in liver is shown in an article published in 1960 (Keeling 1971).

Another pathologist with foresight was HB Marsden who established the first population-based tumor registry in Manchester and wrote a text on children's tumors (Marsden and Steward 1976). Incidentally, the founder of modern chemotherapy, Sydney Farber was also a pathologist.

The still most widely used classifications of pediatric liver tumors are by Ishak and Glunz (1967), Kasai and Watanabe (1970) and L Dehner Gonzales Crussi. An updated and more unified and internationally accepted system including genetic profiling is necessary.

2.6 Pioneers in Surgical Anatomy and Liver Surgery

The techniques of liver surgery are not essentially different in adults and children, and since adult disease is far more common, it is not suprising that "adult" surgeons have taken the lead in these developments, but later on, Pediatric Surgeons, especially in the above-mentioned Children's Hospitals, have also performed liver surgery.

Early reports on liver resections in children are by Howat (1971). Of the 14 malignant ones (out of a total of 19) only 3 survived. Operative mortality due to hemorrhage was 31%. However, in another series by (Price et al. 1982) in a series of 11 resections (6 with hepatoblastoma) in children aged 7 days to 14 years, there were no operative deaths but for 1 tumor-related one at 8 months.

The main risks, as seen above (morbidity, mortality), of liver surgery in the early years, i.e., before an accurate description of the segmental vascular and biliary anatomy, as described by Couinaud in 1954 (Couinaud 1954, 1957) were bleeding and biliary fistula. A resection mortality of over 10% was described by Exelby 1971/1974 (Exelby et al. 1971, 1975). Various procedures were used to try and reduce and minimize these, e.g., the Pringle maneuver (Pringle 1908) (clamping of the afferent hepatic vascular pedicle); total vascular occlusion (clamping of the aorta and balloon occlusion of the inferior vena cava with +/– hypothermia (Fortner)/(Fortner et al. 1974); preresection ligation of the hepatic artery portal vein and/or hepatic veins; hypotensive anesthesia. Various techniques for dividing the liver parenchyma to reduce hemorrhage were devised, e.g., "finger fracture," water jet, or ultrasound dissection – CUSA.

But as mentioned above, most of the credit must still go to Couinaud for his ground breaking description of the classical eight segments (sectors) now universally accepted as the gold standard in liver surgery (Couinaud 1954, 1957). Before that, the terminology in hepatic resection was confusing and misleading being based on the anatomical right and left lobes and the umbilical fissure which however do not correspond to the vascular supply and biliary architecture. In recent years, the mortality and morbidity in specialized liver centers and by liver surgeons is well below 5%.

An exhaustive historical review of all these issues is given by Fortner and Blumgardt (2001).

2.7 Liver Transplantation

Liver and other organ transplantation came into their own after the basic research on rejection and its prevention by immunosuppression, was originally done by R. Calne. In children there remained two barriers for a wider use: Organ shortage and the presumed lifelong immunosuppression thought to be necessary. When these were solved, especially with the introduction of the living donor and split liver techniques, overcoming some of the moral dilemmas due to organ scarcity, liver transplantation became more and more important and amenable to children for cure and survival, in HB (basically as an extension of total resection) (Finegold et al. 2008; Otte et al. 2004). All these are rather recent developments and have little place in a historical review, so the details are better left to others (Chap. 10).

2.8 International Oncology Groups

2.8.1 COG

At the outset in North America, there were a number of interrelated institutions treating only leukemia. An NCI panel was responsible for promoting their integration into a more structured entity with L Murphy as chair in 1958: CALGB (Cancer and Leukemia Group B) and SWOG (South West Oncology Group). Eventually, solid tumors were also included; CCG (Children's Cancer Group) was established in 1968 chaired by D. Hammond and POG (Pediatric Oncology Group) was founded in 1980 by Theresa Vietti and J. Ternberg by merging CALGB and SWOG. The CCG had special tumor-related groups earlier, namely the NWTS (National Wilms' Tumor Study, chaired by G D'Angio and H Wolff) and IRS (Intergroup Rhabdomyosarcoma Study, chaired by H. Maurer). At the same time in 1972, the first cooperative study of combination treatment of liver tumors in children was embarked upon.

In 2000, all these amalgamated to become COG (Children's Oncology Group) under one chair (G. Reaman). COG has a liver subcommittee chaired by M. Malogolowkin followed by R. Myers. Representatives of this group participate actively in all other international liver groups "to come and work together" for exchange of information and plan future generation studies.

Although, strictly speaking, initially, all the above were national American societies, other countries could also become associate members – the beginning of international cooperation (O'Leary et al. 2008).

(This is an attempt to give a simplified version of a complicated summary of the early formation years which may not be as accurate as the founders would wish.)

2.8.2 SIOP

In Europe, SIOP (Société International d'Oncologie Pédiatrique) was officially founded in 1969 by Odile Schweisguth from Paris (hence the French name) after, a group of pediatric oncologists met in Madrid (1967) initiated by J. Monoreo and recognizing the need for a special international pediatric cancer organization in Europe also. From this first group, all of them became the founding members. The society has prospered and had some years ago, over 1,000 members. It meets annually alternating between a European and one of the other member countries.

Under the umbrella of SIOP, newer entities and committees were formed (1987), these being SIOPEL, and IPSO, SIOP Asia (including China/Japan/India/Africa/Australasia), and PODC (Pediatric Oncology in Developing Countries).

In their individual ways all of them especially SIOPEL, have made significant contributions nationally and internationally to the management of liver tumors.

2.8.3 SIOPEL (SIOP Epithelial Liver Tumors)

1987 – Jerusalem. A preliminary gathering by a small band of oncologists interested in forming a future cooperative liver tumor study group and attending the annual SIOP meeting was convened by J. Plaschkes and J. Pritchard. A short questionnaire was designed and distributed to find out if there was enough common ground and the possible number of patients who could be recruited to take part a trial.

1988 – There followed three informal meetings with most of the original "working party" members and countries represented previously: In London (GOS), Paris (I Gustav Roussy), and Trondheim (Annual SIOP meeting). A caretaker core committee chaired by J. Plaschkes and a protocol writing committee were formed.

1989 – The first "official" formal meeting was held in Padua where the details such as the administrative structure, and other committee members were finalized. Consensus on a study strategy (preoperative chemotherapy and pretext staging) (Roebuck et al. 2007) was reached.

A draft treatment protocol (six pages!!) was written and sent to the SIOP scientific committee as well as to most national pediatric oncology societies by J. Plaschkes (with approval of the writing committee) for evaluation.

Application for Funds was made to the Swiss Cancer League for a workshop/symposium in Bern and for the first trial office YRCO (Yorkshire Regional Cancer Office) in Leeds.

The approved protocol was activated in July 1989.

1990 – A full 2 day international Liver Study Symposium was held in Bern (Plaschkes 2001). A Newsletter (L. Shafford) and Budget were presented for the first time. Previous to and after this international workshop, others, under the acronym CELTIC (Common Epithelial Liver Tumors International Criteria), were held in 1990 in London (St. Bartholomew's Hospital hosted by J. Kingston), in 1991 in Athens (hosted by H. Kosmides), and in 1992 in Hannover (hosted by D. von Schweinitz), to try and standardize definitions and mostly sponsored by the local hosts and J. Pritchard.

After all these initial activities, regular biannual SIOPEL meetings in a European host country as well as the annual SIOP meetings followed.

What followed is not history anymore.

2.8.4 IPSO

The "International Society of Pediatric Surgical Oncology" originally brought together, in 1989, the small band of pediatric surgeons committed to oncology by J. Plaschkes and D. Hays at the Prague SIOP meeting hosted by J. Snadjauf, where, aptly, the main topic was surgery. Eventually, these preparatory contacts led to the formation of IPSO, officially founded in 1991 in Rhodes with a constitution written by Antonio Gentil-Martins and J. Plaschkes elected as first president. The society runs a rare tumor registry and has a discussion forum for difficult cases. The president and another representative each have a seat on the scientific committee of SIOP. The main annual meetings are held at the SIOP meetings but other ad hoc ones have also taken place.

Their regular meetings have enhanced the surgical inputs and answered questions raised in clinical trials.

2.8.5 SIOP ASIA

It was formed to encompass and include not only the original European founder countries, but also continental Chapters with their own presidents and representatives in all annual meetings. Regular separate meetings are also held in these continents sponsored by SIOP mainly for educational purposes.

2.8.6 PODC (Pediatric Oncology in Developing Countries)

Similarly, to bring in an even wider membership and assist these countries in developing their own oncology services, the Pediatric Oncology in Developing Countries committee was formed in 1996 and regularly sponsors scholarships "for individuals to attend SIOP meetings."

The PODC committee of SIOP (HP Wagner) and its activities also contribute greatly to further the aims mentioned below.

2.8.7 EONS (European Oncology Nursing Specialists)

One must also not forget to mention the nurses (mostly fully integrated into the European Oncology Nursing Specialists societies) whose care and knowledge are important in maintaining the high safety standards required for the often elaborate chemotherapy regimes.

2.9 National Pediatric Oncology Societies

UK (UKCCSG) later (CRUK) 1977 (Hammond 2003)
France (SFOP) (Schaison and Sommelet 1995)
Germany (GPOH) (1991). Formed by the fusion of GPO (1993) with DAL (German working party for Leukemia) (Hertl 1995)
Austria 1974 (Gadner 1992)
Italy (AIEOP) 1974
Switzerland (SPOG) (1964) (Wagner 1994)
Australia/New Zealand (ANZHOG) (1986)
Latin America (SLAOP) (1979)
Japan (1950) (Evans et al. 1973; Bessho and Kobayashi 1993)
America (ASPHO)/COG (see Sect. 2.8.1)

One of the principal aims and efforts of these societies was to enroll sufficient numbers of patients to enable clinical trials to be conducted scientifically with sufficient statistical power. (Most have organ-related studies and trials.) Obviously, because of the relative rarity of pediatric malignancies (even more so, liver tumors) sufficient numbers of children can be enrolled only by national and international cooperation.

2.10 Clinical Liver Trials

Since the introduction of antineoplastic therapy by Sydney Farber in 1948 (Farber et al. 1948) for leukemia, chemotherapy has taken on an increasingly important role for solid tumors in children.

Liver tumors, in particular hepatoblastoma, was, because of its relative rarity, one of the last of the specific pediatric ones to be investigated in prospective clinical trials.

Incidentally, hepatocellular carcinoma, although inherently of a very different nature and being even more rare, was, for practical reasons, also subjected to the same treatment as HB in most studies.

At the outset, the strategy and staging systems chosen by SIOPEL were different from that in the United States. In the USA, traditionally, primary surgery, wherever possible, was the initial step, whereas in SIOPEl preoperative (neoadjuvant) chemotherapy was the rule. (It was chosen for the simple reason that if the tumor became smaller difficult liver surgery would be safer.) This is not the place to repeat or mention all other advantages and even possible disadvantages for this choice.

Some other countries chose their own individual ways, i.e., Germany followed the USA example, whereas Japan mostly preferred preoperative chemotherapy.

Because the overall results of the different strategies were, broadly speaking, similar, each group has continued to adhere to its own original concept. It must however also be said that the chemotherapy agents used were and are quite substantially different as well.

In addition, the various staging systems used can make comparisons questionable and replete with pitfalls.

For that reason, SIOPEL introduced its own system (PRETEXT) specially designed and conceived to reflect the surgical anatomy of the liver (complete surgical resection still being the most important prognostic factor). This system is now being used by all in conjunction with the others, i.e., the classical Stage I–IV, allowing direct comparison of outcomes.

Below is a concise list of most of the past trials and their results (Tables 2.1–2.4)

2.11 Conclusions and Future Outlook

Unless and until a "magic bullet" is discovered or some treatable genetic profile can be identified and screened for, it seems likely that surgical resection will still remain an integral treatment option in the near future. Since the dawn of effective chemotherapy, the demise of surgery has often been predicted, but so far, this has not happened. Laparoscopic and Robot and computer-assisted surgery from "afar" will, theoretically, make specialized surgery available to all (Koffron et al. 2006).

Scientific international multidisciplinary trials with their logical stepwise improvements will probably, for some time, remain the aim and gold standard, but some serendipitous unexpected discovery (as in many medical instances, see Cisplatinum) (Rosenberg et al. 1965; Rosenberg et al. 1969) cannot be discarded either.

Because of the ever increasing stratification and differentiation of risk groups, both histologically and genetically, "personalized" treatment will become the rule. For that reason, with the smaller study cohorts, international cooperation will be even more essential to be able to fulfill valid statistical criteria. The large populations in India, China, and other developing countries (see PODC above) will all play an increasingly important role in enhancing future developments more rapidly. They will and can initiate their own trials and still be able to participate in the already established ones.

HCC prevention by hepatitis B immunization will substantially reduce the incidence.

Although trying to end on an optimistic note, one cannot fail to mention that the increasing burden of national and international administrative regulations and directives will severely hamper the possibility of international cooperation, and delay, if not make impossible, the development of scientific trials especially in very rare pediatric liver tumors. Future historical reviews will give us an answer to this prediction.

Table 2.1 Pediatric liver trials. North America

Study	Chemotherapy	Number of patients	Outcome	Author
CCG 862/SWOG 7,695 1976–1978	VCR+CPM+DOXO alternating with VCR+CPM+5FU	61 patients All liver tumors	3 year OS Group I - 94% Group II - 57% Group III - 20% Group IV - 14%	Evans [49s]
CCG 823F 1986–1951	CDDP+DOXO	33 patients All liver tumors	2 year OS Stage II - 86% Stage III - 58% Stage IV - 32%	Ortega et al. (2000)
POG 8,697 1986–1989	C5V	60 patients Hepatoblastoma	4 year OS Stage I/PFH - 100% (surgery only) Stage I/II - 90% Stage III - 67% Stage IV (8 pts) - 12%	Douglass et al. (1991)
INT-0098 (CCG-8,881/ POG-8,945) 1989–1992	C5V vs. CDDP+DOXO	Stage I/II: 50 patients Stage III: 83 patients Stage IV: 40 patients All liver tumors	4 year OS I/II = 100% versus 96% III = 68% versus 71% IV = 33% versus 42%	Ortega et al. (2000)
P9545[a] 1993–1995	C5V vs. CDDP+CARBO	Stage I PFH: 17 patients Stage III: 38 patients Stage IV: 50 patients Hepatoblastoma	3 year OS Stage I PFH: 100% Stage III/IV: 74% versus 56%	Malogolowkin et al. (2008)
COG-P9645 1999–2003 **Preliminary results**	Stage I/PFH surgery only Stage I/II randomized to C5V+-amifostine; Stage III/IV randomized CDDP+CARBO versus C5V +/– Amifostine	270 patients Hepatoblastoma	Stage I/PFH (n 16) OS 4 year 100% Stage I/II +/– Ami OS 4 year 96% Stage III OS 4 year 88% Stage III/IV CC (n 56) EFS 3 year 38% C5V(n53) EFS 3 year 60% Stage IV (n10) OS 4 year 67%	Malogolowkin et al. (2008)

Abbreviations: VCR: vincristine; CPM: Cyclophosphamide; DOXO: doxorubicin; 5FU: fluorouracil; CDDP: cisplatin; C5V: cisplatin, fluorouracil and vincristine; CARBO: carboplatin; OS: overall survival.

[a] Final study analysis is still pending.

Table 2.2 Germany

Study	Strategy	Number of patients	Chemotherapy	Stage	Outcome	References
CGPOH-HB89 1988–1993	Primary surgery	72	Ifosfamide Cisplatin Doxorubicin		DFS 75% median FU 64 month	Von Schweinitz et al. (1997)
				I	100%	
				II	50%	
				III	71%	
				IV	29%	
CGPOH-HB94 1994–99	Primary surgery	48	Ifosfamide Cisplatin Doxorubicin	Standard risk	OS Median FU 58 months 77%	Fuchs et al. (2002)
		18	Etoposide Carboplatin	Advanced or recurrent		Fuchs et al. (1999)
HB99 1999–2008	Mixed		IPA/ Carboplatin-VP16		Preliminary results only	Häberle et al. (2003)

Table 2.3 JAPAN

Study	Strategy	Number of patients	Chemotherapy	Stage	Outcome	References
JPLT-1 1991–1999	Mixed PRETEXT	145 HB	Cisplatin THP		3/6 year OS 77.8%/73.4%	Sasaki et al. (2002)
			Adriamycin[a]	I	100%/100%	
				II	100%/95.7%	
				IIIA	76.6%/73.8%	
				IIIB	50.3%/50.3%	
				IV	64.8%/38.9%	
JPLT-2 1999–2004	All preop done except PRETEXT 1	144 HB			3 year OS	Preliminary results
			PRETEXT 1	I	100%	
			PRETEXT 2	II	88%	
			PRETEXT 3	III	68%	
				IV	42%	

[a] Japanese Adriamycin THP = Tetrahydropyranil

Table 2.4 SIOPEL

Study	Strategy	Number of patients	Chemotherapy	Stage	Outcome	References
SIOPEL 1 1990–94	Primary Chemotherapy[a]	154	Cisplatin Doxorubicin		3 year OS 79% 3 year EFS 67% 3 year EFS by PRETEXT	Pritchard et al. (2000))
				I	100%	
				II	83%	
				III	59%	
				IV	44%	
				and metastases	28%	
SIOPEL 2 1995–98	Primary Chemotherapy	Standard risk 77	Cisplatin		3 year OS 91% PFS 89%	Perilongo et al. (2004)
		High risk 58	Alternating Cisplatin, Carboplatin/Doxorubicin		3 year OS 53% PFS 48%	
SIOPEL3 Standard Risk (SR) 1998–2006	Primary Chemotherapy Randomized SR versus HR	SR126:HR129	CDDP vs. CDDP+DOXO	All Stages	3 year EFS/OS CDDP 83%:85% CDDP+DOXO 89%:93%	Perilongo et al. (2009)
SIOPEL 3 High risk (HR) 1989–2004	Primary Chemotherapy	151	Alternating CDDP+Carbo-platin+DOXO	All Stages	3 year EFS/OS 65%:69%	Zsiros et al. (2010)

[a] PRETEXT I were eligible for primary surgery

References

Papers

Anderson DH (1951) Tumors of infancy and childhood. Survey of those seen in the pathology laboratory of the Babies Hospital (NY) during 1935–1950. Cancer 4:890–906

Bessho F, Kobayashi N (1993) A historical sketch of pediatric hematology and oncology in Japan. Pediatr Hematol Oncol 10:5–8

Borman JB, Harbott AJ, Morris D (1961) Hepatic lobectomy in infancy for hepatoblastoma. Br J Surg 49:11–13

Browne M, Sher D, Grant D et al (2008) Survival after liver transplantation for hepatoblastoma: a 2-center experience. J Pediatr Surg 43:1973–1981

Claireaux A (1972) Solid tumors in children. Postgrad Med J 48:451–464

Clatworthy HW, Schiller M, Grossfeld JL (1974) Primary liver tumors in infancy and childhood. 41 cases variously treated. Arch Surg 109:143–147

Clavien PA, Petrowski H, De Oliviera ML et al (2007) Strategies for safer liver surgery and partial liver transplantation. N Engl J Med 365:1545–1559

Coppes-Zantinga AR, Zucker JM, Coppes MJ (2000) Odile Schweisguth, alma mater of pediatric oncology. Med Pediatr Oncol 34:59–60

Couinaud C (1954) Lobes et segmentes hepatiques. Presse Méd 62:709–712

Couinaud C (1957) Etudes anatomiques et chirurgales. Masson, Paris, pp 400–409

Czauderna P, Mackinlay G, Perilongo G et al (2002) Hepatocellular carcinoma in children: results of the first prospective study of the SIOPEL group. J Clin Oncol 15:2798–2804

Evans AE, Borns P, Donaldson M et al (1973) Cure of the child with cancer. Pa? Med 9:53–57

Evans AE, Borns P, Koop CE (1974) The place of combination treatment. Semin Oncol 1:77–80

Evans AE, D'Angio GJ, Koop CE (1976) Childhood cancer: basic considerations in diagnosis and treatment. Pediatr Clin North Am 1:3–9

Exelby PR, El-Domeri A, Huvos AG et al (1971) Primary tumors of the liver in Children. J Pediatr Surg 6:272–276

Exelby PR, Filler RM, Grossfeld JR (1975) Liver tumors in children with particular reference to hepatoblastoma and hepatocellular carcinoma: American Academy of Pediatric Surgical Section Survey – 1974. J Pediatr Surg 10:329–337

Farber S, Diamond LK, Mercer RD et al (1948) Temporary remissions in acute leukemia in children produced by folic acid antagonists, 4 aminopteroglutaminacid (aminopterin). N Engl J Med 238:787–826

Finegold MJ, Egler RA, Goss JA et al (2008) Liver tumors: pediatric population. Liver Transpl 11:1545–1556

Fortner JG, Shiu MH, Kinne J et al (1974) Major hepatic resection using vascular isolation and hypothermic perfusion. Ann Surg 180:644–652

Fortner JG, Blumgardt LH (2001) Historical perspective of liver surgery at the end of the millenium. J Am Coll Surg 193: 210–212

Gadner H (1992) The history of pediatric hematology and oncology in Austria. Pediatr Hematol Oncol 9:3–6

Gale GB, D'Angio GJ, Uri A et al (1982) Cancer in neonates: the experience at the children's hospital of Philadelphia. Pediatrics 3:409–413

Hammond D (2003) Quest for cure – UK Children's Cancer Study Group – the first 25 years. J Pediatr Hematol Oncol 25:989 (book review)

Hertl M (1995) History and present organization of pediatric oncology in Germany. Pediatr Hematol Oncol 12:325–331

Horton JD, Lee S, Brown SR et al (2009) Survival trends in children with hepatoblastoma. Pediatr Surg Int 5:407–412

Howat JM (1971) Major hepatic resections in infancy and childhood. Gut 12:212–217

Hünerwadel U (1962) Lebertumoren im Kindesalter. Diss med Basel Karger. Ann Paed 198:44–63

Ishak KG, Glunz PR (1967) Hepatoblastoma and hepatocellular in infancy and childhood. Cancer 20:396–422

Ito J, Johnson WW (1969) Hepatoblastoma and hepatoma in infancy and childhood, light and electron microscopy studied. Arch Pathol 87:259–266

Kasai M, Watanabe I (1970) Histological classification of liver cell carcinoma in infancy and childhood. Cancer 25: 551–563

Keeling JW (1960) Pathology of the liver in young infants. Proc Int Med Clinics, Chicago

Keeling JW (1971) Liver tumors in infancy and childhood. J Pathol 103:69–85

Koffron A, Geller D, Gamblin et al (2006) Laparoscopic liver surgery: shifting the management of liver tumors. Hepatology 44:1694–1700

Koop CE (1965) Malignant tumors in childhood. Clin Proc Child Hosp Dist Columbia 21:149–158

Martin LW, Woodman KS (1969) Hepatic lobectomy for hepatoblastoma in infants and children. Arch Surg 98:1–7

Murphy ML (1990) Pioneers in pediatric oncology. In: Taylor G (ed) University of Texas M.D. Anderson Cancer Centre, Houston, pp 221–234

Nixon HH (1965) Hepatic tumors in childhood and their treatment by major hepatic resection. Arch Dis Child 40: 169–172

O'Leary M, Krailo M, Anderson JR (2008) Progress in childhood cancer: 50 years of research collaboration. A report from the Childrens Oncology Group. Semin Oncol 35:484–493

Plaschkes J (2001) Proceedings of an international research workshop on pediatric liver tumors 18–20 March 1999 in Berne Switzerland – into the year 2000. Med Pediatr Oncol 36:380–382

Price JB, Schullinger JN, Santali TV (1982) Major hepatic resections for neoplasia in children. Arch Surg 117: 1139–1141

Pringle JH (1908) Notes on the arrest of hepatic hemorrhage due to trauma. Ann Surg 48:541–549

Prokurat A, Kluge P, Kosciesza A et al (2002) Transitional liver cell tumors (TLCT) in older children and adolescents: a novel group of aggressive hepatic tumors expressing beta-catenin. Med Pediatr Oncol 39:510–518

Quinn JJ, Altman AJ, Robinson HT (1985) Adriamycin and cisplatin for hepatoblastoma. Cancer 56:1926–1929

Roebuck DJ, Aronson DC, Clapuyt P et al (2007) PRETEXT (preoperative extent) 2005. A revised staging system for primary malignant liver tumors of childhood developed by the SIOPEL group. Pediatr Radiol 37:123–132

Rosenberg B, Van Camp L, Krigas T (1965) Inhibition of cell division of Escheria coli by electrolysis products from a platinum electrode. Nature 205:698–699

Rosenberg B, Van Camp L, Trosko JE et al (1969) Platinum compounds: a new class of potent antitumour agents. Nature 222:385–386

Schaison GS, Sommelet D (1995) Pediatric hematology and oncology in France. Pediatr Hematol Oncol 12:5–12

Wagner HP (1994) Historical notes on pediatric hematology and oncology in Switzerland. Pediatr Hematol Oncol 11:575–586

Wiedermann HR (1994) The pioneers of pediatric medicine (E Potter). Eur J Pediatr 153:471

Ziegler MM, Vega A, Koop CE (1979) Liver modulation of tumour specific antigen: a metastatic mechanism. Surg Forum 30:160–162

Trial Results North America

Evans AE, Land VJ, Newton WA Jr (1982) Combination chemotherapy in the treatment of children with malignant hepatoma. Cancer 50:821

Douglass EC, Reynolds M, Stalen JP (1991) Effectiveness and toxicity of cisplatin, vincristine, and fluorouracil Therapy for hepatoblastoma. A Pediatric Oncology Group Study. J Clin Oncol 11:96–99

Malogolowkin MH, Katzenstein HM, Krailo M et al (2008) Redefining the role of doxorubicin for the treatment of children with hepatoblastoma. J Clin Oncol 26:2379–2383

Ortega JA, Douglass EC, Feusner JH (2000) Randomized comparison of cisplatin/vincristine/fluoruracil and cisplatin/continuous infusion doxorubicin for the treatment of pediatric hepatoblastoma. A report from the Children's Cancer Group and the Pediatric Oncology Group. J Clin Oncol 18:2665–2675

SIOPEL

SIOPEL 1

Pritchard J, Brown J, Shafford E, Perilongo G et al (2000) Cisplatin, doxorubicin, and delayed surgery for childhood hepatoblastoma: a successful approach-results of the first prospective study of the International Society of Pediatric Oncology. J Clin Oncol 18:3819–3828

SIOPEL 1

Otte JB, Pritchard J, Aronson DC et al (2004) Liver transplantation for hepatoblastoma: results from the International Society of Pediatric Oncology (SIOP) study SIOPEL 1 and review of the world experience. Pediatr Blood Cancer 42:74–83

Perilongo G, Brown J, Shafford E et al (2000) Hepatoblastoma presenting with lung metastases. Treatment results of the first cooperative prospective study of the International Society of Pediatric Oncology on childhood liver tumors. Cancer 89:1845–1853

SIOPEL 2

Perilongo G, Shafford E, Maibach R et al (2004) Risk-adapted treatment for childhood hepatoblastoma, final report of second study of the International Society of Pediatric Oncology-SIOPEL 2. Eur J Cancer 40:411–421

SIOPEL 3 SR (Standard Risk)

Perilongo G, Maibach R, Shafford E et al (2009) Cisplatin versus cisplatin plus doxorubicin for standard-risk hepatoblastoma. N Engl J Med 361:1662–1670

SIOPEL 3 HR (High Risk)

Zsiros J, Maibach R, Shafford E et al (2010) Successful treatment of childhood high-risk hepatoblastoma with dose intensive multiagent chemotherapy and surgery. Final results of the SIOPEL HR study of the International Childhood Liver Tumour Strategy Group (SIOPEL). J Clin Oncol, 28:2584–2590

GERMANY

HB 89

Häberle B, Bode U, von Schweinitz D (2003) Differentiated treatment protocols for high and standard risk hepatoblastoma. An interim report of the German Liver Tumor Study HB99. Klin Pediatrie 215:159–165

Von Schweinitz D et al (1997) Doxorubicin in the treatment of childhood hepatoblastoma. Study Committee of the Cooperative Pediatric Liver Tumour Study HB 89 (?) of the German Society of Paediatric Oncology and Hematology. Eur J Cancer 33:1243–1249

HB 89/HB 94

Fuchs J, Bode U, von Schweinitz D et al (1999) Analysis of treatment efficiency of carboplatin and etoposide in combination with radical surgery in advanced and recurrent childhood hepatoblastoma: a report of the German Cooperative Pediatric Liver Tumor Study HB 89 and HB 94. Klin Pädiatr 211:305–309

HB 94

Fuchs J, Rydzinski J, Von Schweinitz D et al (2002) Pretreatment prognostic factors and treatment results of children with hepatoblastoma: a report from the German Cooperative Pediatric Liver Tumour Study HB 94. Cancer 95:172–182

JAPAN

JPLT-1

Sasaki F, Matsunaga T, Iwafuchi M et al (2002) Outcome of hepatoblastoma treated with the JPLT-1 (Japanese Study Group for the treatment of Pediatric Liver Tumor Protocol 1). J Pediatr Surg 37:851–856

Textbooks

Hays DM (ed) (1986) Pediatric surgical oncology. Grune and Stratton, Orlando

Jones PG, Campbell PE (1976) Tumors of infancy and childhood (liver Ch 19, p 596–625). Blackwell, Oxford

Keeling JW (1989) Pathology of the fetus and newborn, 3rd edn. Butterworth, London

Levine AS (ed) (1982) Cancer in the young. Masson, New York

Marsden HB, Steward JK (1976) Tumors in children, 2nd edn. Springer, Heidelberg/New York

Michel P (1964) Tumors of infancy and childhood. Lippincott, Philadelphia

Peller S (1960) Cancer in childhood and youth. Wright, Bristol

Potter EL (1952) Pathology of the fetus and newborn. Year Book Publishers, Chicago

Willis RA (1962) The pathology of the tumours of children. In: Cameron R, Payling Wright G (eds) Pathological monographs No 2. Oliver and Boyd, Edinburgh

Schweisguth O (1979) Tumeurs Solides de L'Enfant. Flammarion, Paris

Sutow WW, Vietti TJ, Fernbach DJ (1977) Clinical pediatric oncology. Mosby, St. Louis

Epidemiology of Pediatric Liver Tumors

3

Jillian M. Birch

Contents

J.M. Birch
Cancer Research UK Paediatric and Familial Cancer Research Group, The Medical School, Stopford Building, Room 1.900, University of Manchester, Oxford Road, M13 9PT Manchester, United Kingdom
e-mail: jillian.birch@manchester.ac.uk

3.1 Introduction

Epidemiology has been defined as: "the study of the occurrence and distribution of health-related states or events in specified populations, including the study of the determinants influencing such states, and the application of this study to control the health problems" (Porta 2008). Thus, the concern of epidemiology is disease in populations or groups of people as opposed to individuals. Furthermore, it is essential to note that for epidemiological studies of specific diseases, those within the population who do not have the disease are as important as those who do. This distinction marks a fundamental difference between epidemiology and clinical medicine.

Control of health problems can be achieved by adopting strategies to limit or prevent development of disease. These strategies may include screening for early detection, vaccination, and chemoprevention and reduction or elimination of exposure to environmental risk factors for the disease. The aim is to reduce mortality and morbidity within populations and ultimately prevent disease.

Epidemiological studies of pediatric liver tumors have been hindered by the rarity of these conditions. Very large populations of children and/or many years of study are required to generate sufficient number of cases for statistically significant observations to be made. However, in recent years, a number of observations have emerged, which have paved the way for preventative strategies for at least a proportion of cases within the foreseeable future.

A. Zimmermann et al. (eds.), *Pediatric Liver Tumors*, Pediatric Oncology,
DOI: 10.1007/978-3-642-14504-9_3, © Springer-Verlag Berlin Heidelberg 2011

3.2 Descriptive Epidemiology of Pediatric Liver Tumors

The measurement of disease incidence within populations and over time provides essential information to health care providers. Descriptive epidemiological studies also provide a starting point for hypothesis generation about etiology. Demographic patterns of incidence, geographical variations, and changes in incidence with time can all provide clues about etiology. The cornerstone of descriptive epidemiology is the population-based cancer registry.

3.2.1 Spectrum and Frequency of Liver Tumors in Children

Detailed population-based incidence data on the full spectrum of primary malignant liver tumors in children are lacking. This is in part due to the application of the International Classification of Childhood Cancer (ICCC) to national and international cancer registration data in published incidence rates (Steliarova-Foucher et al. 2005, 2006; Linabery and Ross 2008; Parkin et al. 1998). The ICCC defines diagnostic groups using combinations of morphology and primary site codes derived from the International Classification of Diseases for Oncology, second and third editions (Percy et al. 1990; Fritz et al. 2000). ICD-O is used by cancer registries to code diagnoses. Group VII, hepatic tumors, includes hepatoblastoma (HB), hepatic carcinoma, and unspecified malignant hepatic tumors. Other primary liver tumors are distributed among other diagnostic groups, e.g., Group IX, soft tissue, and other extraosseous sarcomas. Therefore, published incidence rates are underestimates of the true incidence of liver tumors in children and relative proportions of different liver tumors in populations cannot be derived from published data. Information on the range of childhood liver tumors in general comes from clinical and histopathological series.

To overcome this lack of data, incident cases of all malignant primary liver tumors in children aged 0–14 years, derived from national cancer registration data for England, have been analyzed (Birch and Alston, in preparation). All cases diagnosed with a site code of liver (C22.0), and any morphology code, were eligible for analysis. There were 213 cases, 1995–2006, comprising: 154 (72.3%) HB; 22 hepatocellular carcinoma (HCC) including 5 fibrolamellor (10.3%); 6 rhabdomyosarcoma, 14 embryonal sarcoma, 5 rhabdoid sarcoma, 1 mesenchymoma, 3 haemangiosarcoma/haemangioendothelial sarcoma, 4 soft tissue sarcoma (STS) not otherwise specified (total STS 15.0%); 1 yolk sac tumor (0.5%) and 4 unspecified malignant liver tumors (1.9%). Therefore, over 16% of specified cases were tumors other than HB and HCC (Fig. 3.1a). The percentage distribution of these varied markedly with age. In 0–4 year olds 85.5% of cases were HB and only 1% HCC. 3.1% and 2.5% were rhabdoid tumors and rhabdomyosarcoma, respectively. 3.8% were other soft tissue tumors (Fig. 3.1b). Figure 3.1c shows the distribution among 5–14 year olds. In this age group, 35.2% of cases were HB, 33.3% were HCC, and 31.5% were soft tissue tumors, among which embryonal sarcoma predominates. Therefore, in 5–14 year olds, nearly one-third were tumors other than HB and HCC. These proportions are consistent with the Armed Forces Institute of Pathology series, 0–20 year old, quoted by Stocker et al. (1998).

Incidence rates of HB, HCC, and other specified and unspecified liver tumors for age groups under 1, 1–4, 5–9, and 10–14 years were calculated for all malignant liver tumors diagnosed in England in the years 1990–2006. Cases were extracted from national cancer registrations and population counts for England using methods described by Alston et al. (2008). HB dominated the under 1 and 1–4 year age groups with low rates for other tumors. In 5–9 and 10–14 year olds there was a more even distribution of rates between the tumor groups but HCC had a higher rate than other tumors in 10–14 year olds, albeit still very low in absolute terms (Table 3.1). Table 3.2 shows that rates for HB were higher in males than females ($p=0.01$). Rates for other liver tumors did not vary significantly by sex, but the number of cases was very low. In some datasets, an excess of males with HCC as well as HB has been reported (Stiller et al. 2006; Chen et al. 2005).

3.2.2 International Variations in Incidence

For reasons discussed above, international comparisons are only possible for HB and HCC. The International Incidence of Childhood Cancer Vol II presents incidence data from registries around the world mainly

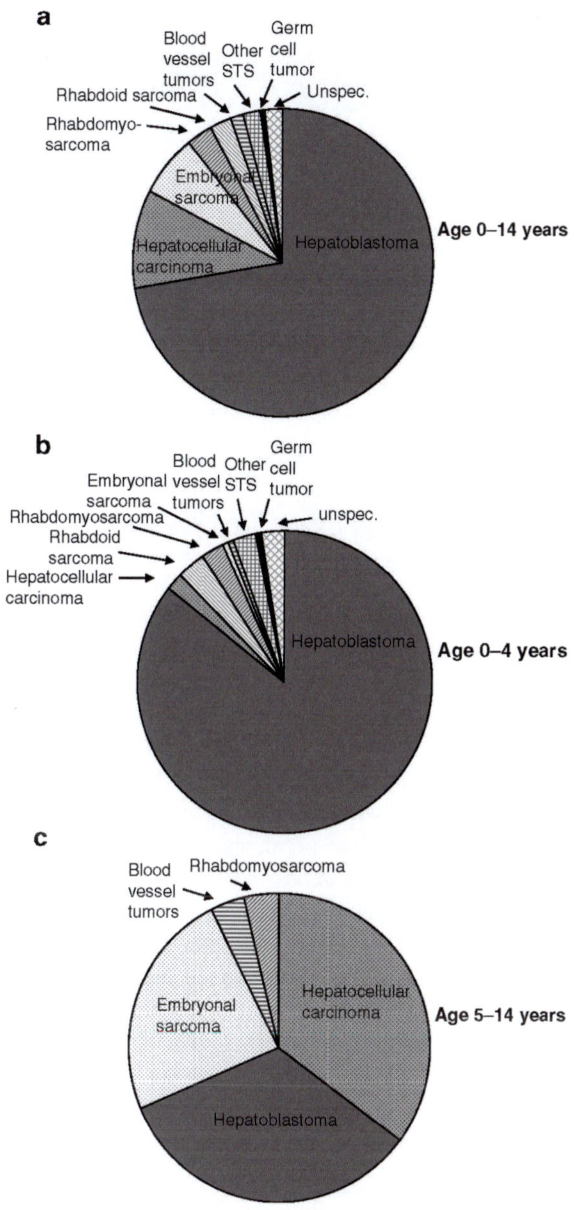

Fig. 3.1 Relative frequencies of specific liver tumours in children by age group

from the early 1980s to early 1990s (Parkin et al. 1998). However, many registries had too few cases to provide stable rates, especially for HCC. Furthermore, a number of registries reported only the "unspecified" category. However, working with the data as presented, there appear to be higher rates of hepatic tumors overall in the Far East than in Western countries and Australia. Highest rates for HB were seen in parts of the USA and Japan. Only six registries reported ten or more cases of HCC. The highest rate was seen in Cuba.

There have been more recent publications from Europe and the USA. European data, 1988–1997, derived from the Automated Childhood Cancer Information System (ACCIS) found overall rates for 0–14 year olds across European registries of 1.2 per million for HB and 0.2 per million for HCC (Stiller et al. 2006). Over 90% of HB cases occurred under age 5, but HCC was distributed fairly evenly across age groups. Highest rates for HB were reported by registries in East (1.4) and North (1.5) Europe and lowest in the British Isles (1.0). Rates for HCC showed little variation.

The most recently published figures from the USA cover 2001–2003 and include incidence data from 39 National Program of Cancer Registries and 5 Surveillance Epidemiology and End Results (SEER) statewide registries, representing over 90% of the US population (Li et al. 2008). The overall rate for HB was 1.44 per million and 1.00 per million for HCC. Rates for HB were significantly higher in males (1.57) than in females (1.09) but there were no differences by sex for HCC. Rates during a comparable time period, 2001–2006, in England were 1.7 for HB overall (1.9 in males and 1.7 in females) and 0.2 for HCC (Birch and Alston, in preparation). Therefore, rates for HCC appear to be higher in the USA than in Europe, but similar for HB.

Table 3.1 Incidence per million person – years of malignant tumors of the liver in children aged 0–14 years in England 1990–2006, by age group at diagnosis

Age group (years)	Hepatoblastoma	Hepatocellular carcinoma	Other specified tumors	Unspecified tumors	All tumors
Under 1	6.2	0	1.5	0.1	7.8
1–4	2.7	0.2	0.3	0.1	3.3
5–9	0.2	0.2	0.2	0.1	0.7
10–14	0.2	0.4	0.2	0	0.7
0–14	1.3	0.2	0.3	0.1	1.9

Table 3.2 Incidence per million person – years of malignant tumors of the liver in children aged 1–14 years in England 1990–2006, by sex

	Hepatoblastoma	Hepatocellular carcinoma	Other specified tumors	Unspecified tumors	All tumors
Males	1.5	0.2	0.4	0.1	2.2
Females	1.0	0.2	0.2	0.1	1.5
Males + females	1.3	0.2	0.3	0.1	1.9

3.2.3 Time Trends in Incidence

Trends in incidence of HB and HCC over time have been reported for the USA and Europe. The ACCIS report found no change in incidence over the time period 1978–1997 in hepatic tumors overall, HB, and HCC either in any country or in Europe as a whole (Kaatsch et al. 2006; Stiller et al. 2006). In contrast, the SEER Pediatric Monograph (Bulterys et al. 1999) covering the years 1975–1995 reported a marked increase in HB in children aged 0–14 years from 0.8 per million in 1975–1979 to 1.5 per million for 1990–1995. This trend was confirmed in a more recent report covering the years, 1992–2004, with an annual change of 4.3% for HB (Linabery and Ross 2008). National cancer registration data for England show a statistically significant increase in incidence of HB between 1990 and 2006 from 1.0 per million in 1990–1995 to 1.7 per million in 2001–2006 ($p = 0.0004$). The trend was significant in males and females and did not differ by age group (Birch and Alston, in preparation).

In the SEER monograph, a decrease in incidence of HCC was reported while no change in incidence of HCC over time was found in the English data. Changes in incidence of HCC in the Far East following the introduction of national vaccination programs are discussed in Sect. 3.4.

3.3 Analytical Epidemiology of Hepatoblastoma and Hepatocellular Carcinoma in Children

In contrast to descriptive studies of incidence patterns, analytical epidemiology seeks to identify and quantify causative risk factors. Often, such studies test hypotheses about causation generated by previous descriptive or observational studies. For rare diseases, the research approach of choice is the case-control study.

3.3.1 Overview of Environmental Risk Factors

There have been very few case-control studies of HB specifically, although certain comprehensive studies of childhood cancer have included cases of HB. Small numbers of cases have hindered progress. One case-control study in the USA, which included 75 cases, reported elevated odds ratios with maternal occupational exposures to paints or pigments, oil or coal products, and metals before or during pregnancy (Buckley et al. 1989). A subsequent nationwide study of childhood cancer in the UK (UKCCS) did not corroborate these findings. However, the UKCCS included only 28 cases of HB (McKinney et al. 2003; Birch 2000).

There have been anecdotal reports of the HB cases following: maternal exposure to steroid hormones (Otten et al. 1977; Melamed et al. 1982); maternal liver transplantation (Roll et al. 1997), and fetal alcohol syndrome (Khan et al. 1979).

HCC, at all ages, often has a viral etiology involving hepatitis B and C viruses (HBV, HCV) (IARC 1994) (see Sect. 3.3.5). The involvement of hepatitis viruses in HB has been investigated but appears not to be a factor (Wiwanitkit 2005; Hsiao et al. 2009; Chen et al. 2005). Other viruses have also been considered (Buckley et al. 1989) and HB has been reported in a child with vertically acquired HIV infection (Pollock et al. 2003). Known viruses do not seem to make a major contribution to HB etiology.

A consistent finding in a number of countries is a strong association between very low birth weight (VLBW) and risk of HB (Tanimura et al. 1998; Ansell et al. 2005; Reynolds et al. 2004). Speculations on, and investigations of, the etiological basis of these observations are ongoing but the improved survival of premature and VLBW infants during the past 3 decades may account for the observed increases in HB incidence in industrialized countries (Spector et al. 2004).

A second consistent finding is an increased risk of HB in the children of mothers who smoke and a higher risk when both parents smoke. This was first reported in an analysis of parental smoking data from the UKCCS (Pang et al. 2003). The association has subsequently been confirmed in three further independent studies from the UK, USA, and China (Sorahan and Lancashire 2004; McLaughlin et al. 2006; Pu et al. 2009). It now seems likely that this association is causal.

The associations between parental tobacco smoking, VLBW, and risk of HB are discussed in detail below (see Sects. 3.3.2 and 3.3.3).

3.3.2 Very Low Birth Weight and Hepatoblastoma

A statistically significant association between VLBW (<1,500 g) and increased risk of HB was first published by a Japanese group (Ikeda et al. 1997). A systematic review of HB cases included in the Japan Children's Cancer Registry revealed nine with VLBW, representing 4% of 231 HB cases over a 9 year period compared with 0.4% among children in the registry overall.

Several reports followed that confirmed and refined the risk of HB in VLBW infants. Reynolds et al. (2004) compared birth registration data on 99 cases of HB from California with 396 control children randomly selected from the same birth certificate files. The odds ratio (OR) for HB in children with birth weight <1,500 g was 50.6 (95% CI 6.6–388.0). A plot of the case distribution by birth weight showed a peak for birth weight <1,000 g. A similar case-control study design was used by McLaughlin et al. (2006) based on New York State Cancer Registry and electronic birth records. In this study, 11 of 58 HB cases had birth weight <1,000 g compared with 24 of 65,056 controls, relative risk (RR) 56.9% (95% CI 24.0, 130.7). Spector et al. (2008) found hazard ratios of 25.6 (95% CI 7.7, 85.0) and 9.2 (95% CI 3.1, 27.1) for birth weights <1,000 and 1,000–1,999 g, respectively, among 36 HB cases and 7,788 comparison children ascertained from Minnesota cancer surveillance and birth records. In the UKCCS, 3 of 22 children with HB weighed <1,500 g (OR = 69.0; 95% CI 12.0, 397.2) (Ansell et al. 2005).

Estimates of risk vary between studies. This is probably due to variations in study design and data sources, and also geographical differences in medical practice regarding the management of VLBW infants. However, these studies establish that there is a substantially increased risk of HB in children with VLBW, especially those with birth weights <1,000 g. This finding begs the question as to the identity of the associated causal factors.

Three subsequent studies from Japan investigated perinatal factors in VLBW infants with HB. The first of these (Maruyama et al. 1999) reviewed the medical records of 15 HB patients with birth weights <1,500 g and a median gestational age of 25 weeks. Nothing remarkable was found in the prenatal histories but oxygen therapy was given to 13 patients. The duration of assisted ventilation was significantly longer in patients with late stage tumors. In addition, furosemide therapy, which was also given to 13 patients, was significantly longer in patients with advanced tumors. The authors concluded that an environmental rather than a genetic etiology was suggested by these results.

These findings prompted a case-control study of 12 HB patients with birth weight <1,000 g and 75 birth weight-matched controls randomly selected from 3 neonatal centers. Medical records of mothers and infants were abstracted systematically for a predetermined range of pre- and postnatal factors. Univariate Cox regression analysis demonstrated durations of oxygen and furosemide therapies, and time taken to regain body weight at birth were significantly associated with HB development. However, in a multivariate analysis, only the duration of oxygen therapy emerged as a significant independent risk factor (Maruyama et al. 2000). These findings were supported by a subsequent smaller case-control study (Oue et al. 2003).

Studies of birth certificate records linked to cancer registry records found a statistically significant trend toward being diagnosed at a later age in those HB cases with birth weight <1,000 g (Reynolds et al. 2004). This finding was supported by an earlier study, which found a similar trend although statistical significance was not reached (Tanimura et al. 1998). Other possible prenatal risk factors derived from birth records include infertility treatment, higher maternal body mass index (McLaughlin et al. 2006; Pu et al. 2009; Spector et al. 2008).

3.3.3 Parental Tobacco Smoking and Hepatoblastoma

Paternal and maternal preconceptional and gestational smoking as possible risk factors for childhood cancer have been extensively studied. In general, analyses have focused on leukaemia, brain tumors, and all childhood cancers combined with equivocal results (Boffetta et al. 2000). Analyses of parental smoking data from the UKCCS considered each childhood cancer diagnostic group separately. After adjustment for parental age and socioeconomic factors, risk of HB was significantly increased for children whose mothers smoked preconceptionally, OR 2.7 (95% CI 1.16, 6.21), and was also elevated for paternal preconceptional smoking with borderline significance, OR 2.2 (95% CI 0.94, 5.12). However, the highest risk was seen when both parents smoked compared with neither, OR 4.7 (95% CI 1.7, 13.4). The association was confined to cases diagnosed at older ages. For maternal smoking in cases diagnosed at the median age or above, the OR was 12.0 (95% CI 2.5, 56.8) (Pang et al. 2003). The association remained after adjustment for birthweight (Pang and Birch 2003). Pang et al. interpreted their results as indicating a possible transplacental carcinogenic effect of tobacco products, rather than a preconceptional effect on germ cells.

Strong support for this finding was published soon after by Sorahan and Lancashire (2004) who analyzed the Oxford Survey of Childhood Cancer (OSCC) data on parental cigarette smoking. The OSCC was an earlier study in the UK and there was no overlap of cases with the UKCCS. They reported an RR of 2.3 (95% CI 1.02, 5.09) for hepatoblastoma in children if both parents smoked relative to neither. Since then, two other reports have corroborated the findings with respect to maternal smoking based on data from birth registrations and medical records for HB cases and other children. ORs for maternal smoking of 2.9 (95% CI 1.1., 4.2) and 2.1 (95% CI 1.0, 4.2) were found in Changqing, China, and New York State, USA, respectively (Pu et al. 2009; McLaughlin et al. 2006). Furthermore, in the study by McLaughlin et al., the risk was found to be stronger for cases diagnosed at later ages and appeared to be limited to children with normal birth weight thereby adding weight to similar findings by Pang et al. (2003) and Pang and Birch (2003).

On the basis of these four studies, the International Agency for Research on Cancer (IARC) has recently classified tobacco smoke (via parental smoking) as a human carcinogen for childhood hepatoblastoma (Secretan et al. 2009).

3.3.4 Associations with Heritable Cancer Predisposition, Congenital Malformation Syndromes, and Anomalies

A wide spectrum of congenital malformation syndromes and isolated anomalies have been reported in cases of HB. The overall frequency of anomalies among children with HB appears to be higher than for any pediatric tumor other than Wilms' (Hartley et al. 1990; Mann et al. 1990; Narod et al. 1997; Ansell et al. 2003). Case reports include children with progressive familial cholestasis, myelodysplasia, Noonan Syndrome, Fragile X Syndrome, Sotos Syndrome, Cardio-Facio-Cutaneous Syndrome, Prader-Willi Syndrome, Goldenhar Syndrome, and neurofibromatosis type 1 (Corona-Rivera et al. 2006; Richter et al. 2005; Neas et al. 2006; Yoshida et al. 2008; Wirojanan et al. 2008; Kato et al. 2009; Hashizume et al. 1991; Gripp et al. 2007; Uçar et al. 2005). The etiological significance of these various syndromes is uncertain but possible links with prematurity/low birth weight and neonatal care should be considered as well as genetic links.

In addition to occasional case reports of HB in syndromic children, three conditions have been established as conferring an increased risk of HB: trisomy 18, Beckwith Wiedemann syndrome (BWS), and familial adenomatous polyposis (FAP). Trisomy 18 or Edwards syndrome (ES) is associated with multiple congenital anomalies including heart defects, craniofacial abnormalities, limb and other skeletal abnormalities, microcephaly, mental retardation, intrauterine growth retardation, and short stature, among others. The incidence of ES is reported as 1 in 3,000 to 7,000 births. Survival past the first year is rare (Edwards et al. 1960; Root and Carey 1994; Taylor 1968; Rasmussen et al. 2003). There have now been at least seven published cases of HB in children with ES. This suggests an etiological association between these two conditions rather than chance (Kitanovski et al. 2009; Maruyama et al. 2001).

BWS, which predisposes to a number of embryonal tumors, is characterized by somatic overgrowth, abdominal wall defects, macroglossia, and ear anomalies, and is associated with imprinting defects of genes located on chromosome 11p15. The overall percentage of children with BWS who developed tumors, and whose molecular defects had been characterized, was 7.5–13.5%. However, tumor risk varies according to the specific defect. The most frequent tumor types are Wilms and HB (Weksberg et al. 2001; Cooper et al. 2005; Rump et al. 2005; De Baun et al. 2002).

The association between FAP and HB was first reported by Kingston et al. (1983). Subsequently, there have been numerous reports and the risk of HB in FAP carriers has been estimated to be as high as 800-fold above sporadic population rates (Giardello et al. 1991; Hughes and Michels 1992). There may be genotype-phenotype links between specific mutations to the APC gene, which is mutated in FAP, and development of HB (Hirschman et al. 2005). This is supported by the occurrence of HB in siblings from FAP families (Thomas et al. 2003; Hirschman et al. 2005). Given the overall rarity of the two conditions, this suggests that penetrance for HB may be increased in certain FAP families in association with specific APC mutations. HB may be the first phenotypic manifestation of APC mutation in a kindred (Thomas et al. 2003).

3.3.5 Etiology of Hepatocellular Carcinoma in Children

The majority of HCC cases across all ages in developing countries are due to hepatitis B virus infection (HBV) and aflatoxin exposure and to alcohol abuse and smoking in developed countries (Hirohashi et al. 2000). Hepatitis C virus (HCV) is also a factor, especially in Japan. Worldwide, the incidence varies according to the prevalence of these risk factors.

There is a particularly high incidence in sub-Saharan Africa and the Far East in HBV hyperendemic areas. HBV specifically infects and replicates in liver cells, and clonally integrated viral DNA sequences are detected in tumor cells (IARC 1994; Levy et al. 2002). In general, tumors arise following decades of chronic infection with HBV, with peak incidence of HCC in fourth, fifth, and sixth decades of life depending on geographical location. HCV, in contrast to HBV, is an RNA virus. It is less prevalent than HBV and accounts for a much smaller proportion of cases worldwide. Similar to HBV, it damages liver cells resulting in continual regrowth. HCV is the etiological agent in most patients with post-transfusion hepatitis.

Aflatoxins are produced by the fungi *Aspergillus flavus* and *Aspergillus parasiticus*. In humans, main exposure comes from contaminated foods including peanuts, corn, and cassava. The fungi proliferate particularly in warm, damp conditions. The carcinogenic potential of aflatoxin is substantially greater in individuals with chronic HBV infection. Reduction of food contamination in populations with a high incidence of HBV infection will reduce HCC rates (Henry et al. 2002).

Although rates of HCC in children are extremely low compared with older adults, childhood HCC is an important tumor in areas of the world with high HBV carrier rates. HCC constitutes between 35% and 70% of childhood liver tumors in such areas (Chen et al. 2005; Hsiao et al. 2009; Moore et al. 2004). Although clearly there is only limited exposure time in children, HBV appears to be the etiologic agent in these cases. The incidence of HCC in HBV hyperendemic areas in China and Thailand appears to have fallen dramatically following the introduction of national HBV vaccination programs. Such programs have been successful in reducing rates of chronic HBV infection in children (Chen et al. 1996; Chang et al. 1997, 2005; Hsiao et al. 2009; Wichajarn et al. 2008). Nevertheless, even after the introduction of vaccination HBV infection was still the most important factor in childhood HCC in Taiwan (Hsiao et al. 2009). It has been suggested that vaccination against HBV would reduce the potency of aflatoxins and reduce risk of HCC (Henry et al. 2002).

In other parts of the world, HCC may arise in children with various metabolic disorders but HBV infection may still be an important etiological factor in a proportion of cases. In a study based on HCC cases in the Kiel pediatric Tumor Registry, 64% of those investigated demonstrated positivity for HBV surface antigen (Leuschner et al. 1988). Such children may be inherently susceptible to the carcinogenic effects of the virus.

3.4 Implications of Findings from Analytical Studies of Pediatric Liver Tumors

There is a paucity of comprehensive studies of etiology and none that includes substantial case numbers. However, studies of HB focused on prenatal and birth characteristics have yielded a number of positive findings; principally, associations with VLBW and prenatal exposure to parental tobacco smoking. Both findings are likely to reflect causation. In addition, HB risk is increased in children with certain heritable conditions. Therefore, there are examples of causative factors for HB acting in the preconceptional, gestational, and postnatal time periods.

Regarding the increased risk of HB in children with VLBW, especially those with birth weights below 1,000 g, the evidence points to factors linked to neonatal intensive care (Spector et al. 2008). Duration of oxygen therapy emerged as the only independent risk factor in a multivariate analysis of data from a case-control study of children. Prolonged oxygen therapy, perhaps in combination with other therapies, e.g., furosemide, is plausible as a causative agent given the probable sensitivity to oxidative damage of immature and rapidly proliferating tissues and cells in the preterm infant (Maruyama et al. 2000). This must be one of the prime hypotheses to be tested in future and ongoing studies of HB etiology.

An alternative hypothesis was suggested by Latini (2004) who proposed that exposure to di-(2-ethylhexyl)phthalate (DEHP) may be a factor. DEHP is a plasticizer widely used in polyvinyl chloride (PVC), medical, and many consumer products. Leaching of DEHP from these products is known to occur and prenatal exposure appears to be associated with shorter gestation (Whyatt et al. 2009; Latini et al. 2003). Furthermore, in experimental models DEHP is a rodent hepatocarcinogen (Maloney and Waxman 1999). The US Food and Drug Administration, Center for Devices and Radiological Health, considered that infants in neonatal intensive care units constituted a population at increased risk of toxicity due to multiple medical device-related exposure to DEHP (US Food and Drug Administration, accessed April 2010).

A question for future studies is whether postnatal exposures are only of etiological significance in the setting of neonatal intensive care of the extremely premature infant, or might apply to related exposures in more mature infants, but perhaps with a lower associated risk. Even in babies weighing less than 1,000 g, although the RR of HB is high, the absolute risk is still quite small and probably of the order of about 0.5% (Oue et al. 2003; Tanimura et al. 1998). Monitoring of these infants during their early years should be considered with a view to early detection.

The association with maternal prenatal tobacco smoke and stronger association when both parents are smokers can be interpreted as a transplacental carcinogenic effect of tobacco products. These exposures, although involuntary, involve direct exposure of the fetal liver, and potential levels of exposure to tobacco products are therefore higher than those associated with passive smoking. Tobacco smoke contains over 60 substances classified by IARC as carcinogenic to humans. Many of these are known to cross the placenta and impact on pregnancy outcome (Wu et al. 2007; Windham et al. 1992, 2000).

Tobacco carcinogens include: N-nitroso compounds, aromatic amines, and polycyclic aromatic hydrocarbons. These interact with DNA and mutations, which are directly attributable to tobacco carcinogens, are detected in smokers' lung cancers. The most likely candidates as transplacental liver carcinogens are N-nitroso compounds that have been shown to induce malignant liver tumors following transplacental exposure in experimental animals (Anderson et al. 1989; Beebe et al. 1993). The identification of a causal link between parental tobacco smoking and HB provides a model of human transplacental liver carcinogenesis. Transplacental carcinogens from other sources, e.g., dietary N-nitroso compounds, should be the focus of future studies.

The proportion of total HB cases attributable to heritable and sporadic and isolated congenital malformations is uncertain. Also uncertain is whether and how frequently new germline mutations, arising in parental germ cells, occur. If these do occur, then the question of whether they are due to endogenous processes or to parental exposures must be addressed.

It might be predicted that cases of HB associated with syndromes and congenital anomalies would occur at the younger end of the HB age-incidence distribution. However, a review of published cases cited in this chapter shows a broad range of ages at diagnosis from soon after birth to nearly 10 years. Although some of this variation may be due to differences in genetic basis of the various conditions, even among cases associated with APC mutations, there is a difference of almost 10 years between the youngest and oldest cases (Hirschman et al. 2005). Different APC mutations may be more or less penetrant for HB but other endogenous and environmental factors may also influence if and when HB develops in APC mutation carriers and in children with other predisposing conditions. Risk and age of onset of HB may vary with polymorphic variants in metabolic and other genes in mothers (transplacental exposures) and case children (Pakakasama et al. 2003, 2004; Wu et al. 2007).

Epigenetic changes are found in many cases including those associated with BWS (Weksberg et al. 2003, 2005; DeBaun et al. 2002). Exogenous factors may lead to epigenetic modifications early in pre- and postnatal life, especially at critical periods in development (Jirtle and Skinner 2007; Waterland and Michels 2007; Heijmans et al. 2008). Assisted reproductive technologies (ART) may be a special example of this and some data on rates of occurrence of imprinting disorders, including BWS, among children conceived by ART, suggest an increased risk (Gosden et al. 2003; Weksberg et al. 2003). The possibility of environmentally induced epigenetic modification is clearly another area for consideration in future studies of HB etiology.

While the etiology of HCC is largely known, there are still some outstanding questions regarding childhood cases. The proportion of cases due to HBV, HCV, and known constitutional disorders requires clarification. Whether there are residual cases of currently unknown etiology needs to be determined and generation of hypotheses about causation will be necessary. Reasons for the development of this usually adult-onset cancer at very young ages should be sought, and genetic variations in susceptibility to exogenous risk factors such as HBV should be investigated. The possibility that risk factors for HB might also apply to HCC and other pediatric liver tumors should be considered.

3.5 Conclusions

In spite of the rarity of pediatric liver tumors and the lack of comprehensive studies of etiology, a number of substantive risk factors have emerged. These include VLBW and parental prenatal tobacco smoking, both of which involve environmental exposures. The classification by IARC of tobacco smoking as a carcinogen for hepatoblastoma provides another strong reason for discouraging cigarette smoking among parents of young children and those approaching parenthood. Mention of this association should be included in governmental and other tobacco control strategies aimed at improving the health of children as well as adults.

Although we do not yet understand the mechanisms involved in the increased risk for the HB associated with VLBW, the association is apparently causal and appears to involve aspects of neonatal intensive care. The risk, though greatly increased above population levels, is still very small and until mechanisms are elucidated, there is no justification for modifying clinical practice. However, VLBW infants should be monitored to ensure early diagnosis of HB wherever possible (Maruyama et al. 2000).

In children with congenital malformations and other predisposition syndromes with an established increased risk of HB, surveillance protocols already exist (Rao et al. 2008; Zarate et al. 2009). Implementation of such protocols should be considered in centers where this is not already the practice. Successful vaccination programs for HBV have been established in some hyperendemic areas and have demonstrated their effectiveness in the control of HCC. In the future, it may be possible to enhance the control of HCC worldwide.

The challenges for future and ongoing studies of etiology are to understand the mechanisms associated with currently known risk factors and to consider whether these explain more cases than currently recognized. Given the inherent vulnerability of the fetal and infant liver, timing, route of exposure, and individual genetic make up may affect the outcome in terms of specific tumor development and age of onset. Large cooperative international studies are required to explore these issues further. Population-based cancer registries will continue to play a vital role in monitoring incidence internationally.

Acknowledgments Statistical analyses were carried out by Dr. Robert D Alston. Professor Jillian M. Birch is Cancer Research UK Professorial Fellow at the University of Manchester. Data on incident cancers were contributed by the eight regional cancer registries in England and supplied by the Northern and Yorkshire Cancer Registry and Information Service.

References

Alston RD, Geraci M, Eden TOB et al (2008) Changes in cancer incidence in teenagers and young adults (ages 13 to 24 years) in England 1979–2003. Cancer 113:2807–2815

Anderson LM, Hecht SS, Dixon DE et al (1989) Evaluation of the transplacental tumor-igenecity of the tobacco-specific carcinogen 4-(methylnitrosamino)-1-(3pyridyl)-1-butanone in mice. Cancer Res 49:3770–3775

Ansell P, Mitchell CD, Roman E et al (2005) Relationships between perinatal and maternal characteristics and hepatoblastoma: a report from the UKCCS. Eur J Cancer 41: 741–748

Beebe LE, Kim YE, Amin S et al (1993) Comparison of transplacental and neonatal initiation of mouse lung and liver tumours by N-nitrosodimethylamine (NDMA) and 4-(methylnitrosamino)-1-(3-pyridyl)-1-butanone (NNK) and promotability by a polychlorinated biphenyls mixture (Aroclor 1254). Carcinogenesis 14:1545–1548

Birch JM (2000) Diagnostic review and classification of solid tumours, in the United Kingdom Childhood Cancer Study: objectives, materials and methods. Br J Cancer 82(5): 1073–1102

Birch JM and Alston RD (2010) Incidence, spectrum and relative frequency of liver tumours in children and adolescents in England, 1990–2006 (in preparation)

Boffetta P, Tredaniel J, Greco A (2000) Risk of childhood cancer and adult lung cancer after childhood exposure to passive smoke: a meta-analysis. Environ Health Perspect 108(1): 73–82

Buckley JD, Sather H, Ruccione K et al (1989) A case-control study of risk factors for hepatoblastoma. Cancer 64: 1169–1176

Bulterys M, Goodman MT, Smith MA et al (1999) Cancer incidence, survival among children, adolescents: United States SEER Program 1975–1995. SEER program, NIH Pub No 99-4649:91–97

Chang MH, Chen CJ, Lai MS et al (1997) Universal hepatitis B vaccination in Taiwan and the incidence of hepatocellular carcinoma in children. N Engl J Med 336:1855–1859

Chang MH, Chen TH, Hsu HM et al (2005) Taiwan Childhood HCC Study Group. Prevention of hepatocellular carcinoma by universal vaccination against hepatitis B virus: the effect and problems. Clin Cancer Res 11:7953–7957

Chen HL, Chang MH, Ni YH et al (1996) Seroepidemiology of hepatitis B virus infection in children: ten years of mass vaccination in Taiwan. JAMA 276(906):908

Chen JC, Chang ML, Lin JN et al (2005) Comparison of childhood hepatic malignancies in hepatitis B hyper-endemic area. World J Gastroenterol 11(34):5289–5294

Cooper WN, Luharia A, Evans GA et al (2005) Molecular subtypes and phenotypic expression of Beckwith–Wiedemann syndrome. Eur J Hum Genet 13:1025–1032

Corona-Rivera JR, Sanchez-Zubieta F, Silva-Padilla N et al (2006) Hepataoblastoma in a patient with Goldenhar syndrome born to a diabetic mother. Am J Med Genet A 140A:2834–2837

De Baun MR, Niemitz EL, McNeil DR et al (2002) Epigenetic alterations of H19 and LIT1 distinguish patients with Beckwith–Wiedemann syndrome with cancer and birth defects. Am J Hum Genet 70:604–611

US Food and Drug Administration, Center for devices and radiological health safety assessment of di(2-ethylhexyl) phthalate (DEHP) released from PVC medical devices. http://www.fda.gov/cdrh/ost/dehp-pvc.pdf. Accessed April 2010

Edwards HJ, Harnden DG, Cameron AH et al (1960) A new trisomic syndrome. Lancet 1:787–790

Fritz A, Percy C, Jack A et al (eds) (2000) International classification of diseases for oncology, 3rd edn. World Health Organization, Geneva

Giardello F, Offerhaus G, Krush A et al (1991) Risk of hepatoblastoma in familial adenomatous polyposis. J Pediatr 1(19):766–768

Gosden R, Trasler J, Lucifero D, Faddy M (2003) Rare congenital disorders, imprinted genes, and assisted reproductive technology. Lancet 361:1975–1977

Gripp KW, Lin AE, Nicholson L et al (2007) Further delineation of the phenotype resulting from BRAF or MEK1 germline mutations helps differentiate cardi-facio-cutaneous syndrome from Costello syndrome. Am J Med Genet A 143A:1472–1480

Hartley AL, Birch JM, Kelsey AM et al (1990) Epidemiological and familial aspects of hepatoblastoma. Med Ped Onc 18:103–109

Hashizume K, Nakajo T, Kawarasaki H et al (1991) Prader-Willi syndrome with del(15)(q11, q13) associated with hepatoblastoma. Acta Pediatr Jpn 33:718–722

Heijmans BT, Tobi EW, Stein AD et al (2008) Persistent epigenetic differences associated with prenatal exposure to famine in humans. PNAS 105(44):17046–17049

Henry SH, Bosch FX, Bowers JC (2002) Aflatoxin, hepatitis and worldwide liver cancer risks. Adv Exp Med Biol 504: 229–233

Hirohashi S, Ishak KG, Kojiro M et al (2000) Hepatocellular carcinoma. In: Hamilton SR, Aaltonen LA (eds) Tumours of the digestive system. IARC Press, Lyon

Hirschman BA, Pollock BH, Tomlinson GE (2005) The spectrum of APC mutations in children with hepatoblastoma from familial adenomatous polyposis kindreds. J Pediatr 147:263–266

Hsiao CC, Chuang JH, Tiao MM, Sheen JM, Shieh CH (2009) Patterns of hepatoblastoma and hepatocellular carcinoma in children after universal hepatitis B vaccination in Taiwan. J Pediatr Hematol Oncol 31(2):91–96

Hughes L, Michels V (1992) Risk of hepatoblastoma in familial adenomatous polyposis. Am J Med Genet 43:1023–1025

IARC Monographs on the Evaluation of Carcinogenic Risks to Humans (1994) IARC Monograph Vol 59, Hepatitis Viruses

Ikeda H, Matsuyama S, Tanimura M (1997) Association between hepatoblastoma and very low birth weight: a trend or a chance? J Pediatr 130:557–560

Jirtle RL, Skinner MK (2007) Environmental epigenomics and disease susceptibility. Nat Rev 8:253–262

Kaatsch P, Steliarova-Foucher E, Crocetti E et al (2006) Time trends of cancer incidence in European children (1978–1997): report from the Automated Childhood Cancer Information project. Eur J Cancer 42:1961–1971

Kato M, Takita J, Takahashi K et al (2009) Hepatoblastoma in a patient with Sotos syndrome. J Pediatr 155(6):937–939

Khan A, Bader JL, Hoy GR et al (1979) Hepatoblastoma in child with fetal alcohol syndrome (letter). Lancet 1: 1403–1404

Kingston JE, Herbert A, Draper GJ et al (1983) Association between hepatoblastoma and polyposis coli. Arch Dis Child 58:959–963

Kitanovski L, Ovcak Z, Jazbec J (2009) Multifocal hepatoblastoma in a 6-month-old girl with trisomy 18: a case report. J Med Case Rep 3:8319. doi:10.4076/1752-1947-3-8319

Latini G (2004) Birth characteristics and hepatoblastoma risk in young children. Cancer 101(1):210

Latini G, De Felice C, Presta G et al (2003) In utero exposure to di-(2-ethylyhexyl)phthalate and duration of human pregnancy. Environ Health Perspect 111(14):1783–1785

Leuschner I, Harms D, Schmidt D (1988) The association of hepatocellular carcinoma in childhood with hepatitis B virus infection. Cancer 62:2363–2369

Lévy L, Renard CA, Wei Y, Buendia MA (2002) Genetic alterations and oncogenic pathways in hepatocellular carcinoma. Ann NY Acad Sci 963:21–36

Li J, Thompson TD, Miller W et al (2008) Cancer incidence among children and adolescents in the United States, 2001–2003. Pediatrics 121:e1470–e1477. doi:10.1542/peds.2007-2964

Linabery AM, Ross JA (2008) Trends in childhood cancer incidence in the U.S. (1992–2004). Cancer 112:416–432

Maloney EK, Waxman DJ (1999) Trans-activation of PPARalpha chemicals. Toxicol Appl Pharmacol 161:209–218

Mann JR, Kashuri N, Raafat et al (1990) Malignant hepatic tumours in children: incidence, clinical features and aetiology. Paediatr Perinat Epidemiol 4:276–289

Maruyama K, Ikeda H, Koizumi T, Tsuchida Y (1999) Prenatal and postnatal histories of very low birthweight infants who developed hepatoblastoma. Pediatr Int 41:82–89

Maruyama K, Ikeda H, Koizumi T et al (2000) Case-control study of perinatal factors and hepatoblastoma in children with an extremely low birthweight. Pediatr Int 42:492–498

Maruyama K, Ikeda H, Koizumi T (2001) Hepatoblastoma associated with trisomy 18 syndrome: a case report and a review of the literature. Pediatr Int 43:302–305

McKinney PA, Fear NT, Stockton D (2003) Parental occupation at periconception: findings from the United Kingdom Childhood Cancer Study. Occup Environ Med 60:901–909

McLaughlin CC, Baptiste MS, Schymura MJ et al (2006) Maternal and infant birth characteristics and hepatoblastoma. Am J Epidemiol 163(9):818–828

Melamed I, Bujanover Y, Hammer J et al (1982) Hepatoblastoma in an infant born to a mother after hormonal treatment for sterility (letter). N Engl J Med 307:820

Moore SW, Millar AJW, Hadley GP et al (2004) Hepatocellular carcinoma and liver tumors in South African children – a case for increased prevalence. Cancer 101:642–649

Narod SA, Hawkins MM, Robertson CM, Stiller CA (1997) Congenital anomalies and childhood cancer in Great Britain. Am J Hum Genet 60:474–485

Neas K, Peters G, Jackson J et al (2006) Chromosome 7 aberrations in a young girl with myelodysplasia and hepatoblastoma: an unusual association. Clin Dysmorphol 15:1–8

Otten J, Smets R, De Jager R et al (1977) Hepatoblastoma in an infant after contraceptive intake during pregnancy (letter). N Engl J Med 297:222

Oue OT, Kubota A, Okuyama H et al (2003) Hepatoblastoma in children of extremely low birth weight: a report from a single perinatal center. J Pediatr Surg 38:134–137

Pakakasama S, Chen TT-L, Frawley W et al (2003) Myeloperoxidase promotor and polymorphism and risk of hepatoblastoma. Int J Cancer 106:205–207

Pakakasama S, Chen TT-L, Frawley W et al (2004) CCND1 polymorphism and age of onset of hepatoblastoma. Oncogene 23:4789–4792

Pang D, Birch JM (2003) Smoking and hepatoblastoma: confounding by birth weight? Br J Cancer 89(3):602–603

Pang D, McNally R, Birch JM (2003) Parental smoking and childhood cancer: results from the United Kingdom Childhood Cancer Study. Br J Cancer 88:373–381

Parkin DM, Kramárová E, Draper GJ et al (eds) (1998) International incidence of childhood cancer, vol II. IARC Scientific Publications, Lyon

Percy C, Van Holten V, Muir C (eds) (1990) International classification of diseases for oncology, 2nd edn. World Health Organization, Geneva

Pollock BH, Jenson HB, Charles T et al (2003) Risk factors for pediatric human immunodeficiency virus-related malignancy. JAMA 289(18):2393–2399

Porta M (ed) (2008) A dictionary of epidemiology, 5th edn. Oxford University Press, New York

Pu CL, Jin XQ, Deng C et al (2009) Retrospective analysis of maternal and infant birth features of hepatoblastoma patients. Zhonghua Gan Zang Bing Za Zhi 17(6):459–461

Rao A, Rothman J, Nichols KE (2008) Genetic testing and tumor surveillance for children with cancer predisposition syndromes. Curr Opin Pediatr 20:1–7

Rasmussen SA, Wong LY, Yang Q et al (2003) Population-based analyses of mortality in trisomy 13 and trisomy 18. Pediatrics 111:777–784

Reynolds P, Urayama KY, Von Behren J, Feusner J (2004) Birth characteristics and hepatoblastoma risk in young children. Cancer 100:1070–1076

Richter A, Grabhorn E, Schulz A et al (2005) Hepatoblastoma in a child with progressive familial intrahepatic cholestasis. Pediatr Trans 9:805–808

Roll C, Luboldt HF, Winter A et al (1997) Hepatoblastoma in a 2-year-old child of a liver-transplanted mother. Lancet 349:103

Root S, Carey JC (1994) Survival in trisomy 18. Am J Med Genet 49:170–174

Rump P, Zeegers MPA, van Essen AJ (2005) Tumor risk in Beckwith–Wiedemann syndrome: a review and meta-analysis. Am J Hum Genet 136A:95–104

Secretan B, Straif K, Baan R et al (2009) A review of human carcinogens – Part E: tobacco, areca nut, alcohol, coal smoke and salted fish. Lancet Oncol 10(11):1033–1034

Sorahan T, Lancashire RJ (2004) Parental cigarette smoking and childhood risks of hepatoblastoma: OSCC data. Br J Cancer 90:1016–1018

Spector LG, Feuner JH, Ross JA (2004) Hepatoblastoma and low birth weight (letter). Pediatr Blood Cancer 43:706

Spector LG, Johnson KJ, Soler JT, Puumala SE (2008) Perinatal risk factors for hepatoblastoma. Br J Cancer 98:1570–1573

Steliarova-Foucher E, Stiller C, Lacour B, Kaatsch P (2005) International classification of childhood cancer, third edition. Cancer 103:1457–1467

Steliarova-Foucher E, Coebergh JW, Kaatsch P et al (eds) (2006) Cancer in children and adolescents in Europe. Eur J Cancer 42(13):1913–2190

Stiller C, Pritchard J, Steliorova-Foucher E (2006) Liver cancer in European children: incidence and survival, (1978–1997). Report from the Automated Childhood Cancer Information System project. Eur J Cancer 42:2115–2123

Stocker JT, Conran RM, Selby DM (1998) Tumors and pseudotumors of the liver. In: Stocker JT, Askin FB (eds) Pathology of solid tumors in children. Chapman and Hall, London

Tanimura M, Matsui I, Abe J et al (1998) Increased rick of hepatoblastoma among immature children with a lower birth weight. Cancer Res 58:3032–3035

Taylor A (1968) Autosomal trisomy syndrome: a detailed study of 17 cases of Edwards Syndrome. J Med Genet 5:227–252

Thomas D, Pritchard J, Davidson R et al (2003) Familial hepatoblastoma and APC gene mutations: renewed call for molecular research. Eur J Cancer 39:2200–2204

Uçar C, Calişkan Ű, Toy H, Gűnel E (2005) Hepatoblastoma in a child with Neurofibromatosis Type 1. Pediat Blood Cancer 49(3):357–359

Waterland RA, Michels KB (2007) Epigenetic epidemiology of the developmental origins hypothesis. Annu Rev Nutr 27: 363–388

Weksberg R, Nishikawa J, Caluseriu O et al (2001) Tumor development in the Beckwith–Wiedemann syndrome is associated with a variety of constitutional molecular 11p15 alterations including imprinting defects of KCNQ1OT1. Hum Mol Genet 10(26):2989–3000

Weksberg R, Smith AC, Squire J, Sadowski P (2003) Beckwith–Wiedemann syndrome demonstrates a role for epigenetic control of normal development. Hum Mol Genet 12(1): R61–R68

Weksberg R, Shuman C, Smith AC (2005) Beckwith–Wiedemann syndrome. Am J Hum Genet 137C:12–23

Whyatt RM, Adibi JJ, Calafat AM et al (2009) Prenatal di(2-ethylhexyl)phthalate exposure and length of gestation among an inner-city cohort. Pediatrics 124:e1213–e1220. doi: 10.1542/peds.2009-0325

Wichajarn K, Kosalaraksa P, Wiangnon S (2008) Incidence of hepatocellular carcinoma in children in Khon Kaen before and after national hepatitis B vaccine program. Asian Pac J Cancer Prev 9(3):507–509

Windham GC, Swan SH, Fenster L (1992) Parental cigarette smoking and the risk of spontaneous abortion. Am J Epidemiol 135:1394–1403

Windham GC, Hopkins B, Fenster et al (2000) Prenatal active or passive smoke exposure and the risk of preterm delivery or low birth weight. Epidemiology 11:427–433

Wirojanan J, Kraff J, Douglas S et al (2008) Two boys with fragile X syndrome and hepatic tumors. J Pediat Hematol Oncol 30(3):239–241

Wiwanitkit V (2005) Hepatitis virus B is not a risk factor in hepatoblastoma patients. Asian Pac J Cancer Prev 6(2):213–214

Wu T, Chen C, Yang F et al (2007) Passive smoking, metabolic gene polymorphisms and infant birth weight in a Prospective Cohort Study of Chinese women. Am J Epidemiol 166: 313–322

Yoshida R, Ogata T, Masawa N, Nagai T (2008) Hepatoblastoma in a Noonan syndrome patient with a PTPN11 mutation. Pediatr Blood Cancer 50:1274–1276

Zarate YA, Mena R, Martin LJ et al (2009) Experience with hemihyperplasia and Beckwith–Wiedemann syndrome surveillance protocol. Am J Med Genet 149A:1691–1697

Molecular Aspects of Hepatoblastoma

4

Roland Kappler and Dietrich von Schweinitz

Contents

R. Kappler (✉)
Kinderchirurgische Klinik, Dr. von Haunersches Kinderspital, Ludwig-Maximilians-Universität München, Lindwurmstrasse 2a, 80337 München, Germany
e-mail: roland.kappler@med.uni-muenchen.de

D. von Schweinitz
Kinderchirurgische Klinik im Dr. von Haunerschen Kinderspital, Universität München, Lindwurmstrasse 4, D-80337 München, Germany
e-mail: dietrich.schweinitz@med.uni-muenchen.de

4.1 Introduction

The purpose of this chapter is to describe briefly the molecular features of hepatoblastoma (HB), the most common hepatic malignancy in early childhood. As this tumor replicates the phenotypic and biological features of the developing liver, many processes known to be essential in early embryonic development are implicated in the genesis of HB. Today's knowledge of the molecular components and mechanisms by which these liver tumors develop and progress is currently used to establish accurate tumor-specific diagnostic tools, systems for predicting prognosis and response to therapy and, ultimately, potential novel therapeutic strategies. Promising approaches integrating molecular and genetic information into traditional morphology-based classification schemes are now on the brink of providing the basis for a risk-adapted and clinically meaningful stratification of patients who either benefit from conventional therapies or are amenable to more targeted forms of treatment.

4.2 Basics of Hepatoblastoma

HB is a rare malignancy of the liver affecting about 1/1,000,000 children under the age of 15 in Western countries (Mann et al. 1990). Although relatively rare, it is still the most common liver tumor of childhood, comprising 50–60% of all hepatic neoplasms in this age group and particularly affecting infants and toddlers between 6 months and 3 years of age, preferentially males (Weinberg and Finegold 1983). Serum alpha fetoprotein (AFP) is currently the most important tumor marker in HB, as it is elevated in approximately 80% of the patients (von Schweinitz et al. 1994), but patients

A. Zimmermann et al. (eds.), *Pediatric Liver Tumors*, Pediatric Oncology,
DOI: 10.1007/978-3-642-14504-9_4, © Springer-Verlag Berlin Heidelberg 2011

with low or negative AFP exist and fare worse than those with elevated AFP levels (von Schweinitz et al. 1997). Although the etiology of HB remains unknown, disturbance of normal differentiation during hepatogenesis is thought to give rise to a wide spectrum of HB subtypes comprising epithelial phenotypes (differentiated fetal and less differentiated embryonal) and mesenchymal elements such as immature fibrous tissue or spindle cells and osteoid (Weinberg and Finegold 1983). In addition, a small fraction of HB with a small cell undifferentiated subtype exists, which is associated with a worse prognosis (Haas et al. 2001; Trobaugh-Lotrario et al. 2009).

4.3 Familial Forms of Hepatoblastoma

Although most HB are sporadic, this tumor has been described in association with a variety of inherited cancer syndromes (Table 4.1). The Beckwith–Wiedemann syndrome (BWS) is a well-recognized overgrowth syndrome characterized by macroglossia, macrosomia, omphalocele, hepatomegaly, nephromegaly, and hemihypertrophy (Engstrom et al. 1988). Besides these complications, a major issue of BWS is cancer predisposition with highest risk of neoplasia in the first decade of life. The most commonly reported tumors in BWS are Wilms' tumor (43%), HB (20%), and adrenocortical carcinoma (7%), although most children with BWS do not develop cancer (Lapunzina 2005). Due to the relative high incidence of HB in children with BWS, sonographic surveillance and serum AFP screening has been considered (Clericuzio et al. 2003). Imprinting defects involving the short arm of chromosome 11 at 11p15.5 have been implicated as a possible pathogenic mechanism in these patients (Weksberg et al. 1993a, b). This locus contains several genes involved in growth regulation including the *insulin-like growth factor 2* (*IGF2*) gene, a maternally imprinted fetal growth factor gene regulating cellular proliferation and differentiation (Pollak 2008).

Familial adenomatous polyposis (FAP) is an autosomal-dominant cancer predisposition syndrome caused by germ-line mutations in the tumor suppressor gene *adenomatous polyposis coli* (*APC*) (Rustgi 2007). Affected individuals characteristically develop hundreds to thousands of colorectal adenomas, a small proportion of which will invariably progress to colorectal carcinoma if not surgically removed. The incidence of HB in children of FAP patients is estimated to be between 0.42% and 0.75%, with a median age at diagnosis similar to that of sporadic HB (Hughes and Michels 1992). Gardner syndrome representing a variant of FAP in which desmoid tumors and osteomas occur together with multiple adenomas of the colon and rectum (Nishisho et al. 1991) is also related to the *APC* gene and consistently presents with HB (Krush et al. 1988). As for BWS, it has been suggested that children at risk for FAP should be closely monitored by measurement of serum AFP levels and abdominal ultrasound (Aretz et al. 2006).

Li–Fraumeni syndrome (LFS) is an autosomal dominant inherited cancer predisposition syndrome characterized by leukemia as well as multiple tumors of soft tissue, bone, breast, brain, and kidney at early ages (Li et al. 1988). LFS patients carry germ-line mutations in the tumor suppressor gene *TP53* and present in 1% of all cases with HB (Nichols et al. 2001). Interestingly, *TP53* mutations are also detected in 24% of sporadic HB (Curia et al. 2008).

Simpson–Golabi–Behmel syndrome (SGBS) is an X-linked overgrowth disorder comprising multiple congenital abnormalities and increased risk for the

Table 4.1 Congenital or genetic syndromes with presentations of hepatoblastoma

Genetic syndrome	Gene/locus	Cytogenetic locus	Presumed function
Beckwith–Wiedemann syndrome	*IGF2/H19*	11p15.5	Fetal growth factor/noncoding RNA
Familial adenomatous polyposis/ Gardner syndrome	*APC*	5q21-q22	Antagonist of Wnt signaling
Li–Fraumeni syndrome	*TP53*	17p13.1	Inducer of cell cycle arrest, apoptosis, senescence, and DNA repair
Simpson–Golabi–Behmel syndrome	*GPC3*	Xq26	Regulator of cell division and growth
Sotos syndrome	*NSD1*	5q35	Histone methyltransferase
Neurofibromatosis type 1	*NF1*	17q11.2	Negative regulator of ras signaling

development of cancer (Behmel et al. 1984; Golabi et al. 1984). Besides Wilms' tumor, the occurrence of HB has been reported for single SGBS patients, who frequently carry mutations in the *glypican 3* (*GPC3*) gene (Li et al. 2001).

Sotos syndrome is an autosomal dominant inherited childhood overgrowth disease characterized by accelerated growth, macrocephaly, distinctive facial features, and developmental delay (Cole and Hughes 1994). Malignant neoplasias associated with this syndrome comprise neuroblastoma, Wilms' tumor, and teratoma. There is a single case of a 21-month-old boy diagnosed with Sotos syndrome, who developed HB (Kato et al. 2009). Interestingly, the tumor displayed a microdeletion of 5q35 in the region of the *nuclear receptor binding SET domain protein 1* (*NSD1*) gene, which is characteristic for Sotos syndrome.

The hallmark of *neurofibromatosis type 1* (NF1) is the development of benign tumors, including peripheral and plexiform neurofibromas (Matsui et al. 1993). There is a single case of a 9-month-old boy diagnosed with NF1 by the existence of numerous café-au-lait spots throughout the trunk and extremities, who developed a well-differentiated fetal HB (Ucar et al. 2007). However, a screen for mutations in the neurofibromatosis-related *NF1* gene has not been performed in this patient.

4.4 Chromosomal Abnormalities in Hepatoblastoma

Analysis of chromosomal and genomic aberrations has become a crucial factor in the description of genes and signaling pathways driving development and progression of human cancers. The first attempts to elaborate on the biology of HB have made use of conventional cytogenetics by analyzing chromosomes prepared from short time cultures of disaggregated tumor tissue. These studies have so far analyzed more than 150 tumor karyotypes and revealed that HB cells are often diploid or hyperdiploid, and usually harbor a limited number of chromosomal abnormalities (summarized in Tomlinson et al. (2005)). The most common chromosomal alterations found in HB are trisomy 2, 8, and 20 (Fig. 4.1a). Other numerical abnormalities in order of decreasing frequency are extra copies of chromosomes 7, 19, 5, 6, 22, 12, 17, 16, 13, 14, 1, 15, 21, and 10 (Tomlinson et al. 2005). Chromosomal losses are less frequent in HB and occur as monosomies 4, 9, 14, 15, 18, and 21 (Fig. 4.1b). Structural aberrations predominantly involve chromosomes 1, 2, and 4, with 1q12-q21, 2q35-q37, and 4q34 being the most common chromosomal breakpoints (Schneider et al. 1997; Tomlinson et al. 2005; Yeh et al. 2000). However, the seven permanent HB cell lines published so far are cytogenetically heterogeneous, except for the gain of chromosome 20 (Scheil et al. 2003).

Comparative genomic hybridization (CGH), which allows for the detection of genomic imbalances within a tumor genome in a single fluorescence in situ hybridization experiment, has proven a valuable tool to further narrow down chromosomal regions identified in HB by classical cytogenetics (Gray et al. 2000b; Scheil et al. 2003; Stejskalova et al. 2009; Weber et al. 2000). On the basis of CGH, gains were frequently found on 2q (47%) and 1q (43%), followed by 8q (15%), 17q (15%; Fig. 4.1c) and 20 (25%). Losses are much rarer and mainly affect the chromosomal arm 4q (9%). Interestingly, chromosomal gains on 8q and 20 can serve as a predictor of poor outcome, since both alterations when taken together occur in 75% of patients who died from disease, compared to 12% in patients who survived (Weber et al. 2000). Another advantage of CGH is that it could provide information on chromosomal sites harboring amplified DNA sequences. The existence of high-level gene amplifications in HB was already known from cytogenetic analyses by the detection of so-called double-minute chromosomes, small fragments of extrachromosomal material. The most relevant regions detected by CGH and suspected to contain HB-relevant genes are 1q25.21-q44, 2q24, 8q11.2-q13, 8q11.2-q21.3, and 10q24-q26 (Gray et al. 2000b; Scheil et al. 2003; Weber et al. 2000).

The recent development of whole-genome DNA chip-based technologies has further advanced the detection limit of chromosomal aberrations in HB (Adesina et al. 2007; Cairo et al. 2008; Stejskalova et al. 2009; Suzuki et al. 2008). One of the first studies was performed on a bacterial artificial chromosome (BAC) array depicting frequent gains at the 14q12 locus, which harbors the *forkhead box G1* (*FOXG1*) gene (Adesina et al. 2007). By using high-density single-nucleotide polymorphism microarrays, three high-grade amplifications were detected at 7q34, 11q22.2, and 14q11.2 (Suzuki et al. 2008). Genes that map to these regions include *ephrin receptor B6* (*EPHB6*), three matrix metallopeptidases (*MMP1*, *MMP7*, *MMP20*), and

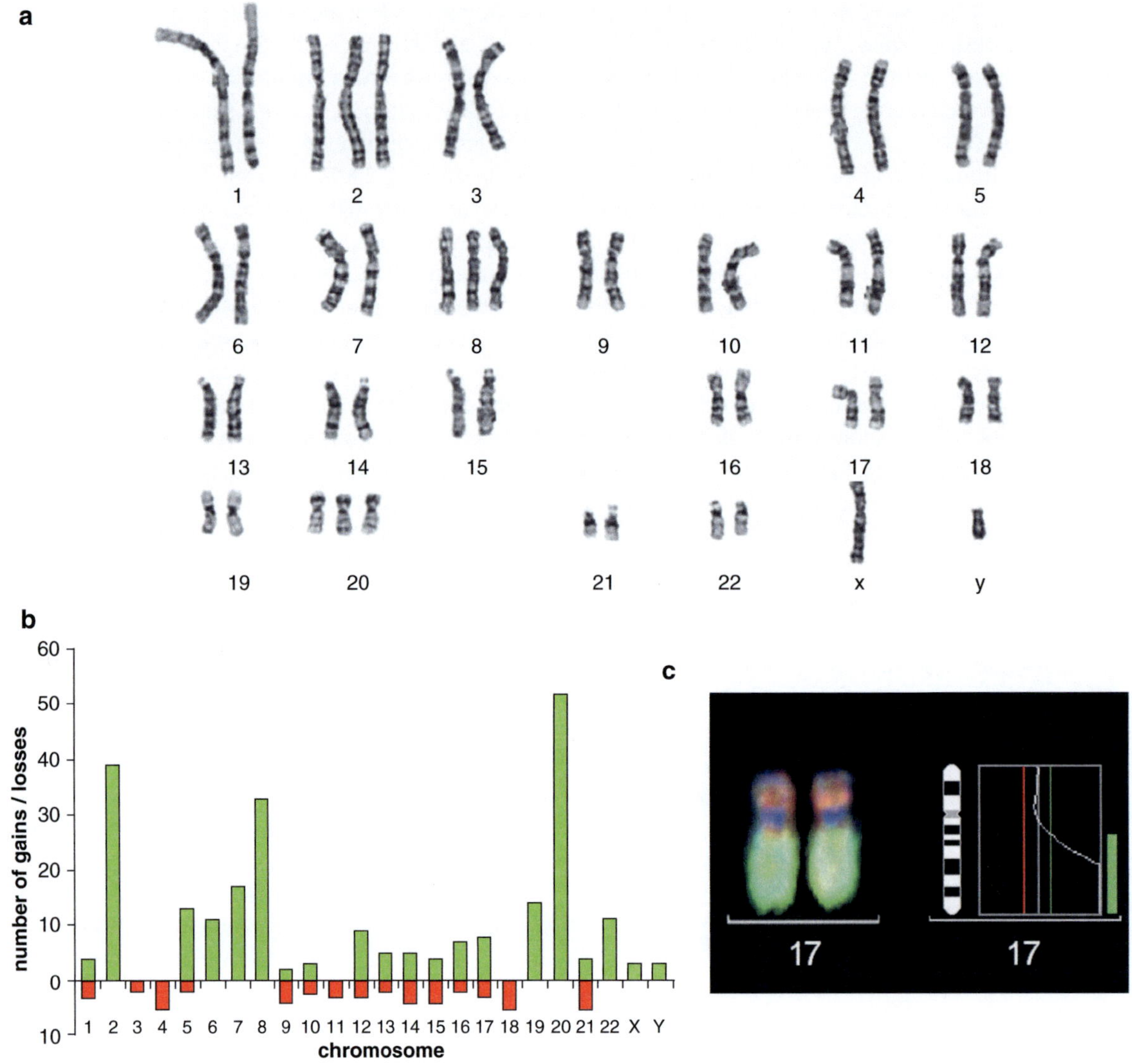

Fig. 4.1 Chromosomal abnormalities in HB. **(a)** Trisomy 3, 8, and 20; **(b)** compilation of cytogenetic findings (gains, *green*; losses, *red*); **(c)** gain of 17q (increased green fluorescence by CGH)

defender against cell death 1 (*DAD1*). However, the candidate genes representing the targets of these gains and/or amplifications identified so far have neither been validated in independent cohorts of HB, nor tested for their relevance in HB development. Using oligonucleotide arrays, three regions of chromosome 2, namely, 2q13-q22, 2q36-37, and the entire 2p arm, were found to have significantly gained in a subclass of HB, which is tightly associated with features of advanced tumor stage, such as vascular invasion and extrahepatic metastasis (Cairo et al. 2008).

Another approach to define chromosomal regions altered in tumor cells is the loss of heterozygosity (LOH) analysis, which makes use of so-called microsatellite markers, DNA sequence polymorphisms that are dispersed all over the genome and can be detected by means of polymerase chain reaction (PCR). By comparing DNA of normal and tumor tissue at various heterozygous loci, tumor-specific deletions of allelic sequences and their expansion can be precisely mapped for the genomic locus of interest. Several studies report on frequent LOH on chromosome 1p32, 1p36.3, and 11p15.5, sites suspected to harbor tumor suppressor genes involved in the genesis of HB (Albrecht et al. 1994; Kraus et al. 1996; Little et al. 1988). Interestingly, lost alleles at 11p15.5

in HB are exclusively of maternal origin (Albrecht et al. 1994), a well-known phenomenon common to a variety of embryonal tumors, including Wilms' tumor and rhabdomyosarcoma (Feinberg 1993). The 11p15.5 locus contains several imprinted genes that are monoallelically expressed, namely, *IGF2*, *H19*, and *KIP2*, the latter two of which are expressed from the maternal allele (Hartmann et al. 2000). Although the exact mechanism is still not clear, it is generally assumed that loss of the tumor suppressor *H19* leads to activation of the reciprocally imprinted and normally silent maternally derived copy of *IGF2* (Albrecht et al. 1994). Moreover, epigenetic silencing of the maternal *H19* allele and activation of both parental *IGF2* alleles has already been deduced from analyses on BWS patients in whom HB development has been described earlier (Weksberg et al. 1993a).

In summary, many analyses have been performed using a variety of different methodologies, generating evidence on the existence of several chromosomal abnormalities, which might play a role in the development of HB, but the identification of tumor-initiating and/or propagating genes by these approaches has not been successful up to now.

4.5 Altered Developmental Signaling Pathways in Hepatoblastoma

Childhood solid tumors are thought to arise from immature cells that harbor defects in molecular mechanisms controlling normal development (Scotting et al. 2005). During the last 2 decades, several signal transduction pathways that govern proliferation, differentiation, and maturation during embryonic development have been implicated in cancer (Birchmeier et al. 2003; Klaus and Birchmeier 2008; Pollak 2008; Ruiz et al. 2002). It is generally assumed that defects in any of the pathways could promote transformation making developing cells prone to tumorigenesis.

4.5.1 *The Wnt Signaling Pathway*

Wnt signaling plays a critical and evolutionary conserved role in directing cell fates during embryogenesis. In addition, inappropriate activation of the Wnt signal transduction pathway is known to drive the development of various cancers (Klaus and Birchmeier 2008; Polakis 2000). A key molecule of Wnt signaling is β-catenin, which is under physiological conditions localized at the plasma membrane of epithelial cells in a complex together with E-cadherin and α-catenin ensuring cell-cell contact as adherens junctions (Fig. 4.2a). The regular fate of β-catenin is phosphorylation at four N-terminal serine-threonine residues by glycogen synthase kinase 3 (GSK3β) and caseine kinase 1 (CK1), which are located together with APC and AXIN in a cytoplasmic multi-protein complex. Upon phosphorylation and subsequent ubiquitinylation, β-catenin is degraded by the proteasomal pathway. However, binding of Wnt ligands to frizzled (FZD) receptors vitally changes the scenario by inhibiting GSK3β activity and stabilizing β-catenin, which, on its part, translocates to the nucleus. Together with the transcription factors TCF and LEF, β-catenin activates the transcription of several target genes, such as *MYC* and *cyclin D1* (He et al. 1998; Shtutman et al. 1999).

There are several mechanisms by which canonical Wnt signaling gets activated during cancer development, generally leading to inappropriate stabilization of β-catenin in the cytoplasm (Klaus and Birchmeier 2008; Polakis 2000). The most prominent one in HB is the oncogenic activation of β-catenin itself, an alteration present in approx. two-thirds of all patients analyzed so far (Cairo et al. 2008; Koch et al. 1999; Taniguchi et al. 2002; Wei et al. 2000). This is the highest mutation frequency of all tumor types known to carry oncogenic β-catenin mutations, including colorectal carcinoma and melanoma (Klaus and Birchmeier 2008). Mutations in HB preferentially affect exon 3 of the *β-catenin* gene either by point mutation in codons 32, 34, 37, 41, and 45 (Fig. 4.2b and c), or, more frequently, by deletion of part of or the entire exon 3 (Fig. 4.2b). This proportion of the *β-catenin* gene encodes four amino acids (serines and threonine) that have been implicated in the down-regulation of β-catenin through phosphorylation by the GSK3β kinase (Yost et al. 1996). Nevertheless, there is no clear correlation between *β-catenin* mutation and loss of membrane localization. Extensive immunohistological analyses revealed that a large proportion of tumors present with nuclear or cytoplasmic accumulation of the protein, irrespective of their β-catenin mutational status, suggesting alternative activation mechanisms (Wei et al. 2000). This is particularly

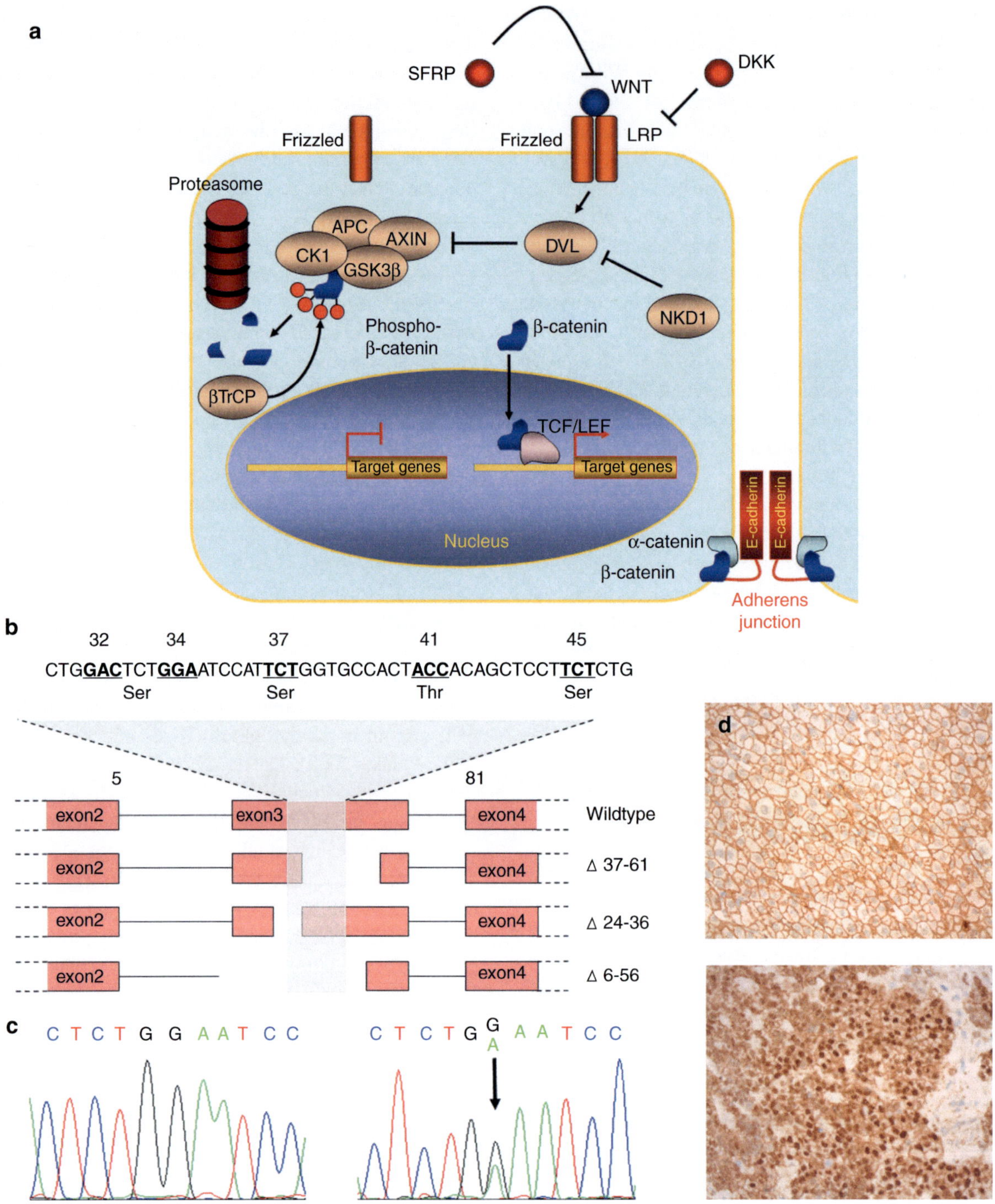

Fig. 4.2 Wnt signaling in HB. **(a)** The Wnt signaling cascade; **(b)** most commonly affected region of the *β-catenin* gene; **(c)** point mutation in codon 34; **(d)** membraneous (*upper panel*) and nuclear (*lower panel*) β-catenin by immunohistochemistry

intriguing in view of the predominant occurrence of nuclear β-catenin in the embryonal subtype that has a more immature appearance (Fig. 4.2d), whereas the fetal subtype characteristically exhibits a membranous localization with an additional E-cadherin expression (Wei et al. 2000).

Loss of APC function has been suggested to display another activation mechanism of Wnt signaling (Klaus and Birchmeier 2008). Accordingly, truncating mutations of the *APC* gene have been characterized in both familial FAP-related HB and about 5% of sporadic HB cases (Cairo et al. 2008; Giardiello et al. 1996; Kurahashi et al. 1995; Oda et al. 1996). However, controversy exists on the relevance of *APC* mutations in HB development, as several comprehensive studies failed to detect any *APC* mutation (Koch et al. 1999; Wei et al. 2000).

Moreover, constitutive activation of β-catenin in cancer cells could also be achieved by loss-of-function mutations of the Wnt negative regulators AXIN1 and conductin (AXIN2) (Salahshor and Woodgett 2005). Of note, mutations in both the *AXIN1* and *AXIN2* gene have been identified in single cases of HB (Cairo et al. 2008; Koch et al. 2004; Taniguchi et al. 2002).

Accumulated experimental evidence moreover indicates that several inhibitors of the Wnt signaling pathway, which are regularly induced by activation of canonical Wnt signaling to facilitate its own regulation, are frequently activated in HB. The genes encoding NKD1 that targets the pathway upstream of β-catenin by interfering with disheveled (DVL), βTrCP that is part of the ubiquitin ligase complex responsible for targeting β-catenin for proteasomal degradation as well as dickkopf proteins (DKK1 and DKK3) that antagonize Wnt signals by blocking the LRP6-frizzled complex are frequently over-expressed in HB (Koch et al. 2005; Pei et al. 2009; Wirths et al. 2003). It has been suggested that the biological capability of these antagonists to inhibit Wnt signaling through a negative feedback loop is abrogated in HB, most likely because genetic alterations disrupt the central multi-protein complex that controls the stability of β-catenin (Koch et al. 2005).

Collectively, these data clearly show that aberrant Wnt signaling is a hallmark of HB. It is tempting to speculate that future efforts will deal with the identification of specific inhibitors of Wnt signaling that could be used in therapeutic strategies to treat HB.

4.5.2 The Hedgehog Signaling Pathway

Hedgehog (HH) signaling plays a crucial role in a variety of aspects of vertebrate development, including pattern formation, proliferation, and differentiation of numerous cell types (Ruiz et al. 2002). The association between the HH pathway and cancer was initially depicted in a human cancer predisposition disease, the Gorlin–Goltz or nevoid basal cell carcinoma syndrome, by identifying germ-line mutations in the HH receptor gene *Patched* (*PTCH*), which results in inappropriate activation of the HH pathway thereby leading to the development of basal cell carcinoma and embryonal tumors such as medulloblastoma and rhabdomyosarcoma (Gorlin 1987). In the physiological state of differentiated cells, the HH signaling pathway (Fig. 4.3a) is expected to be in the off state. This is achieved by the absence of the secreted HH ligands, which leads to the inhibition of the smoothened (SMO) protein by the cell surface receptor PTCH. This results in the sequential phosphorylation of GLI family transcription factors and subsequent degradation by the proteasome. Binding of HH ligands to PTCH leads to loss of the inhibitory activity of PTCH on SMO, which initiates an intracellular signaling cascade by acting on a multi-protein complex consisting of fused (FU), suppressor of fused (SUFU), kinesins (KIF), and GLI. This leads to stabilization and nuclear localization of GLI, which drives transcriptional activation of HH target genes, such as *BCL2* (Bigelow et al. 2004; Regl et al. 2004), *FOXM1* (Teh et al. 2002), *CCND1* (Kenney and Rowitch 2000), *MYCN* (Kenney et al. 2003), *IGF2* (Hahn et al. 2000), and *PTCH* itself (Goodrich et al. 1996), which leads to a negative feedback ensuring precise regulation of the pathway.

Two types of HH pathway activation have been described in human cancers: mutational activation by loss-of-function of repressors (*PTCH* and *SUFU*) or gain-of-function of activators (*SMO* and *GLI1*), and overabundance of HH ligands (Rubin and de Sauvage 2006). The second category of HH-associated tumors have been described to be driven by either an autocrine or paracrine stimulation of HH ligands secreted by the tumor cells themselves or the stromal surrounding. HB is believed to belong to the ligand-driven group of HH-associated tumors, as high mRNA or protein levels of HH ligands have been found in approximately 65% of HB cases (Eichenmuller et al. 2009; Oue et al. 2010). Consequently, upregulation of the downstream targets *GLI1*, *BCL2*, and *PTCH* is present in a large proportion of HB tumors, as compared to normal fetal and adult liver. Interestingly, a dramatic downregulation of the hedgehog interacting protein (HHIP) was also detected in HB (Eichenmuller et al. 2009), which is a well-established negative regulator of hedgehog signaling (Chuang and McMahon 1999). It is important to emphasize that comparative genomic approaches have revealed common deletions at the *HHIP* locus on chromosome 4q28–32 in 10–18% of HB cases, thus

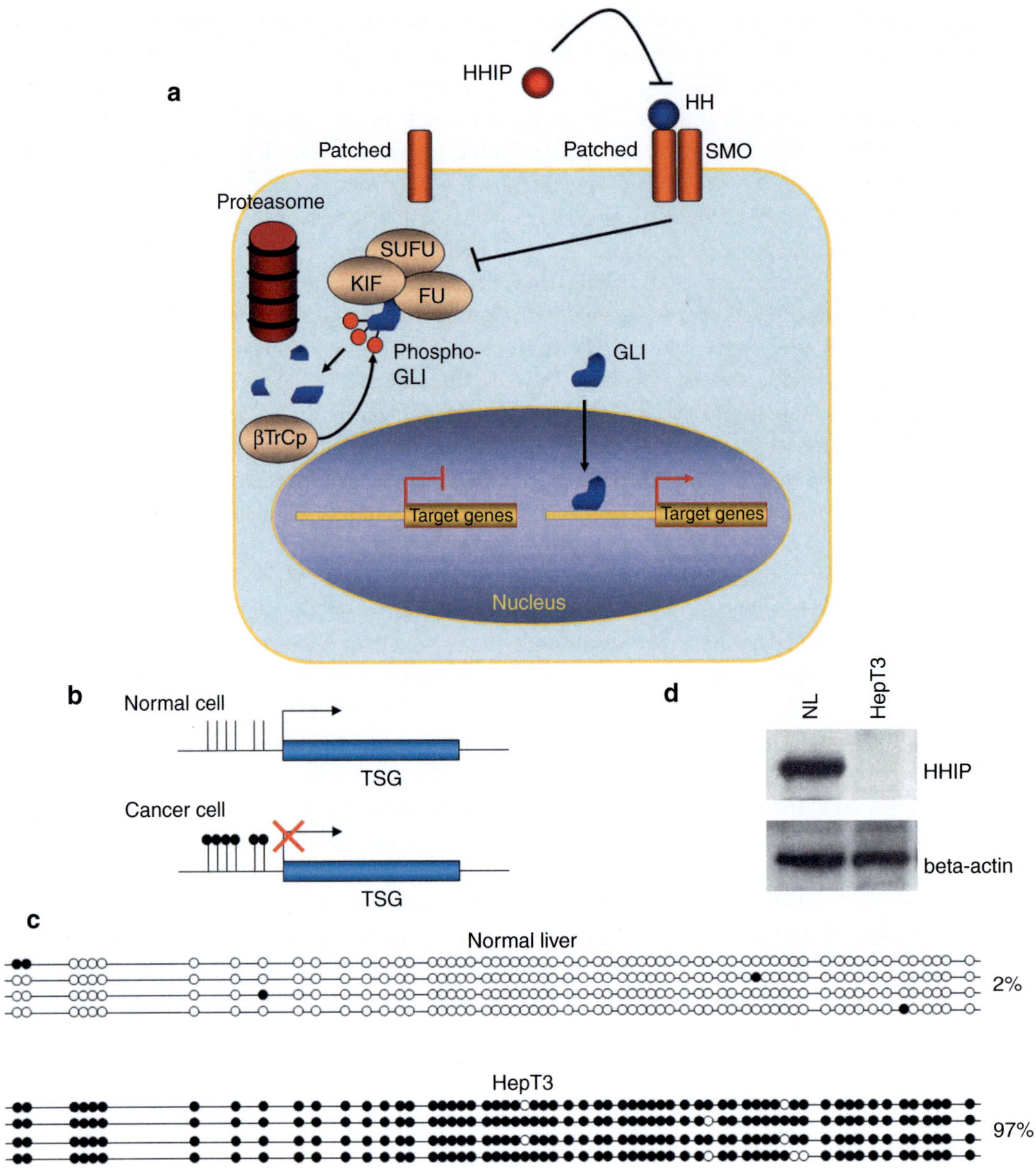

Fig. 4.3 HH signaling in HB. **(a)** The HH signaling cascade; **(b)** promoter methylation and transcriptional silencing of tumor suppressor genes; **(c)** methylation status of the *HHIP* gene in normal liver and HB cells; **(d)** HHIP protein expression in normal liver and HB cells

making downregulation of *HHIP* through genomic alterations in a subset of tumors conceivable (Gray et al. 2000b; Suzuki et al. 2008; Weber et al. 2000).

Collectively, these studies clearly bolster the relevance of an activated HH signaling pathway in HB. Although a comprehensive sequencing analysis of HH components is lacking, autocrine stimulation through endogenous expression of HH ligands in tumor cells along with downregulation of the *HHIP* gene can be anticipated as the driving forces for HH activation in HB. In line with this, blocking HH signaling by the SMO inhibitor cyclopamine has already been shown to successfully induce growth inhibition and apoptosis in HB cells (Eichenmuller et al. 2009).

4.5.3 The Insulin-Like Growth Factor Axis

Activation of the IGF signaling pathway is a well-known aspect in the genesis of embryonal tumors such as Wilms' tumor, rhabdomyosarcoma, and HB (Scotting et al. 2005). Activation of the IGF axis is initiated by binding of the ligands IGF1 and IGF2 to and subsequent activation of the type 1 insulin-like growth factor receptor (IGF1R), which in turn triggers inactivation of proapoptotic factors and confers a survival advantage to a wide range of cell types (Manning and Cantley 2007). Consequently, aberrant up-regulation of IGF1R and/or its ligands IGF1 and IGF2 is known from a variety of human cancers (Pollak et al. 2004). The prevailing mechanism for IGF pathway activation in HB has been allocated to the over-expression of *IGF2*, which is a result of genetic and epigenetic alterations at the *IGF2/H19* locus (Gray et al. 2000a; Hartmann et al. 2000; Li et al. 1995) and causes activation of the downstream survival factor AKT (Manning and Cantley 2007; Pollak et al. 2004).

Since early studies on Wilms' tumor and rhabdomyosarcoma have suggested that loss of imprinting (LOI) and subsequent biallelic expression of the gene is a major cause for *IGF2* upregulation in these embryonal tumors (Anderson et al. 1999; Taniguchi et al. 1995), several attempts have been made to prove this mechanistic basis for HB (Albrecht et al. 1994; Eriksson et al. 2001; Hartmann et al. 2000; Li et al. 1995). However, these studies have scarcely detected LOI due to a limited number of tumors with informative polymorphisms in the *IGF2/H19* locus, ending up with the suggestion that molecular mechanisms other than LOI must cause the frequently observed over-expression of *IGF2* in HB. One explanation came from the finding that the *PLAG1* gene, which codes for a positive regulator of IGF2 (Voz et al. 2000), is frequently amplified and thus over-expressed in HB (Zatkova et al. 2004). However, a recent study came up with the analysis of 54 HB that reports on a frequency of LOI of 17% in their HB collection (Honda et al. 2008a). These data suggest that disruption of the methylation-dependent enhancer competition model of the *IGF2/H19* locus reported for Wilms' tumor and rhabdomyosarcoma may also apply for HB.

Oncogenic mutations affecting the *PI3KCA* gene, which encodes the p110α phosphatidylinositol-3′-kinase (PI3K) catalytic subunit, have been described to be an alternative activation mechanism of the IGF/PI3K/AKT pathway (Samuels et al. 2004). Interestingly, a single case of HB with a *PI3KCA* mutation has recently been described (Hartmann et al. 2009). The same study has convincingly shown that the downstream targets of the IGF2 axis, namely, AKT and mTOR, are strongly expressed and activated by phosphorylation in the vast majority of HB. Moreover, it seems that HB cells strongly depend on an activated IGF/PI3K/AKT pathway, as in vitro experiments clearly demonstrate a dramatic loss of viability upon the addition of PI3K inhibitors (Hartmann et al. 2009). This approach is especially interesting in view of the finding that inhibition of IGF/PI3K/AKT signaling sensitizes HB cells for chemotherapeutic treatments (Hartmann et al. 2009).

Altogether, these data clearly indicate that HB strongly depends on the activation of the IGF/PI3K/AKT pathway, although the exact causing mechanism for the aberrant activation still remains elusive.

4.5.4 The Hepatocyte Growth Factor/c-Met Pathway

The hepatocyte growth factor/scatter factor (HGF) is a pleiotropic molecule that stimulates a variety of cellular responses including angiogenesis, cellular motility, growth, invasion, morphological differentiation, embryological development, tissue regeneration, and wound healing (Birchmeier et al. 2003). HGF is mainly expressed by mesenchymal cells and acts as the natural ligand for the receptor tyrosine kinase c-Met, which is consistently expressed on epithelial cells. Deletion of either gene causes lethal disruption to embryogenesis and widespread expression persists throughout adulthood (Birchmeier et al. 2003). The HGF/c-Met signal is transmitted via the PI3K/AKT and mitogen-activated protein kinase (MAPK) signaling pathways (Potempa and Ridley 1998).

Highly elevated serum levels of HGF are a striking feature in HB patients at the time of diagnosis (von Schweinitz et al. 1998, 2000; Weinberg and Finegold 1983). Interestingly, an increase of up to fourfold in HGF was detected in 10 out of 12 children as early as 24–72 h after liver resection (von Schweinitz et al. 2000). This pre- and post-operative increase of HGF serum levels is suspected to promote growth and progression of residual tumor cells after incomplete resection in HB patients. However, data suggest that HGF has no direct impact on overall cell viability and proliferation of HB cells, although signal transduction occurs downstream of HGF, such as c-Met phosphorylation and activation of PI3K/AKT and MAPK signaling

(Grotegut et al. 2010). Instead of being mitogenic, HGF confers anti-apoptotic properties upon serum starvation and moreover protects HB cells against strong apoptotic inducers such as cisplatin and camptothecin, thereby contributing to chemotherapeutic resistance. This effect is mainly dependent on the PI3K/AKT signaling pathway, since inhibition by wortmannin results in abrogation of HGF-mediated survival, whereas inhibition of the MAPK pathway has no effect.

New data convincingly demonstrate that HGF is also implicated in cell scattering, migration, and invasion of HB cells (Grotegut et al. 2006). HGF mediates downregulation of the adhesion-ensuring genes *E-cadherin* and *claudin-3* via the zinc-finger transcription factor Snail, thereby highlighting its importance in tumor progression. Interestingly, HGF and c-Met have been recently proposed as potential targets for therapeutic intervention in hepatocellular carcinoma (Son et al. 2006).

Altogether, these findings highlight the importance of HGF in tumor cell survival and suggest that HGF and its cognate receptor c-Met should be considered as a candidate for combined therapeutic strategies of advanced HB.

4.6 Epigenetically Altered Tumor Suppressor Genes in Hepatoblastoma

Epigenetics is defined as heritable cellular information that is encoded by mechanisms other than the DNA sequence itself (Feinberg and Tycko 2004). There are three main types of epigenetic information: DNA methylation, genomic imprinting, and histone modification. The most prominent epigenetic mechanism described to play a role in cancer formation and progression displays hypermethylation of promoter regions (Fig. 4.3b), which results in transcriptional silencing of the respective genes (Baylin and Ohm 2006). DNA methylation may inactivate tumor suppressor genes alone or in concert with classical genetic mechanisms such as point mutations or deletions (Esteller 2002). Extensive work has been conducted to study the role of epigenetically silenced genes in HB, mainly focusing on genes known to be involved in the developmental signaling pathways and apoptosis (Eichenmuller et al. 2009; Harada et al. 2002; Honda et al. 2008b; Nagai et al. 2003; Sakamoto et al. 2010; Shih et al. 2007; Shim et al. 2003; Sugawara et al. 2007). However, only for some of these genes an aberrant methylation has been proven (Table 4.2), of which two might serve as markers for poor prognosis.

Secreted frizzled-related proteins (SFRPs) are a family of secreted glycoproteins that have been identified as negative regulators of the Wnt signaling pathway by competing with frizzled for binding of Wnt ligands (Jones and Jomary 2002). Promoter hypermethylation and subsequent silencing of *SFRP* genes is a well-known mechanism to activate Wnt signaling (Suzuki et al. 2004). The *SFRP1* gene is the first candidate of this family, which has been shown to be epigenetically silenced in liver cancers, namely, hepatocellular carcinoma (Shih et al. 2006), HB (Sakamoto et al. 2010), and the two HB cell lines, HUH6 and HepG2 (Shih et al. 2007). Interestingly, restoring SFRP function is suggested to attenuate Wnt signaling even in the presence of downstream mutations in β-catenin (Suzuki et al. 2004). Other family members such as *SFRP2*, *SFRP4*, and *SFRP5* seem to lack promoter methylation in primary HB (Sugawara et al. 2007).

Another inhibitory component of Wnt signaling encoded by the *APC* gene is known to be mutated in about 5% of sporadic HB cases (Cairo et al. 2008; Giardiello et al. 1996; Kurahashi et al. 1995; Oda et al. 1996). New data report on *APC* promoter methylation in 30% of sporadic HB thereby suggesting an alternative mechanism by which *APC* expression could be down-

Table 4.2 Epigenetically silenced genes in hepatoblastoma

Gene	Description	Locus	Methylation frequency (%)
SFRP1	Secreted frizzled-related protein 1	8p11.21	20
APC	Adenomatous polyposis coli	5q21-q22	30
HHIP	Hedgehog interacting protein	4q28–32	26
SOCS1	Suppressor of cytokine signaling 1	16p13.13	40–47
CASP8	caspase 8	2q33-q34	15
MT1G	metallothionein 1G	16q13	55
RASSF1A	ras association domain family protein 1 isoform A	3p21.3	19–80

regulated, which culminates in Wnt signaling activation (Sakamoto et al. 2010).

The HHIP protein functions as a negative regulator of hedgehog signaling by competitively binding HH ligands (Chuang and McMahon 1999). The *HHIP* promoter is methylated in a large proportion of HB, whereas normal liver tissue is unmethylated (Eichenmuller et al. 2009). Interestingly, promoter methylation of the *HHIP* gene (Fig. 4.3c) is strongly associated with a decreased expression in the respective tumors (Fig. 4.3d). Aberrant *HHIP* methylation and subsequent low expression of *HHIP* strengthen the importance of a mechanism by which the negative regulatory feedback loop of HHIP might be lost or abolished in HB by promoter methylation.

The *suppressor of cytokine signaling 1* (*SOCS1*) gene encodes a Janus kinase (JAK)-binding protein that regulates the JAK/STAT signal transduction pathway (Naka et al. 1997). Inactivation of this gene by promoter methylation is present in hepatocellular carcinoma (Yoshikawa et al. 2001) and HB tumors (Nagai et al. 2003; Sakamoto et al. 2010), and the restoration of SOCS1 leads to suppression of growth and induction of apoptosis in liver cancer cells (Yoshikawa et al. 2001). Of note, *SOCS1* methylation is associated with the fetal histological type of HB (Honda et al. 2008b).

Caspase 8 belongs to the caspase family of proteases and plays a key role in the regulation of apoptosis (Fulda 2009). Inactivation of *CASP8* by promoter methylation is known to promote tumor progression as well as resistance to current treatment approaches in a variety of human cancers. Hypermethylation of the *CASP8* promoter is found in a small proportion of HB and is associated with recurrent disease (Honda et al. 2008b).

MT1G codes for the 1G subtype of metallothionein, which belongs to a cysteine-rich protein family that binds various heavy metals. Expression of metallothioneins can be used as a prognostic factor for tumor progression and drug resistance in a variety of malignancies (Eckschlager et al. 2009). Methylation of *MT1G* is a common feature of hepatocellular carcinoma (Kanda et al. 2009) and HB (Sakamoto et al. 2010). Interestingly, *MT1G* methylation level is correlated with poor outcome in HB (Sakamoto et al. 2010).

Ras association domain family 1 isoform A (RASSF1A) is a tumor suppressor exhibiting epigenetic silencing in many human cancers (Avruch et al. 2009), including hepatocellular carcinoma (Schagdarsurengin et al. 2003) and HB (Harada et al. 2002; Honda et al. 2008b; Sakamoto et al. 2010; Sugawara et al. 2007). Consequently, reexpression of *RASSF1A* relays pro-apoptotic and anti-proliferative effects on tumor cells. *RASSF1A* is the gene with the highest methylation rate in HB, with reported frequencies ranging from 19% up to 80%. Remarkably, it seems that *RASSF1A* promoter methylation is a promising marker for predicting prognosis of HB patients (Honda et al. 2008b; Sugawara et al. 2007). *RASSF1A* methylation is significantly associated with age ≥2 years, advanced tumor stage, poor outcome, and tends to be associated with refractoriness to cisplatin-based chemotherapy (Sugawara et al. 2007). Thus, the *RASSF1A* methylation status could be useful to identify patients who are likely to suffer recurrences or death from disease (Honda et al. 2008b).

In summary, increasing evidence demonstrates that promoter hypermethylation is a common feature of HB, especially affecting genes involved in survival and apoptosis processes. Thus, it should be considered that demethylating drugs, which have already been under clinical evaluation (Sigalotti et al. 2007), might be introduced into future treatment protocols as a novel therapeutic option for high-risk HB.

4.7 Gene Signatures as Predictors of Outcome

Increasing evidence indicates that gene expression information generated by DNA microarray analysis of human tumors can provide molecular phenotyping that identifies distinct tumor classifications not evident by traditional histopathological methods. The promise of such information lies in the potential to improve clinical decisions and strategies used to treat cancer patients. Indeed, traditional methods of phenotypic characterization do not have the ability to discern subtle differences that may be of importance for developing a better understanding of the tumor and advancing therapeutic strategies for the treatment of disease.

The first attempts to study gene expression in HB in a more holistic fashion were based on comparisons of HB specimens and non-diseased liver tissues by virtue of high-density oligonucleotide DNA arrays (Nagata et al. 2003). Besides confirming *IGF2* as the most prominent upregulated gene in HB, this first screen identified two new interesting candidate genes: *stathmin 1* (*STNM1*), which encodes a protein involved in the disassembly of microtubule filaments, and *insulin-like growth factor binding protein 4* (*IGFBP4*), encoding a multifunctional protein produced by the liver, which mediates growth suppression and induction of apoptosis by competitively binding IGFs (Clemmons 1997). Upregulation of *STNM1* is known from several cancers to be positively associated with metastasis, vascular invasion, advanced tumor stage, and poor outcome, including hepatocellular carcinoma (Gan et al. 2010; Singer et al. 2007). Suppression of IGFBP4 might influence HB cells in a dual fashion by elevating the levels of IGFs and attenuating inhibition of the canonical Wnt pathway (Zhu et al. 2008). Although the exact contribution of these genes in the genesis and progression of HB is still unclear, it might be deduced from these data that other than the above mentioned mechanisms these might also contribute to the activation of the Wnt and IGF developmental signaling pathways.

A much more comprehensive microarray study has recently described a large set of genes significantly deregulated in HB (Cairo et al. 2008). Strikingly, Wnt signaling components such as *AXIN2*, *LEF1*, *DVL2*, *DVL3*, *DKK1*, and *DKK4* are largely upregulated in HB compared to normal liver tissue. Moreover, several imprinted genes abundantly expressed in fetal liver, such as *IGF2*, *DLK1*, *PEG3*, *PEG10*, *BEX1*, *NDN*, and *MEG3* are strongly elevated in tumor tissues, suggesting a prominent role of epigenetic derailment in the development of HB. More interestingly, expression profiling and subsequent statistical analyses were able to discriminate two distinct HB subtypes: the so-called C1 tumors comprising predominantly the fetal phenotype, and the C2 tumors that show a more immature pattern with embryonal or crowded fetal histotypes and a high proliferation rate (Table 4.3). Consistently, C2 tumors show increased levels of markers for proliferation (Ki67, *MYCN*, Survivin) and hepatic progenitors (*AFP* and *KRT19*, Ep-CAM), whereas markers for mature hepatocytes such as *ALDH2*, *ALAS1*, and *UGT2B4* are markedly downregulated. Interestingly, the β-catenin mutation status as well as presence of the mesenchymal histotype is not associated with a distinct subgroup. An additional intriguing result of this study is that a molecular classifier consisting of only 16 genes (Table 4.3) is able to predict prognosis with an even better accuracy than the currently used procedure using tumor stage defined by pretreatment extent of disease (PRETEXT), vascular invasion, and extrahepatic metastases as criteria. C2 tumors were associated with a markedly impaired overall survival for these patients with a probability at 2 years of 44% versus 92% for patients with C1 tumors (Cairo et al. 2008). Collectively, recent data clearly demonstrate that expression profiling could be efficiently used to disclose molecular subclasses of HB that discriminate between different developmental tumor stages and more promising clinical behavior. Thus, the 16-gene signature will be implemented in future clinical trials not only to monitor the biology of HB, but also to stratify patients into risk-adapted treatment groups.

Table 4.3 Molecular features of hepatoblastoma subclasses

Subtype	C1	C2
Histology	Well differentiated (fetal)	Poorly differentiated (embryonal or crowded fetal)
Markers	Alike mature hepatocytes (ALDH2, ALAS1 and UGT2B4)	Alike immature liver tissue (CK19, AFP, EpCAM)
Clinic	Rarely adverse tumor characteristics, better prognosis	Vascular invasion, extrahepatic metastasis, impaired survival
Proliferation	Low	High (Ki67, *MYCN*, Survivin)
β-catenin localization	Predominantly membranous and cytoplasmic	Predominantly nuclear
16-gene signature	ALDH2↑, APCS↑↑, APOC4↑↑, AQP9↑, C1S↑, CYP2E1↑, GHR↑↑, HPD↑	AFP↑↑, BUB1↑, DLG7↑↑, DUSP9↑↑, E2F5↑, IGSF1↑↑, NLE1↑, RPL10A↑

↑↑, very strong expression; ↑, strong expression

References

Adesina AM, Nguyen Y, Guanaratne P, Pulliam J, Lopez-Terrada D, Margolin J, Finegold M (2007) FOXG1 is overexpressed in hepatoblastoma. Hum Pathol 38:400–409

Albrecht S, von Schweinitz D, Waha A, Kraus JA, von Deimling A, Pietsch T (1994) Loss of maternal alleles on chromosome arm 11p in hepatoblastoma. Cancer Res 54:5041–5044

Anderson J, Gordon A, McManus A, Shipley J, Pritchard-Jones K (1999) Disruption of imprinted genes at chromosome region 11p15.5 in paediatric rhabdomyosarcoma. Neoplasia 1:340–348

Aretz S, Koch A, Uhlhaas S, Friedl W, Propping P, von Schweinitz D, Pietsch T (2006) Should children at risk for familial adenomatous polyposis be screened for hepatoblastoma and children with apparently sporadic hepatoblastoma be screened for APC germline mutations? Pediatr Blood Cancer 47:811–818

Avruch J, Xavier R, Bardeesy N, Zhang XF, Praskova M, Zhou D, Xia F (2009) Rassf family of tumor suppressor polypeptides. J Biol Chem 284:11001–11005

Baylin SB, Ohm JE (2006) Epigenetic gene silencing in cancer – a mechanism for early oncogenic pathway addiction? Nat Rev Cancer 6:107–116

Behmel A, Plochl E, Rosenkranz W (1984) A new X-linked dysplasia gigantism syndrome: identical with the Simpson dysplasia syndrome? Hum Genet 67:409–413

Bigelow RL, Chari NS, Unden AB, Spurgers KB, Lee S, Roop DR, Toftgard R, McDonnell TJ (2004) Transcriptional regulation of bcl-2 mediated by the sonic hedgehog signaling pathway through gli-1. J Biol Chem 279:1197–1205

Birchmeier C, Birchmeier W, Gherardi E, Vande Woude GF (2003) Met, metastasis, motility and more. Nat Rev Mol Cell Biol 4:915–925

Cairo S, Armengol C, De Reynies A, Wei Y, Thomas E, Renard CA, Goga A, Balakrishnan A, Semeraro M, Gresh L, Pontoglio M, Strick-Marchand H, Levillayer F, Nouet Y, Rickman D, Gauthier F, Branchereau S, Brugieres L, Laithier V, Bouvier R, Boman F, Basso G, Michiels JF, Hofman P, Arbez-Gindre F, Jouan H, Rousselet-Chapeau MC, Berrebi D, Marcellin L, Plenat F, Zachar D, Joubert M, Selves J, Pasquier D, Bioulac-Sage P, Grotzer M, Childs M, Fabre M, Buendia MA (2008) Hepatic stem-like phenotype and interplay of Wnt/beta-catenin and Myc signaling in aggressive childhood liver cancer. Cancer Cell 14:471–484

Chuang PT, McMahon AP (1999) Vertebrate Hedgehog signalling modulated by induction of a Hedgehog-binding protein. Nature 397:617–621

Clemmons DR (1997) Insulin-like growth factor binding proteins and their role in controlling IGF actions. Cytokine Growth Factor Rev 8:45–62

Clericuzio CL, Chen E, McNeil DE, O'Connor T, Zackai EH, Medne L, Tomlinson G, DeBaun M (2003) Serum alpha-fetoprotein screening for hepatoblastoma in children with Beckwith-Wiedemann syndrome or isolated hemihyperplasia. J Pediatr 143:270–272

Cole TR, Hughes HE (1994) Sotos syndrome: a study of the diagnostic criteria and natural history. J Med Genet 31: 20–32

Curia MC, Zuckermann M, De Lellis L, Catalano T, Lattanzio R, Aceto G, Veschi S, Cama A, Otte JB, Piantelli M, Mariani-Costantini R, Cetta F, Battista P (2008) Sporadic childhood hepatoblastomas show activation of beta-catenin, mismatch repair defects and p53 mutations. Mod Pathol 21:7–14

Eckschlager T, Adam V, Hrabeta J, Figova K, Kizek R (2009) Metallothioneins and cancer. Curr Protein Pept Sci 10: 360–375

Eichenmuller M, Gruner I, Hagl B, Haberle B, Muller-Hocker J, von Schweinitz D, Kappler R (2009) Blocking the hedgehog pathway inhibits hepatoblastoma growth. Hepatology 49:482–490

Engstrom W, Lindham S, Schofield P (1988) Wiedemann–Beckwith syndrome. Eur J Pediatr 147:450–457

Eriksson T, Frisk T, Gray SG, von Schweinitz D, Pietsch T, Larsson C, Sandstedt B, Ekstrom TJ (2001) Methylation changes in the human IGF2 p3 promoter parallel IGF2 expression in the primary tumor, established cell line, and xenograft of a human hepatoblastoma. Exp Cell Res 270: 88–95

Esteller M (2002) CpG island hypermethylation and tumor suppressor genes: a booming present, a brighter future. Oncogene 21:5427–5440

Feinberg AP (1993) Genomic imprinting and gene activation in cancer. Nat Genet 4:110–113

Feinberg AP, Tycko B (2004) The history of cancer epigenetics. Nat Rev Cancer 4:143–153

Fulda S (2009) Caspase-8 in cancer biology and therapy. Cancer Lett 281:128–133

Gan L, Guo K, Li Y, Kang X, Sun L, Shu H, Liu Y (2010) Up-regulated expression of stathmin may be associated with hepatocarcinogenesis. Oncol Rep 23:1037–1043

Giardiello FM, Petersen GM, Brensinger JD, Luce MC, Cayouette MC, Bacon J, Booker SV, Hamilton SR (1996) Hepatoblastoma and APC gene mutation in familial adenomatous polyposis. Gut 39:867–869

Golabi M, Ito M, Hall BD (1984) A new X-linked multiple congenital anomalies/mental retardation syndrome. Am J Med Genet 17:367–374

Goodrich LV, Johnson RL, Milenkovic L, McMahon JA, Scott MP (1996) Conservation of the hedgehog/patched signaling pathway from flies to mice: induction of a mouse patched gene by Hedgehog. Genes Dev 10:301–312

Gorlin RJ (1987) Nevoid basal-cell carcinoma syndrome. Medicine (Baltimore) 66:98–113

Gray SG, Eriksson T, Ekstrom C, Holm S, von Schweinitz D, Kogner P, Sandstedt B, Pietsch T, Ekstrom TJ (2000a) Altered expression of members of the IGF-axis in hepatoblastomas. Br J Cancer 82:1561–1567

Gray SG, Kytola S, Matsunaga T, Larsson C, Ekstrom TJ (2000b) Comparative genomic hybridization reveals population-based genetic alterations in hepatoblastomas. Br J Cancer 83:1020–1025

Grotegut S, von Schweinitz D, Christofori G, Lehembre F (2006) Hepatocyte growth factor induces cell scattering through MAPK/Egr-1-mediated upregulation of Snail. EMBO J 25:3534–3545

Grotegut S, Kappler R, Tarimoradi S, Lehembre F, Christofori G, Von Schweinitz D (2010) Hepatocyte growth factor protects hepatoblastoma cells from chemotherapy-induced apoptosis by AKT activation. Int J Oncol 36: 1261–1267

Haas JE, Feusner JH, Finegold MJ (2001) Small cell undifferentiated histology in hepatoblastoma may be unfavorable. Cancer 92:3130–3134

Hahn H, Wojnowski L, Specht K, Kappler R, Calzada-Wack J, Potter D, Zimmer A, Muller U, Samson E, Quintanilla-Martinez L (2000) Patched target Igf2 is indispensable for the formation of medulloblastoma and rhabdomyosarcoma. J Biol Chem 275:28341–28344

Harada K, Toyooka S, Maitra A, Maruyama R, Toyooka KO, Timmons CF, Tomlinson GE, Mastrangelo D, Hay RJ, Minna JD, Gazdar AF (2002) Aberrant promoter methylation and silencing of the RASSF1A gene in pediatric tumors and cell lines. Oncogene 21:4345–4349

Hartmann W, Waha A, Koch A, Goodyer CG, Albrecht S, von Schweinitz D, Pietsch T (2000) p57(KIP2) is not mutated in hepatoblastoma but shows increased transcriptional activity in a comparative analysis of the three imprinted genes p57(KIP2), IGF2, and H19. Am J Pathol 157:1393–1403

Hartmann W, Kuchler J, Koch A, Friedrichs N, Waha A, Endl E, Czerwitzki J, Metzger D, Steiner S, Wurst P, Leuschner I, von Schweinitz D, Buettner R, Pietsch T (2009) Activation of phosphatidylinositol-3′-kinase/AKT signaling is essential in hepatoblastoma survival. Clin Cancer Res 15:4538–4545

He TC, Sparks AB, Rago C, Hermeking H, Zawel L, da Costa LT, Morin PJ, Vogelstein B, Kinzler KW (1998) Identification of c-MYC as a target of the APC pathway. Science 281: 1509–1512

Honda S, Arai Y, Haruta M, Sasaki F, Ohira M, Yamaoka H, Horie H, Nakagawara A, Hiyama E, Todo S, Kaneko Y (2008a) Loss of imprinting of IGF2 correlates with hypermethylation of the H19 differentially methylated region in hepatoblastoma. Br J Cancer 99:1891–1899

Honda S, Haruta M, Sugawara W, Sasaki F, Ohira M, Matsunaga T, Yamaoka H, Horie H, Ohnuma N, Nakagawara A, Hiyama E, Todo S, Kaneko Y (2008b) The methylation status of RASSF1A promoter predicts responsiveness to chemotherapy and eventual cure in hepatoblastoma patients. Int J Cancer 123:1117–1125

Hughes LJ, Michels VV (1992) Risk of hepatoblastoma in familial adenomatous polyposis. Am J Med Genet 43: 1023–1025

Jones SE, Jomary C (2002) Secreted frizzled-related proteins: searching for relationships and patterns. Bioessays 24: 811–820

Kanda M, Nomoto S, Okamura Y, Nishikawa Y, Sugimoto H, Kanazumi N, Takeda S, Nakao A (2009) Detection of metallothionein 1G as a methylated tumor suppressor gene in human hepatocellular carcinoma using a novel method of double combination array analysis. Int J Oncol 35:477–483

Kato M, Takita J, Takahashi K, Mimaki M, Chen Y, Koh K, Ida K, Oka A, Mizuguchi M, Ogawa S, Igarashi T (2009) Hepatoblastoma in a patient with sotos syndrome. J Pediatr 155:937–939

Kenney AM, Rowitch DH (2000) Sonic hedgehog promotes G(1) cyclin expression and sustained cell cycle progression in mammalian neuronal precursors. Mol Cell Biol 20: 9055–9067

Kenney AM, Cole MD, Rowitch DH (2003) Nmyc upregulation by sonic hedgehog signaling promotes proliferation in developing cerebellar granule neuron precursors. Development 130:15–28

Klaus A, Birchmeier W (2008) Wnt signalling and its impact on development and cancer. Nat Rev Cancer 8:387–398

Koch A, Denkhaus D, Albrecht S, Leuschner I, von Schweinitz D, Pietsch T (1999) Childhood hepatoblastomas frequently carry a mutated degradation targeting box of the beta-catenin gene. Cancer Res 59:269–273

Koch A, Weber N, Waha A, Hartmann W, Denkhaus D, Behrens J, Birchmeier W, von Schweinitz D, Pietsch T (2004) Mutations and elevated transcriptional activity of conductin (AXIN2) in hepatoblastomas. J Pathol 204:546–554

Koch A, Waha A, Hartmann W, Hrychyk A, Schuller U, Wharton KA Jr, Fuchs SY, von Schweinitz D, Pietsch T (2005) Elevated expression of Wnt antagonists is a common event in hepatoblastomas. Clin Cancer Res 11:4295–4304

Kraus JA, Albrecht S, Wiestler OD, von Schweinitz D, Pietsch T (1996) Loss of heterozygosity on chromosome 1 in human hepatoblastoma. Int J Cancer 67:467–471

Krush AJ, Traboulsi EI, Offerhaus JA, Maumenee IH, Yardley JH, Levin LS (1988) Hepatoblastoma, pigmented ocular fundus lesions and jaw lesions in Gardner syndrome. Am J Med Genet 29:323–332

Kurahashi H, Takami K, Oue T, Kusafuka T, Okada A, Tawa A, Okada S, Nishisho I (1995) Biallelic inactivation of the APC gene in hepatoblastoma. Cancer Res 55:5007–5011

Lapunzina P (2005) Risk of tumorigenesis in overgrowth syndromes: a comprehensive review. Am J Med Genet C Semin Med Genet 137C:53–71

Li FP, Fraumeni JF Jr, Mulvihill JJ, Blattner WA, Dreyfus MG, Tucker MA, Miller RW (1988) A cancer family syndrome in twenty-four kindreds. Cancer Res 48:5358–5362

Li X, Adam G, Cui H, Sandstedt B, Ohlsson R, Ekstrom TJ (1995) Expression, promoter usage and parental imprinting status of insulin-like growth factor II (IGF2) in human hepatoblastoma: uncoupling of IGF2 and H19 imprinting. Oncogene 11:221–229

Li M, Shuman C, Fei YL, Cutiongco E, Bender HA, Stevens C, Wilkins-Haug L, Day-Salvatore D, Yong SL, Geraghty MT, Squire J, Weksberg R (2001) GPC3 mutation analysis in a spectrum of patients with overgrowth expands the phenotype of Simpson–Golabi–Behmel syndrome. Am J Med Genet 102:161–168

Little MH, Thomson DB, Hayward NK, Smith PJ (1988) Loss of alleles on the short arm of chromosome 11 in a hepatoblastoma from a child with Beckwith–Wiedemann syndrome. Hum Genet 79:186–189

Mann JR, Kasthuri N, Raafat F, Pincott JR, Parkes SE, Muir KR, Ingram LC, Cameron AH (1990) Malignant hepatic tumours in children: incidence, clinical features and aetiology. Paediatr Perinat Epidemiol 4:276–289

Manning BD, Cantley LC (2007) AKT/PKB signaling: navigating downstream. Cell 129:1261–1274

Matsui I, Tanimura M, Kobayashi N, Sawada T, Nagahara N, Akatsuka J (1993) Neurofibromatosis type 1 and childhood cancer. Cancer 72:2746–2754

Nagai H, Naka T, Terada Y, Komazaki T, Yabe A, Jin E, Kawanami O, Kishimoto T, Konishi N, Nakamura M, Kobayashi Y, Emi M (2003) Hypermethylation associated with inactivation of the SOCS-1 gene, a JAK/STAT inhibitor, in human hepatoblastomas. J Hum Genet 48:65–69

Nagata T, Takahashi Y, Ishii Y, Asai S, Nishida Y, Murata A, Koshinaga T, Fukuzawa M, Hamazaki M, Asami K, Ito E, Ikeda H, Takamatsu H, Koike K, Kikuta A, Kuroiwa M, Watanabe A, Kosaka Y, Fujita H, Miyake M, Mugishima H (2003) Transcriptional profiling in hepatoblastomas using high-density oligonucleotide DNA array. Cancer Genet Cytogenet 145:152–160

Naka T, Narazaki M, Hirata M, Matsumoto T, Minamoto S, Aono A, Nishimoto N, Kajita T, Taga T, Yoshizaki K, Akira S, Kishimoto T (1997) Structure and function of a new STAT-induced STAT inhibitor. Nature 387:924–929

Nichols KE, Malkin D, Garber JE, Fraumeni JF Jr, Li FP (2001) Germ-line p53 mutations predispose to a wide spectrum of early-onset cancers. Cancer Epidemiol Biomarkers Prev 10:83–87

Nishisho I, Nakamura Y, Miyoshi Y, Miki Y, Ando H, Horii A, Koyama K, Utsunomiya J, Baba S, Hedge P (1991) Mutations of chromosome 5q21 genes in FAP and colorectal cancer patients. Science 253:665–669

Oda H, Imai Y, Nakatsuru Y, Hata J, Ishikawa T (1996) Somatic mutations of the APC gene in sporadic hepatoblastomas. Cancer Res 56:3320–3323

Oue T, Yoneda A, Uehara S, Yamanaka H, Fukuzawa M (2010) Increased expression of the hedgehog signaling pathway in pediatric solid malignancies. J Pediatr Surg 45:387–392

Pei Y, Kano J, Iijima T, Morishita Y, Inadome Y, Noguchi M (2009) Overexpression of Dickkopf 3 in hepatoblastomas and hepatocellular carcinomas. Virchows Arch 454:639–646

Polakis P (2000) Wnt signaling and cancer. Genes Dev 14: 1837–1851

Pollak M (2008) Insulin and insulin-like growth factor signalling in neoplasia. Nat Rev Cancer 8:915–928

Pollak MN, Schernhammer ES, Hankinson SE (2004) Insulin-like growth factors and neoplasia. Nat Rev Cancer 4:505–518

Potempa S, Ridley AJ (1998) Activation of both MAP kinase and phosphatidylinositide 3-kinase by Ras is required for hepatocyte growth factor/scatter factor-induced adherens junction disassembly. Mol Biol Cell 9:2185–2200

Regl G, Kasper M, Schnidar H, Eichberger T, Neill GW, Philpott MP, Esterbauer H, Hauser-Kronberger C, Frischauf AM, Aberger F (2004) Activation of the BCL2 promoter in response to Hedgehog/GLI signal transduction is predominantly mediated by GLI2. Cancer Res 64:7724–7731

Rubin LL, de Sauvage FJ (2006) Targeting the Hedgehog pathway in cancer. Nat Rev Drug Discov 5:1026–1033

Ruiz I, Altaba A, Sanchez P, Dahmane N (2002) Gli and hedgehog in cancer: tumours, embryos and stem cells. Nat Rev Cancer 2:361–372

Rustgi AK (2007) The genetics of hereditary colon cancer. Genes Dev 21:2525–2538

Sakamoto LH, DEC B, Cajaiba M, Soares FA, Vettore AL (2010) MT1G hypermethylation: a potential prognostic marker for hepatoblastoma. Pediatr Res 67:387–393

Salahshor S, Woodgett JR (2005) The links between axin and carcinogenesis. J Clin Pathol 58:225–236

Samuels Y, Wang Z, Bardelli A, Silliman N, Ptak J, Szabo S, Yan H, Gazdar A, Powell SM, Riggins GJ, Willson JK, Markowitz S, Kinzler KW, Vogelstein B, Velculescu VE (2004) High frequency of mutations of the PIK3CA gene in human cancers. Science 304:554

Schagdarsurengin U, Wilkens L, Steinemann D, Flemming P, Kreipe HH, Pfeifer GP, Schlegelberger B, Dammann R (2003) Frequent epigenetic inactivation of the RASSF1A gene in hepatocellular carcinoma. Oncogene 22:1866–1871

Scheil S, Hagen S, Bruderlein S, Leuschner I, Behnisch W, Moller P (2003) Two novel in vitro human hepatoblastoma models, HepU1 and HepU2, are highly characteristic of fetal-embryonal differentiation in hepatoblastoma. Int J Cancer 105:347–352

Schneider NR, Cooley LD, Finegold MJ, Douglass EC, Tomlinson GE (1997) The first recurring chromosome translocation in hepatoblastoma: der(4)t(1;4)(q12;q34). Genes Chromosom Cancer 19:291–294

Scotting PJ, Walker DA, Perilongo G (2005) Childhood solid tumours: a developmental disorder. Nat Rev Cancer 5: 481–488

Shih YL, Shyu RY, Hsieh CB, Lai HC, Liu KY, Chu TY, Lin YW (2006) Promoter methylation of the secreted frizzled-related protein 1 gene SFRP1 is frequent in hepatocellular carcinoma. Cancer 107:579–590

Shih YL, Hsieh CB, Lai HC, Yan MD, Hsieh TY, Chao YC, Lin YW (2007) SFRP1 suppressed hepatoma cells growth through Wnt canonical signaling pathway. Int J Cancer 121: 1028–1035

Shim YH, Park HJ, Choi MS, Kim JS, Kim H, Kim JJ, Jang JJ, Yu E (2003) Hypermethylation of the p16 gene and lack of p16 expression in hepatoblastoma. Mod Pathol 16:430–436

Shtutman M, Zhurinsky J, Simcha I, Albanese C, D'Amico M, Pestell R, Ben-Ze'ev A (1999) The cyclin D1 gene is a target of the beta-catenin/LEF-1 pathway. Proc Natl Acad Sci USA 96:5522–5527

Sigalotti L, Fratta E, Coral S, Cortini E, Covre A, Nicolay HJ, Anzalone L, Pezzani L, Di Giacomo AM, Fonsatti E, Colizzi F, Altomonte M, Calabro L, Maio M (2007) Epigenetic drugs as pleiotropic agents in cancer treatment: biomolecular aspects and clinical applications. J Cell Physiol 212:330–344

Singer S, Ehemann V, Brauckhoff A, Keith M, Vreden S, Schirmacher P, Breuhahn K (2007) Protumorigenic overexpression of stathmin/Op18 by gain-of-function mutation in p53 in human hepatocarcinogenesis. Hepatology 46: 759–768

Son G, Hirano T, Seki E, Iimuro Y, Nukiwa T, Matsumoto K, Nakamura T, Fujimoto J (2006) Blockage of HGF/c-Met system by gene therapy (adenovirus-mediated NK4 gene) suppresses hepatocellular carcinoma in mice. J Hepatol 45:688–695

Stejskalova E, Malis J, Snajdauf J, Pycha K, Urbankova H, Bajciova V, Stary J, Kodet R, Jarosova M (2009) Cytogenetic and array comparative genomic hybridization analysis of a series of hepatoblastomas. Cancer Genet Cytogenet 194:82–87

Sugawara W, Haruta M, Sasaki F, Watanabe N, Tsunematsu Y, Kikuta A, Kaneko Y (2007) Promoter hypermethylation of the RASSF1A gene predicts the poor outcome of patients with hepatoblastoma. Pediatr Blood Cancer 49: 240–249

Suzuki H, Watkins DN, Jair KW, Schuebel KE, Markowitz SD, Chen WD, Pretlow TP, Yang B, Akiyama Y, Van Engeland M, Toyota M, Tokino T, Hinoda Y, Imai K, Herman JG, Baylin SB (2004) Epigenetic inactivation of SFRP genes allows constitutive WNT signaling in colorectal cancer. Nat Genet 36:417–422

Suzuki M, Kato M, Yuyan C, Takita J, Sanada M, Nannya Y, Yamamoto G, Takahashi A, Ikeda H, Kuwano H, Ogawa S, Hayashi Y (2008) Whole-genome profiling of chromosomal aberrations in hepatoblastoma using high-density single-nucleotide polymorphism genotyping microarrays. Cancer Sci 99:564–570

Taniguchi T, Sullivan MJ, Ogawa O, Reeve AE (1995) Epigenetic changes encompassing the IGF2/H19 locus associated with relaxation of IGF2 imprinting and silencing of H19 in Wilms tumor. Proc Natl Acad Sci USA 92:2159–2163

Taniguchi K, Roberts LR, Aderca IN, Dong X, Qian C, Murphy LM, Nagorney DM, Burgart LJ, Roche PC, Smith DI, Ross JA, Liu W (2002) Mutational spectrum of beta-catenin, AXIN1, and AXIN2 in hepatocellular carcinomas and hepatoblastomas. Oncogene 21:4863–4871

Teh MT, Wong ST, Neill GW, Ghali LR, Philpott MP, Quinn AG (2002) FOXM1 is a downstream target of Gli1 in basal cell carcinomas. Cancer Res 62:4773–4780

Tomlinson GE, Douglass EC, Pollock BH, Finegold MJ, Schneider NR (2005) Cytogenetic evaluation of a large series of hepatoblastomas: numerical abnormalities with recurring aberrations involving 1q12-q21. Genes Chromosom Cancer 44:177–184

Trobaugh-Lotrario AD, Tomlinson GE, Finegold MJ, Gore L, Feusner JH (2009) Small cell undifferentiated variant of hepatoblastoma: adverse clinical and molecular features similar to rhabdoid tumors. Pediatr Blood Cancer 52:328–334

Ucar C, Caliskan U, Toy H, Gunel E (2007) Hepatoblastoma in a child with neurofibromatosis type I. Pediatr Blood Cancer 49:357–359

von Schweinitz D, Burger D, Bode U, Weinel P, Erttmann R, Hecker H, Mildenberger H (1994) Results of the HB-89 Study in treatment of malignant epithelial liver tumors in childhood and concept of a new HB-94 protocol. Klin Pädiatr 206:282–288

von Schweinitz D, Hecker H, Schmidt-von-Arndt G, Harms D (1997) Prognostic factors and staging systems in childhood hepatoblastoma. Int J Cancer 74:593–599

von Schweinitz D, Fuchs J, Gluer S, Pietsch T (1998) The occurrence of liver growth factor in hepatoblastoma. Eur J Pediatr Surg 8:133–136

von Schweinitz D, Faundez A, Teichmann B, Birnbaum T, Koch A, Hecker H, Gluer S, Fuchs J, Pietsch T (2000) Hepatocyte growth-factor-scatter factor can stimulate post-operative tumor-cell proliferation in childhood hepatoblastoma. Int J Cancer 85:151–159

Voz ML, Agten NS, Van de Ven WJ, Kas K (2000) PLAG1, the main translocation target in pleomorphic adenoma of the salivary glands, is a positive regulator of IGF-II. Cancer Res 60:106–113

Weber RG, Pietsch T, von Schweinitz D, Lichter P (2000) Characterization of genomic alterations in hepatoblastomas. A role for gains on chromosomes 8q and 20 as predictors of poor outcome. Am J Pathol 157:571–578

Wei Y, Fabre M, Branchereau S, Gauthier F, Perilongo G, Buendia MA (2000) Activation of beta-catenin in epithelial and mesenchymal hepatoblastomas. Oncogene 19:498–504

Weinberg AG, Finegold MJ (1983) Primary hepatic tumors of childhood. Hum Pathol 14:512–537

Weksberg R, Shen DR, Fei YL, Song QL, Squire J (1993a) Disruption of insulin-like growth factor 2 imprinting in Beckwith-Wiedemann syndrome. Nat Genet 5:143–150

Weksberg R, Teshima I, Williams BR, Greenberg CR, Pueschel SM, Chernos JE, Fowlow SB, Hoyme E, Anderson IJ, Whiteman DA et al (1993b) Molecular characterization of cytogenetic alterations associated with the Beckwith–Wiedemann syndrome (BWS) phenotype refines the localization and suggests the gene for BWS is imprinted. Hum Mol Genet 2:549–556

Wirths O, Waha A, Weggen S, Schirmacher P, Kuhne T, Goodyer CG, Albrecht S, von Schweinitz D, Pietsch T (2003) Overexpression of human Dickkopf-1, an antagonist of wingless/WNT signaling, in human hepatoblastomas and Wilms' tumors. Lab Invest 83:429–434

Yeh YA, Rao PH, Cigna CT, Middlesworth W, Lefkowitch JH, Murty VV (2000) Trisomy 1q, 2, and 20 in a case of hepatoblastoma: possible significance of 2q35-q37 and 1q12-q21 rearrangements. Cancer Genet Cytogenet 123:140–143

Yoshikawa H, Matsubara K, Qian GS, Jackson P, Groopman JD, Manning JE, Harris CC, Herman JG (2001) SOCS-1, a negative regulator of the JAK/STAT pathway, is silenced by methylation in human hepatocellular carcinoma and shows growth-suppression activity. Nat Genet 28:29–35

Yost C, Torres M, Miller JR, Huang E, Kimelman D, Moon RT (1996) The axis-inducing activity, stability, and subcellular distribution of beta-catenin is regulated in Xenopus embryos by glycogen synthase kinase 3. Genes Dev 10: 1443–1454

Zatkova A, Rouillard JM, Hartmann W, Lamb BJ, Kuick R, Eckart M, von Schweinitz D, Koch A, Fonatsch C, Pietsch T, Hanash SM, Wimmer K (2004) Amplification and overexpression of the IGF2 regulator PLAG1 in hepatoblastoma. Genes Chromosom Cancer 39:126–137

Zhu W, Shiojima I, Ito Y, Li Z, Ikeda H, Yoshida M, Naito AT, Nishi J, Ueno H, Umezawa A, Minamino T, Nagai T, Kikuchi A, Asashima M, Komuro I (2008) IGFBP-4 is an inhibitor of canonical Wnt signalling required for cardiogenesis. Nature 454:345–349

Ontogenetic Aspects of Liver Tumors 5

Arthur Zimmermann

Contents

A. Zimmermann
Institute of Pathology of the University, Murtenstrasse 31, CH-3010 Berne, Switzerland
e-mail: zimmerma@patho.unibe.ch

5.1 Introduction

Liver cell tumors, in particular hepatoblastomas and related neoplasms, exhibit histologic features that appear to mimic processes taking place during normal hepatic organogenesis. Epithelial hepatoblastomas consist of cell lineages, which resemble those appearing in distinct ontogenetic phases of the liver, e.g., embryonal and fetal-type hepatoblasts. In mixed hepatoblastomas, specific mesenchymal components develop, which may also exist in early periods of normal liver development (Zimmermann 2002a). The last few years have provided an impressive increase in our understanding of liver ontogeny, including the identification of the complex molecular machinery that drives cell lineages along a pathway from committed endoderm to the mature liver. It is tempting to assume that part of the molecular mechanisms operational in normal morphogenesis is paralleled by respective processes taking place in pediatric liver cell tumors.

5.2 Liver Ontogenesis: Pathways from Endoderm to Liver

5.2.1 Generation of the Hepatoblast and Hepatocyte Lineages

A complex machinery endows the foregut endoderm with the capability to form domains of competence fated to become liver and pancreas. In undifferentiated, multipotent endoderm cells, a network of transcription factors, morphogenetic proteins, and growth factors renders the cells responsive for specific tissue-inductive, hepatogenic signals. These inductive

A. Zimmermann et al. (eds.), *Pediatric Liver Tumors*, Pediatric Oncology,
DOI: 10.1007/978-3-642-14504-9_5, © Springer-Verlag Berlin Heidelberg 2011

factors include FoxA and GATA-4 transcription factors, fibroblast growth factors, and bone morphogenetic proteins (reviews: Zaret 2000; Tremblay and Zaret 2005; McLin and Zorn 2006; Zaret et al. 2008; Lemaigre 2009; Wandzioch and Zaret 2009).

The developing liver contains two main hepatocyte precursor cell systems, i.e., hepatic stem cells proper and hepatoblasts. Hepatic stem cells possess multilineage or bilineage differentiation potentials and self-renewing capability (Theise and Krause 2002; Dan et al. 2006; Michalopoulos 2006). Hepatoblasts are the immediate precursors of hepatocytes, a feature that they seem to share with hepatic stem cells. Therefore, are hepatoblast hepatic stem cells, and where do they come from? Epithelial cells of the liver originate from foregut endoderm, and this crucial structure seems to contain progenitor cells, which are primed to become hepatoblasts. The fated endoderm displays the future liver primordium in the form of thickening of the ventral endoderm epithelium. The source of the later liver is the so-called liver bud, which is derived from the foregut endoderm and gives rise to hepatoblasts, which express alpha-fetoprotein and are located around spaces within the septum transversum mesenchyme. These spaces will become the hepatic sinusoids. The homeobox gene Hex is required for the generation of a liver bud from the endoderm and the production of hepatoblasts (Bort et al. 2006). Hepatoblast survival and expansion requires Prospero-related homeobox 1 (Prox1) (Papoutsi et al. 2007; Kamiya et al. 2008) and the Wnt/beta-catenin signaling pathway, which in turn is activated by fibroblast growth factor 10 secreted by mesenchymal cells (Berg et al. 2007). The growth and maturation of the hepatoblast-containg liver bud depends on associated mesoderm-derived mesenchyme (Zaret 2000). Proliferating hepatoblasts migrate into the septum transversum mesenchyme in a Prox1-dependent manner (Sosa-Pineda et al. 2000).

A differerential expression of hepatocyte nuclear factor 4alpha (HNF4alpha) is essential for the pathway leading from hepatoblasts to mature hepatocytes (Parviz et al. 2003), critically affecting the production of proteins required for cell junction assembly and adhesion (Battle et al. 2006). The lineage restriction of hepatoblasts, i.e., shutting down the cholangiocyte lineage, depends on the repression of the cholangiocyte transcription factors, HNF1b and HNF6, and on the T-box transcriptional repressor Tbx3 (Suzuki et al. 2008; Lüdtke et al. 2009).

5.2.2 Development of the Cholangiocyte Lineage and the Bile Duct System

Morphologically, the extrahepatic biliary tree develops through the lengthening of the caudal part of the hepatic diverticulum and is patent from beginning. In contrast, the construction of the intrahepatic bile duct system requires a unique structure developing at the interface between the hepatoblastic parenchyma and the portal mesenchymal tissue, the ductal plate, which gives rise to intrahepatic bile ducts, which are not patent from the beginning but undergo secondary remodeling. This process proceeds from the liver hilum toward the organ's periphery along the branches of the developing portal venous system (Roskams and Desmet 2008).

In developmental terms, the extrahepatobiliary system shares a common origin with the ventral pancreas and not the liver. The pancreatobiliary progenitor cells of this anlage coexpress the transcription factors PDX1 and SOX17, and the restriction of SOX17+ biliary progenitors to the ventral gut region requires the Notch effector Hes1 (Spence et al. 2009). Intrahepatic cholangiocytes differentiate from hepatoblasts in the vicinity of the future ductal plate, and a network of regulatory factors induces the cells to construct a mature biliary tree, which starts from the ductal plate itself (review: Raynaud et al. 2009). Committment of hepatoblasts to future cholangiocytes is visualized by the expression of cytokeratin 19 in human cells. Biochemically, the earliest biliary lineage committment marker is the HMG box transcription factor Sox9 regulating the timing of the tubulogenic process (Antoniou et al. 2009). Early fating of hepatoblasts to cholangiocytes depends on Foxa transcription factors (Li et al. 2009) and the differentiation regulator, SAL-Like 4 (Sall4) (Oikawa et al. 2009). HNF6 is expressed in hepatoblasts and plays a central role in the development of intrahepatic bile ducts, affecting the expression of a second transcription factor, HNF1beta (Clotman et al. 2002). HNF1beta seems to be required for the generation of a luminal space (Tanimizu et al. 2009).The Notch receptor group (Notch 1–4) is differentially expressed during liver development and plays a role in biliary morphogenesis (Zong et al. 2009). In the fetal liver, Notch3 is expressed in mesenchymal cells adjacent to ductal plate cells expressing Jagged1. Notch2 signaling regulates the differentiation of biliary epithelial cells, the induction of tubulogenesis during development of intrahepatic bile ducts, and biliary cell survival (Geisler et al. 2008; Lozier et al. 2008; Tchorz et al. 2009). Moreover, the Wnt/catenin pathway is involved in biliary morphogenesis. Ductal plate cells strongly express E-cadherin and alpha-catenin, but only weakly beta-catenin, whereas migrating biliary cells and immature bile ducts markedly express beta-catenin in addition to alpha-catenin (Terada et al. 1998).

5.3 Stem Cells in the Pathogenesis of Hepatoblastomas

Important features of stem cells comprise pluripotency, self-renewal with limitless low-level proliferation, a long-lived undifferentiated state, and the capability to be primeable. Several signals and signaling pathways are involved to arrive at and maintain this distinct cellular phenotype. Is there evidence that stem cells are involved in the pathogenesis of hepatoblastomas, and can we detect such cells in the tumors?

A stem cell role and stem cell plasticity may be expected in tumors with several differentiation lineages. In teratoid hepatoblastoma, the presence of several cell lineages representing three germ layers was taken as an argument for the involvement of (tumor) progenitor cells (Kim et al. 2001). In epithelial heptoblastomas, cells in atypical duct-like structures were found to co-express stem cell markers and hepatic lineage markers (Fiegel et al. 2004), and small epithelial cells in hepatoblastomas expressed oval cell markers (OV-1 and OV-6) and had oval cell features by electron microscopy (Ruck et al. 1996; Ruck and Xiao 2002). On the other hand, cells of small cell-undifferentiated hepatoblastoma lacked oval cell markers in another investigation (Badve et al. 2003). A recent investigation showed that DLK1, a marker of bipotential oval cells, is upregulated in hepatoblastoma, suggesting that these neoplasms may originate from a bipotential progenitor cell (Lopez-Terrada et al. 2009).

Are there stem cell features in more differentiated hepatoblastoma cells? Normal fetal human liver epithelial cells display stem cell properties with multilineage gene expression in vitro and are capable of switching into a mesodermal-endodermal phenotype, i.e., generation of mesenchymal lineage cells (including osteogenic cells). This phenotype is genetically regulated through cytokine signaling (Inada et al. 2008). When analyzing epithelial hepatoblastomas, one may note small, more or less spherical, foci of pale cells (Fig. 5.1). We (Zimmermann 2005) found that these cell clusters have a very low proliferative activity, similar to stem cells, while a rim of hepatoblastoma cells surrounding the foci are highly proliferative (Fig. 5.2). The cells of the clusters are poorly differentiated, seen in their low content in mitochondria in comparison with surrounding embryonal/fetal hepatoblastoma

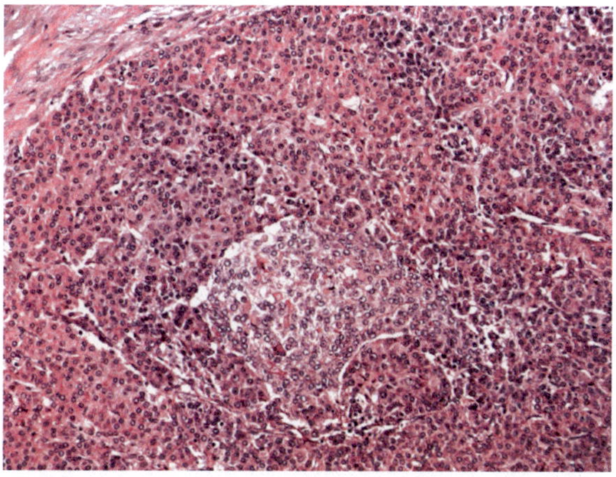

Fig. 5.1 This embryonal/fetal hepatoblastoma displays a focus (cluster) of pale and poorly diferentiated cells (below the *middle* of the figure; hematoxylin and eosin stain)

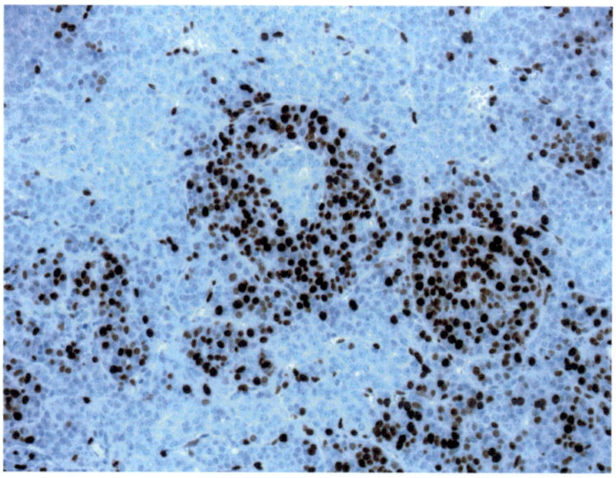

Fig. 5.2 In this immunostain for proliferation (proliferating cells with dark-brown nuclei), the cluster (above the center) exhibits minimal proliferation, whereas the hepatoblastoma cells directly surrounding the cluster show marked proliferative activity (Ki-67 immunostain)

cells (Fig. 5.3). Interestingly, it is these cells that have nuclear reactivity for beta-catenin (likely to represent a mutated phenotype; Fig. 5.4), whereas surrounding hepatoblastoma cells display a membraneous beta-catenin staining pattern (the nonmutated state). These findings suggest that the clustered cells have stem cell features (Zimmermann 2005).

The dilemma in understanding stem cells in mixed hepatoblastomas is the synchronous presence of epithelial and mesenchymal lineages. This phenomenon may involve plasticity of hepatic stem cells (Dan et al. 2006) and/or epithelial-mesenchymal transition, discussed later.

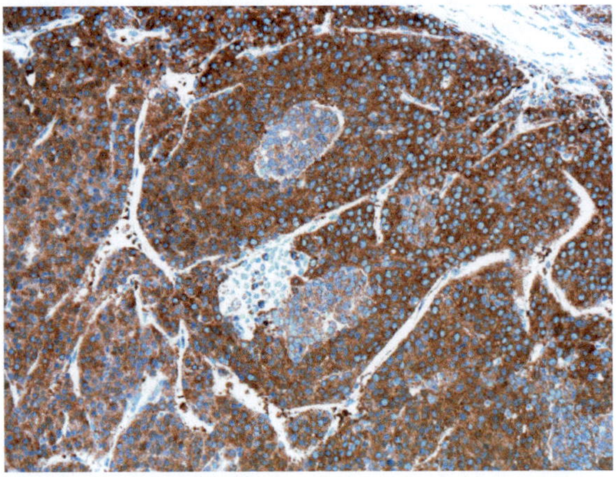

Fig. 5.3 Mitochondrial antigen immunostain. Cluster cells are poor in mitochondria and thus display low differentiation, while hepatoblastoma cells are rich in mitochondria and better differentiated

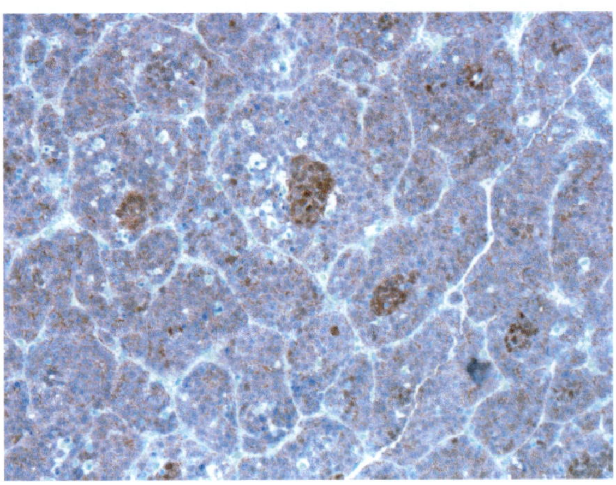

Fig. 5.4 Nuclear positivity for beta-catenin of the cells located in the clusters. In contrast, the surrounding hepatoblastoma cells show membranous beta-catenin expression (beta-catenin immunostain)

5.4 Undifferentiated Epithelial Hepatoblastomas and the Rhabdoid Cell/INI1 Connection

As outlined in Chap. 9, a subset of small cell undifferentiated hepatoblastomas displays rhabdoid features and shares lack of INI1 expression with malignant rhabdoid tumors (MRT) (Trobaugh-Lotrario et al. 2009).

MRTs display a recurrent deletion in the long arm of chromosome 22 (22q11.2) and show mutations of INI1 (review: Roberts and Biegel 2009). The INI1 gene is also known as hSNF5, BAF47, and SMARCB1. The human ortholog is a protein interacting with the HIV-1 integrase (**IN**tegrase **I**nteractor 1 or INI1). The mammalian version of the gene was later renamed Brg1/Brm Associated Factors complex or BAF complex with molecular mass 47 kD (BAF47). The genetic nomenclature committee then proposed the name, SMARCB1, for **SW**I/SNF related, **M**atrix-associated, **A**ctin-dependent **R**egulator of **C**hromatin, subfamily **B**, member **1** (Das et al. 2009; Roberts and Biegel 2009). Immunohistochemistry of INI1/BAF47 is established (Judkins 2007) and loss of INI1 immunostaining and INI1 mutations are correlated (Wu et al. 2008). But what is INI1? INI1 is a guardian of chromatin and DNA stability acting in the chromatin remodeling machinery requiring SWI/SNF complexes, which mobilize nucleosomes and are master regulators of gene expression and chromatin dynamics, and ATP-remodeling enzymes (Martens and Winston 2003; Stojanova and Penn 2009; Weissman and Knudsen 2009).The remodeling complex SNF is a partner of a further complex, ASCOM (activating signal cointegrator2 complex), required for nuclear receptor transactivation (Lee et al. 2009). In cell division, INI1 expression induces cell cycle arrest by blocking S phase entry at the G1/G0 checkpoint, linked to the pRb-E2F/p16Ink4a/cyclinD1 pathways, and to repression of Polo-like kinase 1 (PLK1; spindle checkpoint), which is overexpressed in MRTs and small cell hepatoblastomas lacking INI1 (Morozov et al. 2007; Stojanova and Penn 2009).

The failure of appropriate chromatin remodeling in MRTs and rhabdoid small cell hepatoblastomas deficient in INI1 may be central to the aggressive biology of these tumors. Taken together, these findings suggest a genetic connection between a subset of undifferentiated hepatoblastomas and tumors with a rhabdoid cell lineage. The origin and features of rhabdoid cells remain to be clarified, and this will have an impact on the histogenesis of hepatoblastomas and related tumors.

5.5 Beyond Hepatoblasts: Tumors with More Differentiated Liver Cell Lineages

Hepatoblasts give rise to differentiated liver cells and this process will terminate in mature hepatocytes. In contrast to embryonal and fetal hepatoblastomas showing different steps of hepatoblast development, several other liver cell tumors consist of more differentiated liver cells and even hepatocyte-like cells. They include a subset of macrotrabecular hepatoblastomas, hepatocellular carcinoma (HCC), and the recently described transitional liver cell tumor (TLCT), occuring in older children and young adolescents (see Chap. 9). TLCT is of theoretical significance insofar as its cell lineages synchronously display features of hepatoblast-like cells, cholangiocyte-like cells, and hepatocyte-like cells and, therefore, is thought to represent a transition between hepatoblastoma and HCC. Irrespective of the morphologically more mature phenotype of both HCC and TLCT, most of these tumors are clinically aggressive and behave differently from embryonal and fetal hepatoblastomas, chiefly with regard to treatment responses and prognosis.

In the rare macrotrabecular hepatoblastoma (Chap. 9), the cellular composition comes in two main phenotypes. In the first type, expected to be more aggressive, the cell plates consist of hepatocyte-like cells as seen in HCCs, while the second type consists of a mixture of embryonal and fetal hepatoblasts as seen in other hepatoblastomas (Zimmermann 2005). We have shown that TLCT shares with many hepatoblastomas a deranged beta-catenin signaling system with tumor cell nuclear reactivity for beta-catenin (Prokurat et al. 2002), suggesting a pathogenic role for the Wnt/beta-catenin signaling system in the transition from hepatoblasts to hepatocytes in these tumors. Experimentally produced failure of the beta-catenin axis promotes an immature phenotype of hepatocytes (Tan et al. 2008). A recent study demonstrated that marked deregulation of the Wnt/beta-catenin signaling pathway characterizes aggressive hepatoblastomas (Adesina et al. 2009) and may thus represent a molecular signature for high-grade malignancy. On the other hand, factors known from normal hepatic ontogenesis may be expected to be involved in the neoplastic hepatoblast-hepatocyte switch, including hepatocyte nuclear factor 4alpha (HNF4). It has been shown that loss of HNF4 expression is an important determinant of HCC progression in mice (Lazarevich et al. 2004), and that differentiation of experimental HCCs can be induced by HNF4 (Yin et al. 2008). On the other hand, a recent study showed that HNF4alpha was relatively elevated only in embryonal hepatoblastoma (Lopez-Terrada et al. 2009). Future studies may show whether macrotrabecular hepatoblastomas and TLCTs exhibit a deranged expression of transcription factors and/or homeobox gene products relevant for the generation of mature hepatocytes.

5.6 Bimodal Differentiation: Cholangioblastic Hepatoblastomas and Ductal Plate Tumors May Recapitulate Early Steps of Hepatogenesis

Tissue structures resembling small bile ducts and cholangiocytes are now known to occur in a subset of hepatoblastomas, termed cholangioblastic hepatoblastoma or hepatoblastoma with cholangioblastic features (Zimmermann 2002b; Chap. 9). Mechanisms and factors that induce the formation of neoplastic immature cholangiocytic ("cholangioblastic") lineages are not yet characterized. Specifically, it has not been demonstrated so far whether hepatoblastic and cholangioblastic cells present in these tumors emerge from one set of progenitor cells, but it is tempting to assume that a bipotential precursor cell is involved. As outlined above, periportal stem cells of the normal liver have the capacity to differentiate into both, parenchymal cells and bile duct cells (Fiel et al. 1997; Raynaud et al. 2009). Similar to normal liver, one or several differentiation checkpoints may be present in cholangioblastic hepatoblastomas deciding whether a neoplastic cell will follow the hepatoblast lineage or the cholangiocellular lineage. Molecules operational in these differentation switches have been discussed above and will be the target of future molecular studies of these tumors. In a subset of tumors possessing both hepatocyte and cholangiocyte lineages, the phenocopy with regard to normal ontogeny is striking: these are the tumors where not only immature cholangiocytes but also structures resembling the ductal plate ("ductal plate tumors"; Gornicka et al. 2001) are generated, suggesting that key events in normal morphogenesis can be closely mimicked by tumors.

5.7 Epithelial-Mesenchymal Transition as a Pathogenic Mechanism in Mixed Hepatoblastomas and Related Tumors

Epithelial-mesenchymal transition (EMT) is defined as a process whereby polarized epithelial cells undergo a series of changes enabling them to assume a mesenchymal cell phenotype. EMT has a central role in development, regeneration, remodeling of tissues, and cancerogenesis (reviews: Guarino et al. 2007; Baum et al. 2008).Three types of EMT have been identified, viz., EMT during embryogenesis and organ development (type 1 EMT); EMT associated with the regulation of tissue turnover, inflammation, and regeneration (type 2 EMT); and EMT associated with cancer progression and metastasis (type 3 EMT). EMT is operated via distinct sets of cells that are termed, transitioning cells or cells that undergo partial EMT, with synchronous expression of both epithelial and mesenchymal markers (Zavadil and Bottinger 2005).

Apparent transitions between epithelial and mesenchymal phenotypes are observed in mixed epithelial and mesenchymal hepatoblastomas, most notably in tumor osteoid, where osteoblast-like cells generating bone matrix express a hepatocytic cytokeratin pattern. EMT may be a particularly distinct feature of bimorphic/biphasic hepatic tumors where neoplastic epithelial and mesenchymal components come in close and highly characteristic association, summarized in Table 5.1.

What is the role of EMT in the liver, and how is it regulated? Generally, EMT occurs both in the developing and adult normal liver, but is more active in any process that alters the hepatic cell turnover (review: Choi and Diehl 2009). In principle, three types of adult liver cells, namely, hepatocytes, cholangiocytes, and hepatic stellate cells, can undergo EMT in cell culture. Adult hepatocytes undergoing TGFbeta-induced EMT resemble fibroblastoid cells (Zeisberg et al. 2007; Godoy et al. 2009). EMT of cholangiocytes plays a role in several normal and pathologic processes (Glaser et al. 2009). Several factors have been identified to regulate EMT, and these factors also play a role in tumors showing EMT, where distinct molecular signatures for EMT are specifically found at the cancer invasion front (De Wever et al. 2008). The important downregulation of E-cadherin expression in tumors is a key feature of EMT and is differentially regulated in epithelial cells and mesenchymal cells via activation or inactivation (repression) of the respective E cadherin promoters. During EMT, transcription factors repressing E cadherin promoter induce mesenchymal features in epithelial cells (review: De Wever et al. 2008). A major step ahead was, therefore, the identification of transcriptional repressors, which include Snail, Slug, Smad interacting protein (SIP1), and deltaEF1. Other factors inducing EMT with loss of E cadherin are TWIST, homeobox-B7, FOXC2, TGF-beta1, Krüppel-like factor 8, sonic hedgehog, and the Wnt/beta-catenin signaling pathway.

Table 5.1 Biphasic hepatic tumors which may result from disordered epithelial-mesenchymal transition [EMT] ("EMT tumors"; Zimmermann 2005)

Mixed epithelial and mesenchymal hepatoblastoma
Mesenchymal hamartoma
Undifferentiated (embryonal) sarcoma (UES)
Hepatic carcinosarcomas
Nested epithelial and stromal tumor
Pediatric hepatic stromal tumors

Epithelial hepatoblastomas are commonly poor in stroma, and most of the connective tissue and its extracellular matrix are associated with the tumor's vascular tree. The situation is very different for the second main type of hepatoblastomas, i.e., the mixed epithelial and mesenchymal type. Here, a rich non-epithelial component is typical and may even dominate the tumor mass. This mesenchymal tissue shows a complex composition and derivation because, on the one hand, it is part of the tumor itself (neoplastic mesenchyme, including immature bone), whereas on the other hand, it is non-neoplastic and mainly related to the angiogenic response. Histologically, it is rather easy to allocate osteoid, chondroid tissue, and muscle tissue occurring in mixed hepatoblastoma to the neoplastic compartment, while it may be difficult or impossible to decide whether an immature mesenchyme is tumor or reactive stromal tissue. This will be important when trying to solve the question whether viable tumor is still present after chemotherapy in the absence of tumor epithelia.

What is the evidence that EMT is pathogenically involved in hepatic epithelial tumors? In human hepatocellular carcinomas (HCC), EMT plays a role in stroma formation and correlates with aggressiveness of the tumors and poor survival. The tumor stroma showing transition of fibroblasts into myofibroblasts plays a central role in angiogenesis and invasion (De Wever and Mareel 2003; Ostman and Augsten 2009). Hepatic epithelial tumor cells and stromal cells perform a complex crosstalk that guides EMT at the invasion front (tumor edge; Van Zijl et al. 2009). With regard to the promotion of invasion, more than 50% of HCCs exhibit reduced E-cadherin expression, a hallmark of EMT. In HCCs, the EMT regulator twist has been shown to induce EMT via downregulation of E cadherin expression, promoting cell migration and an invasive phenotype (Lee et al. 2006). A similar E cadherin decrease in HCCs is also caused by the EMT inducer, tetraspanin TM4SF5 (Lee et al. 2008). EMT in HCC is furthermore induced by another factor central to EMT, Snail, which promotes EMT and metastatic spread in HCC (Yang et al. 2009). A potential link between HCC and hepatoblastoma is seen in the form of sarcomatoid HCC with hepatoblastoma-like features (Cho et al. 2004). But are there findings showing that the neoplastic mesenchyme of mixed hepatoblastomas is the result of EMT? So far (and in contrast to HCC), there is only indirect evidence at best. It is noteworthy that the mixed epithelial and mesenchymal phenotype seem to be more frequent after chemotherapy. Whether this observation reflects reality or is just a sampling effect, i.e., mixed components having a greater chance of being detectable in the more numerous and larger histology sections of post-chemotherapy resection specimens in contrast to a pretreatment needle biopsy, is not yet clear. If the phenomenon is real, one may argue that therapy alters the ratio between tumor epithelia and tumor mesenchyme, e.g., favoring a transition from epithelia to mesenchyme (and here in particular bone/osteoid).

5.8 Conclusion

A deeper insight into the distinct morphologies of hepatoblastomas and related tumors shows that this group of tumors reflects several processes taking place during normal liver ontogeny. Apart from mimicking specific cell lineages with increasing differentiation there is evidence that these tumors replicate features of stem cell biology and of epithelial-mesenchymal transition. These morphologic findings are now progressively enlarged by distinct molecular features, again shared between the normal development of the liver and the neoplasms derived thereof. These novel molecular findings will hopefully be suited to be employed for refined molecular classifications of liver cell tumors and for novel therapeutic strategies.

References

Adesina AM, Lopez-Terrada D, Wong KK et al (2009) Gene expression profiling reveals signatures characterizing histologic subtypes of hepatoblastoma and global reregulation in cell growth and survival pathways. Hum Pathol 40:843–853

Antoniou A, Raynaud P, Cordi S et al (2009) Intrahepatic bile ducts develop according to a new mode of tubulogenesis regulated by the transcription factor SOX9. Gastroenterology 136:2325–2333

Badve S, Logdberg L, Lal A et al (2003) Small cells in hepatoblastoma lack "oval" cell phenotype. Mod Pathol 16:930–936

Battle MA, Konopka G, Parviz F et al (2006) Hepatocyte nuclear factor 4alpha orchstrates expression of cell adhesion proteins during the epithelial transformation of the developing liver. Proc Natl Acad Sci USA 103:8419–8424

Baum B, Settleman J, Quinlan MP (2008) Transitions between epithelial and mesenchymal states in development and disease. Semin Cell Dev Biol 19:294–308

Berg T, Rountree CB, Lee L et al (2007) Fibroblast growth factor 10 is critical for liver growth during embryogenesis and controls hepatoblast survival via beta-catenin activation. Hepatology 46:1187–1197

Bort R, Signore M, Tremblay K et al (2006) Hex homeobox gene controls the transition of the endoderm to a pseudostratified, cell emergent epithelium for liver bud development. Dev Biol 290:44–56

Cho MS, Lee SN, Sung SH et al (2004) Sarcomatoid hepatocellular carcinoma with hepatoblastoma-like features in an adult. Pathol Int 54:446–450

Choi SS, Diehl AM (2009) Epithelial-to-mesenchymal transitions in the liver. Hepatology 50:2007–2013

Clotman F, Lannoy VJ, Reber M et al (2002) The onecut transcription factor HNF6 is required for normal development of the biliary tract. Development 129:1819–1828

Dan YY, Riehle KJ, Lazaro C et al (2006) Isolation of multipotent progenitor cells from human fetal liver capable of differentiating into liver and mesenchymal lineages. Proc Natl Acad Sci USA 103:9912–9917

Das S, Cano J, Kalpana GV (2009) Multimerization and DNA binding properties of INI1/hSNF5 and its functional significance. J Biol Chem 284:19903–19914

De Wever O, Mareel M (2003) Role of tissue stroma in cancer cell invasion. J Pathol 200:429–447

De Wever O, Pauwels P, De Craene B et al (2008) Molecular and pathological signatures of the epithelial-mesenchymal transitions at the cancer invasion front. Histochem Cell Biol 130:481–494

Fiegel HC, Glüer S, Roth B et al (2004) Stem-like cells in human hepatoblastoma. J Histochem Cytochem 52:1495–1501

Fiel MI, Antonio LB, Nalesnik MA et al (1997) Characterization of ductular hepatocytes in primary liver allograft failure. Mod Pathol 10:348–353

Geisler F, Nagl F, Mazur PK et al (2008) Liver-specific inactivation of Notch2, but not Notch1, compromises intrahepatic bile duct development in mice. Hepatology 48:607–616

Glaser SS, Gaudio E, Miller T et al (2009) Cholangiocyte proliferation and liver fibrosis. Expert Rev Mol Med 11:e7

Godoy P, Hengstler JG, Ilkavets I et al (2009) Extracellular matrix modultes sensitivity of hepatocytes to fibroblastoid dedifferentiation and transforming growth factor beta-induced apoptosis. Hepatology 49:2031–2043

Gornicka B, Ziarkiewicz-Wroblewska B, Michalowicz B et al (2001) Immature hepatic tumor of bimodal differentiation in a young adult patient: a novel lesion expressing β-catenin and mimicking a distinct phase of hepatogenesis. J Hepatol 34:955–961

Guarino M, Rubino B, Ballabio G (2007) The role of epithelial-mesenchymal transition in cancer pathology 39:305–318

Inada M, Follenzi A, Cheng K et al (2008) Phenotype reversion in fetal human liver epithelial cells identifies the role of an intermediate meso-endodermal stage before hepatic maturation. J Cell Sci 121:1002–1013

Judkins AR (2007) Immunohistochemistry of INI1 expression: a new tool for old challenges in CNS and soft tissue pathology. Adv Anat Pathol 14:335–339

Kamiya A, Kakinuma S, Onodera M et al (2008) Prospero-related homeobox 1 and liver receptor homolog 1 coordinately regulate long-term proliferation of murine fetal hepatoblasts. Hepatology 48:252–264

Kim L, Park YN, Kim SE et al (2001) Teratoid hepatoblastoma: multidirectional differentiation of stem cell of the liver. Yonsei Med J 42:431–435

Lazarevich NL, Cheremnova OA, Varga EV et al (2004) Progression of HCC in mice is associated with a downregulation in the expression of hepatocyte nuclear factors. Hepatology 39:1038–1047

Lee TK, Poon RT, Yuen AP et al (2006) Twist overexpression correlates with hepatocellular carcinoma metastasis through induction of epithelial-mesenchymal transition. Clin Cancer Res 12:5369–5376

Lee SA, Lee SY, Cho IH et al (2008) Tetraspanin TM4SF5 mediates loss of contact inhibition through epithelial-mesenchymal transition in human hepatocarcinoma. J Clin Invest 118: 1354–1366

Lee S, Kim DH, Goo YH et al (2009) Crucial roles for interactions between MLL3/4 and INI1 in nuclear receptor transactivation. Mol Endocrinol 23:610–619

Lemaigre FP (2009) Mechanisms of liver development: concepts for understanding liver disorders and design of novel therapies. Gastroenterology 137:62–79

Li Z, White P, Tuteja G et al (2009) Foxa1 and Foxa2 regulate bile duct development in mice. J Clin Invest 119: 1537–1545

Lopez-Terrada D, Gunaratne PH, Adesina AM et al (2009) Histologic subtypes of hepatoblastoma are characterized by differential canonical Wnt and Notch pathway activation in DLK+precursors. Hum Pathol 40:783–794

Lozier J, McCright B, Gridley T (2008) Notch signaling regulates bile duct morphogenesis in mice. PLoS ONE 3:e1815

Lüdtke TH, Christoffels VM, Petry M et al (2009) Tbx3 promotes liver bud expansion during mouse development by suppression of cholangiocyte differentiation. Hepatology 49:969–978

Martens JA, Winston F (2003) Recent advances in understanding chromatin remodeling by Swi/Snf complexes. Curr Opin Genet Dev 13:136–142

McLin VA, Zorn AM (2006) Molecular control of liver development. Clin Liver Dis 10:1–25

Michalopoulos GK (2006) Flexible lineage specifications of adult hepatic cells, associated molecular pathways, and their relationship to liver cancer. Cell Transplant 15(Suppl 1):S67–S68

Morozov A, Lee SJ, Zhang ZK et al (2007) INI1 induces interferon signaling and spindle checkpoint in rhabdoid tumors. Clin Cancer Res 13:4721–4730

Oikawa T, Kamiya A, Kakinuma S et al (2009) Sall4 regulates cell fate decision in fetal hepatic stem/progenitor cells. Gastroenterology 136:1000–1011

Ostman A, Augsten M (2009) Cancer-associated fibroblasts and tumor growth – bystanders turning into key players. Curr Opin Genet Dev 19:67–73

Papoutsi M, Dudas J, Becker J et al (2007) Gene regulation by homeobox transcription factor Prox1 in murine hepatoblasts. Cell Tissue Res 330:209–220

Parviz F, Matullo C, Garrison WD et al (2003) Hepatocyte nuclear factor 4alpha controls the development of a hepatic epithelium and liver morphogenesis. Nat Genet 34:292–296

Prokurat A, Kluge P, Kosciesza A et al (2002) Transitional liver cell tumors (TLCT) in older children and adolescents: a novel group of aggressive hepatic tumors expressing beta-catenin. Med Pediatr Oncol 39:510–518

Raynaud P, Carpentier R, Antoniou A et al (2009) Biliary differentiation and bile duct morphogenesis in development and disease. Int J Biochem Cell Biol. doi:Doi: 10.1016/j biocel 2009.07.020

Roberts CWM, Biegel JA (2009) The role of SMARCB1/INI1 in development of rhabdoid tumor. Cancer Biol Ther 8:412–416

Roskams T, Desmet V (2008) Embryology of extra-and intrahepatic bile ducts, the ductal plate. Anat Rec (Hoboken) 291:628–635

Ruck P, Xiao JC (2002) Stem-like cells in hepatoblastoma. Med Pediatr Oncol 39:504–507

Ruck P, Xiao JC, Kaiserling E (1996) Small epithelial cells and the histogenesis of hepatoblastoma. Electron microscopic, immunoelectron microscopic, and immunohistochemical findings. Am J Pathol 148:321–329

Sosa-Pineda B, Wigle JT, Olivier G (2000) Hepatocyte migration during liver development requires Prox1. Nat Genet 25:254–255

Spence JR, Lange AW, Lin SC et al (2009) Sox17 regulates organ lineage segregation of ventral foregut progenitor cells. Dev Cell 17:62–74

Stojanova A, Penn LZ (2009) The role of INI1/hSNF5 in gene regulation and cancer. Biochem Cell Biol 87:163–177

Suzuki A, Sekiya S, Büscher D et al (2008) Tbx3 controls the fate of hepatic progenitor cells in liver development by suppressing p19ARF expression. Development 135:1589–1595

Tan X, Yuan Y, Zeng G et al (2008) Beta-catenin deletion in hepatoblasts disrupts hepatic morphogenesis and survival during mouse development. Hepatology 47:1667–1679

Tanimizu N, Miyajima A, Mostov KE (2009) Liver progenitor cells fold up a cell monolayer into a double-layered structure during tubular morphogenesis. Mol Biol Cell 20: 2486–2494

Tchorz JS, Kinter J, Müller M et al (2009) Notch2 signaling promotes biliary epithelial cell fate specification and tubulogenesis during bile duct development in mice. Hepatology 50:871–879

Terada T, Ashida K, Kitamura Y et al (1998) Expression of epithelial-cadherin, alpha-catenin and beta-catenin during human intrahepatic bile duct development: a possible role in bile duct morphogenesis. J Hepatol 28:263–269

Theise ND, Krause DS (2002) Bone marrow to liver: the blood of Prometheus. Semin Cell Dev Biol 13:411–417

Tremblay KD, Zaret KS (2005) Distinct populations of endoderm cells converge to generate the embryonic liver bud and ventral foregut tissues. Dev Biol 280:87–99

Trobaugh-Lotrario AD, Tomlinson GE, Finegold MJ et al (2009) Small cell undifferentiated variant of hepatoblastoma: adverse clinical and molecular features similar to rhabdoid tumors. Pediatr Blood Cancer 52:328–334

Van Zijl F, Mair M, Csiszar A et al (2009) Hepatic tumor-stroma crosstalk guides epithelial to mesenchymal transition at the tumor edge. Oncogene 28:4022–4033

Wandzioch E, Zaret KS (2009) Dynamic signaling network for the specification of embryonic pancreas and liver progenitors. Science 324:1707–1710

Weissman B, Knudsen KE (2009) Hijacking the chromatin remodeling machinery: impact of SWI/SNF perturbations in cancer. Cancer Res 69:8223–8230

Wu X, Dagar V, Algar E et al (2008) Rhabdoid tumour: a malignancy of early childhood with variable primary site, histology and clinical behaviour. Pathology 40:664–670

Yang MH, Chen CL, Chau GY et al (2009) Comprehensive analysis of the independent effect of twist and snail in promoting metastasis of hepatocellular carcinoma. Hepatology 50:1464–1474

Yin C, Lin Y, Zhang X et al (2008) Differentiation therapy of hepatocellular carcinoma in mice with recombinant adenovirus carrying hepatocyte nuclear factor-4alpha gene. Hepatology 48:1528–1539

Zaret KS (2000) Liver specification and early morphogenesis. Mech Dev 92:83–88

Zaret KS, Watts J, Xu J et al (2008) Pioneer factors, genetic competence, and inductive signaling: programming liver and pancreas progenitors from the endoderm. Cold Spring Harb Symp Quant Biol 73:119–126

Zavadil J, Bottinger EP (2005) TGF-β· and epithelial-to-mesenchymal transitions. Oncogene 24:5764–5774

Zeisberg M, Yang C, Martino M et al (2007) Fibroblasts derived from hepatocytes in liver fibrosis via epithelial to mesenchymal transition. J Biol Chem 282:23337–23347

Zimmermann A (2002a) Pediatric liver tumors and hepatic organogenesis: common and distinctive pathways. Med Pediatr Oncol 39:492–503

Zimmermann A (2002b) Hepatoblastoma with cholangioblastic features ('cholangioblastic hepatoblastoma') and other liver tumours with a bimodal differentiation in young patients. Med Pediatr Oncol 39:487–491

Zimmermann A (2005) The emerging family of hepatoblastoma tumors: from ontogenesis to oncogenesis. Eur J Cancer 41:1503–1514

Zong Y, Panikkar A, Xu J et al (2009) Notch signaling controls liver development by regulating biliary differentiation. Development 136:1727–1739

Translational Investigations of Liver Tumors: Sampling Strategies and Banking

6

Michael Grotzer and Tarek Shalaby

Contents

M. Grotzer (✉) and T. Shalaby
Pediatric Neuro-Oncology, University Children's Hospital, Steinwiesstrasse 75, 8032 Zurich, Switzerland
e-mail: Michael.Grotzer@kispi.uzh.ch

6.1 Introduction

Amazing progress has been achieved recently in our knowledge about cancer at the molecular level as a result of advances in molecular technology (Cassidy and Radda 2005; Clements et al. 2006; van der Merwe et al. 2007; Ali-Khan et al. 2009). This knowledge has led to an increased understanding of the complex factors involved in cancer development and progression. To improve cancer management, the scientific discoveries at the cellular and molecular level must be translated into practical clinical applications with the aim of reducing cancer incidence, morbidity, and mortality (Cassidy and Radda 2005; Clements et al. 2006; van der Merwe et al. 2007; Ali-Khan et al. 2009).

Translational research that transforms scientific discoveries into clinical applications involves laboratory investigation on clinical materials (Adams et al. 2009; Arbab et al. 2009; Clermont et al. 2009; Hawkins et al. 2009; Payne et al. 2009). Hence, it requires access to collections of well-preserved tissues accompanied by high-quality clinical data to examine the relationship between molecular changes and clinical variables or outcomes. However, the small number of available tumor tissue samples has disappointingly limited the researcher's outputs in the field of rare tumors (Adams et al. 2009; Arbab et al. 2009; Clermont et al. 2009; Hawkins et al. 2009; Payne et al. 2009) and has brought recognition to the urgent need to improve the access to tissue resources. Tumor collections by single institutions or individual scientists are mostly not sufficient to address these resource problems. Therefore, improved tools such as biobanks, one of the key resources in the fight against cancer, are certainly needed (Adam 2002; Qualman et al. 2004; Herpel et al. 2008). Recently, biobanks have become a critical engine for basic,

A. Zimmermann et al. (eds.), *Pediatric Liver Tumors*, Pediatric Oncology,
DOI: 10.1007/978-3-642-14504-9_6, © Springer-Verlag Berlin Heidelberg 2011

translational, and clinical research and the recent development of different biobanks in a number of countries reflects scientists' and policy-makers' beliefs in the future health benefits to be derived from molecular research (Watson et al. 1996; Anderer et al. 1998; Spinney 2003; Whyte 2003; Bauchet et al. 2007).

However, unlike other research tools such as cell lines and animal models, the boom of biobanks spawned a "boomlet" of regulations and guidelines, which has created controversies, particularly about the importance and definition of informed consent (Chadwick and Berg 2001; Everett 2003; Elger and Caplan 2006). The consent of participants is usually required before biobank samples can be used in research, but the nature of this consent, and how it is obtained, vary widely. Many European guidelines take the view that general consent is acceptable to use samples for future, as yet unspecified research projects; US and Canadian policy follows a more rigorous standard of consent (Elger and Caplan 2006).

Biobanks include the collection of characterized human tumor tissues, associated pathological information, and access to linked clinical patient data. The tissues are collected, processed, and organized in such a way so as to facilitate research (Kerr 2003; Lopez-Guerrero et al. 2006; Rodrigues et al. 2009). The collected samples usually include tumors as well as adjacent normal tissues and blood samples and are associated with a spectrum of information that usually includes the collection time, the tissue composition, and the alterations within that reflect the type and stage of the disease (histopathology). The clinical data comprise information about the donor of the material, such as demographic characteristics, the outcome of the disease, treatment, and so on. Different banks vary in their emphasis on the spectrum of pathologies and related histological data, or the selection and consistency of the patient cohort, to serve different levels of research (Kerr 2003; Lopez-Guerrero et al. 2006; Rodrigues et al. 2009).

6.2 SIOPEL Liver Tumour Storage Programme

Liver tumors of children are rare and comprise approximately 5% of pediatric neoplasms (Isaacs 2007). Hepatoblastoma (HB) is the most common pediatric liver tumor – followed by hepatocellular carcinoma (HCC) – and more than 70% of the tumors are diagnosed in children less than 2 years old (Perilongo and Shafford 1999; Isaacs 2007). HB, which is derived from hepatic precursor cells, is morphologically similar to immature hepatocytes and the prognosis of the patients is variable (Brown et al. 2000; Fuchs et al. 2002). Although high- and low-risk groups in childhood HB have been described (Takayasu et al. 2001; von Schweinitz et al. 2002; Yamada et al. 2004; Yamaoka et al. 2006), the clinical or pathological prognostic factors cannot predict treatment response on an individual basis. Therefore, further efforts aimed at better understanding of HB biology are highly warranted. The ultimate goal is the development of better risk-based stratification systems and more efficacious and less toxic targeted treatment schedules, used alone or in combination with conventional cytotoxic drugs.

One of the primary objectives of the SIOPEL scientific group is to facilitate basic and translational research aimed at a better understanding of the biology of childhood liver tumors. To this end, the SIOPEL Liver Tumour Storage Programme was established in 2005 at the University Children's Hospital of Zurich, Switzerland. The aim of the SIOPEL Liver Tumour Storage Programme is to create a basis for molecular genetic cancer research into children's liver tumors. This goal was planned to be reached through: (1) the central collection and storage of pediatric liver tumor specimens, normal liver tissues (when available), and blood in high quality, for later molecular genetic analysis, (2) the documentation of the conserved material and its tumor of origin in a comprehensive database, and (3) the distribution of the conserved materials and the tumor-derived materials for approved research projects conducted by investigators affiliated with SIOPEL.

6.2.1 Tumor Tissue Collection

Regardless of recent major advances in genetic and other biological techniques, the reliability of biological research depends primarily on the quality of the material that is studied. For this reason, collection and submission of representative tumor material remain key enterprises in the pathway leading to good biological studies (Ambros and Ambros 2001; Parham and Qualman 2001). Accordingly, emphasis has been put

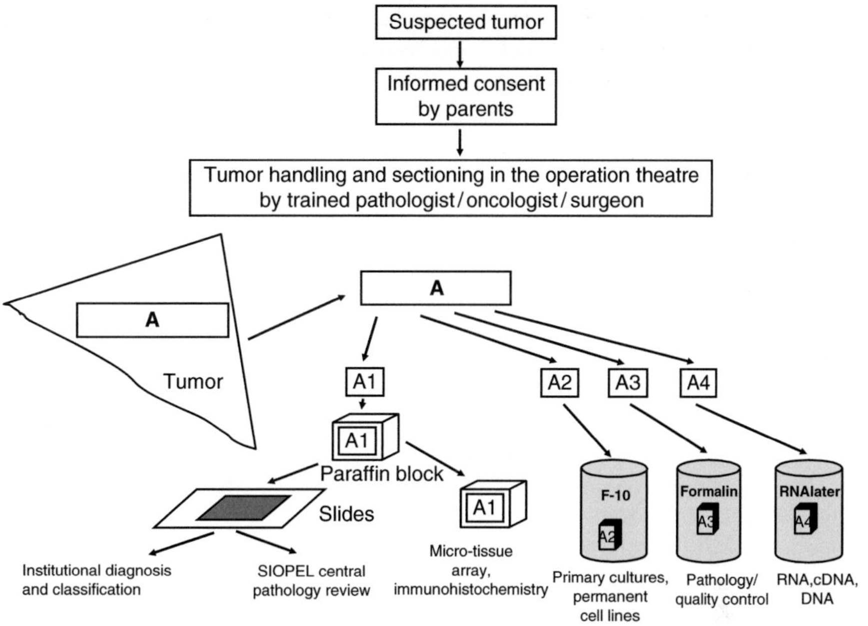

Fig. 6.1 Sample collection and processing for the SIOPEL Liver Tumour Storage Programme

on a detailed description of the tumor collection procedure in the operating theater, which is usually performed by the local surgeon, the pathologist, or a trained pediatric oncologist (Fig. 6.1). After collection, the tumor samples are reversibly (linked) anonymized: a link exists between tumor sample and patient, but the researcher does not have access (Elger and Caplan 2006). Then, the transport tubes with the tumor samples are sent at room temperature by express mail to the centralized SIOPEL Liver Tumour Storage Programme in Zurich, Switzerland.

Diagnostic biopsies can be obtained by closed Tru-cut biopsy or laparoscopic wedge resection. Both approaches allow the surgeon or interventional radiologist to collect sufficient material for an accurate diagnostic classification (by the local pathologist), and for tumor material to be retained for the SIOPEL Liver Tumour Storage Programme. If closed Tru-cut biopsies are taken, an additional pass is recommended for tissue banking. Importantly, the sample should be processed immediately to ensure its viability and to preserve nucleic acids, particularly RNA.

Accurate histopathological diagnosis and staging of tumors are of extreme importance in planning the treatment of patients with cancer. Typically, the tissue from surgical resections is processed through aldehyde-based fixatives (e.g., formalin) and embedded in paraffin. This practice is well suited to immunohistochemic methods at the protein level, but may damage mRNA integrity (Klimecki et al. 1994). Therefore, tumor tissue preservation for subsequent RNA isolation is usually done by freezing biopsy material in liquid nitrogen in the operating room. The rapidly frozen (i.e., snap frozen) biopsy material is then stored at −70°C and shipped from one laboratory to another in dry ice. Use of liquid nitrogen snap freezing and storage at −70°C poses significant logistical problems in many institutions and may preclude their participation in important multi-institutional trials. Moreover, shipping of well-preserved tissue samples from one laboratory to another on dry ice is costly and may be complicated by delays at national borders. To circumvent the logistical difficulties inherent in such procedures, we tested a new RNA stabilization solution (RNA*later*; Ambion) and found that tumor tissue can be stored for a period of up to 7 days at room temperature without significant RNA degradation (Grotzer et al. 2000).

6.2.2 Tumor Tissue Storing

After arrival in Zurich, Switzerland, tumor samples in RNA*later* are cut into smaller pieces, labeled, and stored at −20°C in designated boxes until they are required for a specific project. Amount of tumor tissue and location of the stored samples are then entered in the tumor bank database. All the clinical information including age, gender, staging, treatment, and outcome is stored separately at the SIOPEL Clinical Trial Center in Leicester, UK.

As the refrigerator freezers depend on the electrical power supply network, they require appropriate security measures to minimize the risk of major temperature fluctuations. For this reason, the SIOPEL Liver Tumour Storage Programme freezers are connected to the secure electricity supply of the University Children's Hospital of Zurich, Switzerland, in such a way that in the case of deficiencies in the electrical supply, emergency generators will ensure continuity of the supply.

Stored tumor bank samples usually require review at years 2, 3, and 5 with focus on structural and molecular integrity (Jewell et al. 2002). For quality assessment purposes, the SIOPEL Tumour Storage Programme periodically assesses the molecular integrity of the stored specimens by extracting nucleic acids (DNA and RNA) from randomly chosen RNA*later* preserved tissues. The quality of the isolated nucleic acids is measured by the Agilent bioanalyzer for RNA and by gel electrophoresis for DNA.

6.2.3 Tumor Tissue Distribution

By the end of 2009, the SIOPEL Tumour and Tissue Storage Programme has managed to collect 86 childhood liver tumor samples from 18 different countries (Fig. 6.2). Proposals to use specimens stored in the SIOPEL tumor bank are submitted in writing to the Chair of the SIOPEL in the format shown in Table 6.1; they are reviewed by appropriate members of the SIOPEL Scientific Committee according to the criteria summarized in Table 6.2. Investigators whose proposals are approved are expected to abide by the guidelines shown in Table 6.3 in conducting their research with specimens from the SIOPEL Liver Tumour Storage Programme.

After approval, carefully packed samples are sent to the researchers together with the information about the specimens as quickly as possible (by express mail). The investigators are notified by email on the same day of sending the sample. Copies of the correspondence about the shipped samples are kept in the archive of the SIOPEL Liver Tumour Storage Programme.

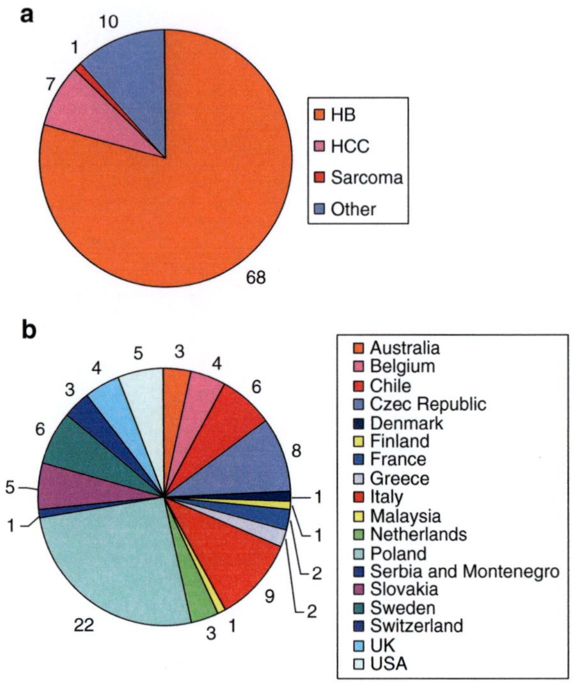

Fig. 6.2 Tumor samples collected for the SIOPEL Liver Tumour Storage Programme (2005–2009) according to histology (**a**) and countries (**b**)

Table 6.1 Format of submission of proposals to obtain specimens from the SIOPEL Liver Tumour Storage Programme

1. Title of project, Principal investigator information
2. Project-specific aims
3. Background and rationale
4. Methods and technical feasibility
5. Preliminary data
6. Statistical considerations
7. Funding available to complete the proposed study
8. References
9. Laboratory shipping address

Table 6.2 Review criteria of the SIOPEL Scientific Committee for access to specimens

1. Will the study move the field forward; is it unique?
2. Does the study require the resources of a cooperative group?
3. Does the investigator have appropriate expertise/ preliminary data?
4. Can the work be done in a timely fashion?
5. Will the results of the study have an impact on patient care?
6. Does the investigator have funding to conduct the work?

Table 6.3 Guidelines for investigators using specimens from the SIOPEL Tumour and Tissue Storage Programme

1. Submit Institutional Review Board approval for the proposed research
2. Present progress reports to the SIOPEL Scientific Committee
3. Use specimens only for approved projects and return unused specimens to the SIOPEL Liver Tumour Storage Programme
4. Submit manuscripts and abstracts to the SIOPEL Scientific Committee for review before submission for presentations/publication
5. The biological materials must not be sold, shared, distributed, or otherwise transferred to third parties without authorization of SIOPEL Scientific Committee
6. The researcher shall not attempt to establish the identity of a donor, but may relay any clinically significant findings to SIOPEL Scientific Committee

6.3 Discussion

Our understanding of cancer biology has expanded dramatically with recent advances in molecular technology. Scientific and technical advances in genomics, proteomics, and bioinformatics make it possible now to do extensive analyses of very small tissue samples (Watson et al. 1996). It has never been more rewarding to collect and store leftover tissues from diagnostic and therapeutic procedures in biobanks (Oosterhuis et al. 2003). We are now beginning to diagnose and treat cancer by identifying markers and critical biological targets in tumors. Biobanks have recently played pivotal roles in identifying predictive biomarkers and in the development of diagnostic and prognostic tools that provide the basis for patient-specific treatments. Furthermore, storage of patient materials will permit analysis at a future time, when the response to treatment is known, thus allowing rapid assessment of new diagnostic or predictive tests (Morente et al. 2006; Riegman et al. 2006; van Veen et al. 2006; Mager et al. 2007; Rodrigues et al. 2009). But, unlike other research tools, biobanks incorporating human tissues and data invoke complex social, medical, and multidisciplinary issues (Oosterhuis et al. 2003; Patel et al. 2005; Elger and Caplan 2006; Cavusoglu et al. 2008).

The long-term research goal in childhood liver malignancies is to define better risk-based stratification systems and to find novel more efficacious and less toxic therapies. It is through translational research that we will gain the knowledge that will eventually lead to better approaches in therapy. With help from the SIOPEL Liver Tumour Storage Programme, it will be possible to examine molecular genetic changes in a large number of pediatric liver tumor patients and to discover relevant pathogenetic steps, molecular diagnostic and prognostic criteria, as well as targets for novel therapies.

References

Adam D (2002) Online tumour bank aims to offer ready route to tissues. Nature 416(6880):464

Adams V, Mobius-Winkler S et al (2009) Basic and translational research: from molecule, to mouse, to man. Eur J Cardiovasc Prev Rehabil 16(Suppl 1):S48–S52

Ali-Khan SE, Daar AS et al (2009) Whole genome scanning: resolving clinical diagnosis and management amidst complex data. Pediatr Res 66(4):357–363

Ambros PF, Ambros IM (2001) Pathology and biology guidelines for resectable and unresectable neuroblastic tumors and bone marrow examination guidelines. Med Pediatr Oncol 37(6):492–504

Anderer U, Nohren H et al (1998) Organization of the pediatric tumor cell bank of the society of pediatric oncology and hematology (GPOH). Klin Pädiatr 210(1):1–9

Arbab AS, Janic B et al (2009) In vivo cellular imaging for translational medical research. Curr Med Imaging Rev 5(1):19–38

Bauchet L, Rigau V et al (2007) French brain tumor data bank: methodology and first results on 10,000 cases. J Neurooncol 84(2):189–199

Brown J, Perilongo G et al (2000) Pretreatment prognostic factors for children with hepatoblastoma – results from the International Society of Paediatric Oncology (SIOP) study SIOPEL 1. Eur J Cancer 36(11):1418–1425

Cassidy PJ, Radda GK (2005) Molecular imaging perspectives. J R Soc Interface 2(3):133–144

Cavusoglu AC, Saydam S et al (2008) A pilot study for human tumor/DNA banking: returned more questions than answers. Med Oncol 25(4):471–473

Chadwick R, Berg K (2001) Solidarity and equity: new ethical frameworks for genetic databases. Nat Rev Genet 2(4): 318–321

Clements MO, Godfrey A et al (2006) Lentiviral manipulation of gene expression in human adult and embryonic stem cells. Tissue Eng 12(7):1741–1751

Clermont G, Auffray C et al (2009) Bridging the gap between systems biology and medicine. Genome Med 1(9):88

Elger BS, Caplan AL (2006) Consent and anonymization in research involving biobanks: differing terms and norms present serious barriers to an international framework. EMBO Rep 7(7):661–666

Everett M (2003) The social life of genes: privacy, property and the new genetics. Soc Sci Med 56(1):53–65

Fuchs J, Rydzynski J et al (2002) Pretreatment prognostic factors and treatment results in children with hepatoblastoma: a report from the German Cooperative Pediatric Liver Tumor Study HB 94. Cancer 95(1):172–182

Grotzer MA, Patti R et al (2000) Biological stability of RNA isolated from RNA*later* – treated brain tumor and neuroblastoma xenografts. Med Pediatr Oncol 34(6):438–442

Hawkins N, de Vries J et al (2009) Planning for translational research in genomics. Genome Med 1(9):87

Herpel E, Koleganova N et al (2008) Tissue bank of the National Center for Tumour Disease. An innovative platform for translational tumour. Pathologe 29(Suppl 2):204–209

Isaacs H Jr (2007) Fetal and neonatal hepatic tumors. J Pediatr Surg 42(11):1797–1803

Jewell SD, Srinivasan M et al (2002) Analysis of the molecular quality of human tissues: an experience from the cooperative human tissue network. Am J Clin Pathol 118(5):733–741

Kerr C (2003) UK launch "virtual" tumour bank to improve treatment research. Lancet Oncol 4(5):264

Klimecki WT, Futscher BW et al (1994) Effects of ethanol and paraformaldehyde on RNA yield and quality. Biotechniques 16:1021–1023

Lopez-Guerrero JA, Riegman PH et al (2006) TuBaFrost 4: access rules and incentives for a European tumour bank. Eur J Cancer 42(17):2924–2929

Mager SR, Oomen MH et al (2007) Standard operating procedure for the collection of fresh frozen tissue samples. Eur J Cancer 43(5):828–834

Morente MM, Mager R et al (2006) TuBaFrost 2: standardising tissue collection and quality control procedures for a European virtual frozen tissue bank network. Eur J Cancer 42(16):2684–2691

Oosterhuis JW, Coebergh JW et al (2003) Tumour banks: well-guarded treasures in the interest of patients. Nat Rev Cancer 3(1):73–77

Parham DM, Qualman SJ (2001) Submission of pathologic material for biologic research and testing – what are the issues? Med Pediatr Oncol 37(6):489–491

Patel AA, Kajdacsy-Balla A et al (2005) The development of common data elements for a multi-institute prostate cancer tissue bank: the cooperative prostate cancer tissue resource (CPCTR) experience. BMC Cancer 5:108

Payne PR, Embi PJ et al (2009) Translational informatics: enabling high throughput research paradigms. Physiol Genomics 39(3):131–140

Perilongo G, Shafford EA (1999) Liver tumours. Eur J Cancer 35:953–958

Qualman SJ, France M et al (2004) Establishing a tumour bank: banking, informatics and ethics. Br J Cancer 90(6):1115–1119

Riegman PH, Dinjens WN et al (2006) TuBaFrost 1: uniting local frozen tumour banks into a European network: an overview. Eur J Cancer 42(16):2678–2683

Rodrigues M, Vito I et al (2009) Establishment of a tumour bank: the experience of the department of pathology of hospital S. Joao (Porto, Portugal). Cell Tissue Bank 10(1):75–77

Spinney L (2003) UK launches tumor bank to match maligned Biobank. Nat Med 9(5):491

Takayasu H, Horie H et al (2001) Frequent deletions and mutations of the beta-catenin gene are associated with overexpression of cyclin D1 and fibronectin and poorly differentiated histology in childhood hepatoblastoma. Clin Cancer Res 7(4):901–908

van der Merwe DE, Oikonomopoulou K et al (2007) Mass spectrometry: uncovering the cancer proteome for diagnostics. Adv Cancer Res 96:23–50

van Veen EB, Riegman PH et al (2006) TuBaFrost 3: regulatory and ethical issues on the exchange of residual tissue for research across Europe. Eur J Cancer 42(17):2914–2923

von Schweinitz D, Kraus JA et al (2002) Prognostic impact of molecular genetic alterations in hepatoblastoma. Med Pediatr Oncol 38(2):104–108

Watson PH, Snell L et al (1996) The NCIC-Manitoba breast tumor bank: a resource for applied cancer research. Cmaj 155(3):281–283

Whyte B (2003) National tumor bank set up in United Kingdom. J Natl Cancer Inst 95(10):706

Yamada S, Ohira M et al (2004) Expression profiling and differential screening between hepatoblastomas and the corresponding normal livers: identification of high expression of the PLK1 oncogene as a poor-prognostic indicator of hepatoblastomas. Oncogene 23(35):5901–5911

Yamaoka H, Ohtsu K et al (2006) Diagnostic and prognostic impact of beta-catenin alterations in pediatric liver tumors. Oncol Rep 15(3):551–556

Clinical Presentation and Diagnosis

7

Laurence Brugières

Contents

Liver tumors are rare in children accounting for less than 2% of all childhood malignancies. Malignant tumors including hepatoblastomas (HB), hepatocellular carcinomas (HCC), rhabdoid tumors, and sarcomas account for the majority of malignant masses in children (Weinberg and Finegold 1983). A variety of benign tumors can also occur in this age group including benign vascular tumors, mesenchymal hamartomas, focal nodular hyperplasias, and adenomas (Fabre et al. 2004). The main elements for diagnosis are age at presentation, the clinical symptoms, the association with an underlying disease, the AFP level, and the radiological characteristics. In most cases, a biopsy is mandatory to confirm the diagnosis.

7.1 Malignant Liver Tumors

7.1.1 Age at Diagnosis

Most cases of HB occur in very young children. More than 80% of the patients are under the age of 2 at diagnosis (Horton et al. 2009). Occasionally, some cases can be diagnosed in neonates or even during the prenatal period. In the main series published in literature, the median age at diagnosis ranges between 12 and 21 months (von Schweinitz et al. 1997; Pritchard et al. 2000; Fuchs et al. 2002; Perilongo et al. 2004, 2009; Zsíros et al. 2010).

Apart from HB, infants and young children may also be diagnosed with a rhabdoid tumor or a rhabdomyosarcoma arising from the biliary ducts.

In older children and adolescents, the main malignant liver tumors are hepatocellular carcinoma and undifferentiated sarcoma of the liver. Hepatocellular

L. Brugières
Dépt. de Pédiatrie, Service d' Oncologie Pédiatrique, Institut Gustave Roussy, 11, Rue Camille Desmoulins, 94805 Villejuif, France
e-mail: Brugieres@igr.fr

A. Zimmermann et al. (eds.), *Pediatric Liver Tumors*, Pediatric Oncology,
DOI: 10.1007/978-3-642-14504-9_7, © Springer-Verlag Berlin Heidelberg 2011

carcinomas (HCC) in this age group are a heterogeneous group of tumors comprising transitional liver tumors with features of both HB and HCC (Prokurat et al. 2002b), hepatocellular carcinomas developing on an underlying liver disease, and fibrolamellar carcinomas (Katzenstein et al. 2003). The median age at diagnosis for HCC is 12 years in the SIOPEL1 series (Czauderna 2002) but HCC has also been described in young children under 5 (Czauderna et al. 2002; Katzenstein et al. 2002).

7.1.2 Clinical Symptoms

Most hepatoblastomas are asymptomatic and the presenting symptom is usually abdominal distension or an abdominal mass discovered either by a parent or a physician. In some patients, the volume of the tumor may induce abdominal pain and/or anorexia. These symptoms are more frequent in HCC than in HB (Exelby et al. 1975). A few patients present with acute abdominal symptoms due to tumor rupture or intra-abdominal hemorrhage (Chan et al. 2002). Jaundice is a rare symptom associated with extensive disease and compression of the major bile duct. It is rare in HB or HCC but commonly present in rhabdomyosarcoma of the biliary tract (Sanz et al. 1997).

In a few patients with HB, early puberty may be the initial symptom in tumors associated with Human Chorionic Gonadotrophin (HCG) production (Navarro et al. 1985).

Generalized osteoporosis has been described in association with HB and may lead to multiple factures (Lack et al. 1982).

Whereas most HCC occur as a complication of an underlying liver disease in adults, the incidence of childhood HCC associated with chronic liver disease is lower in western countries. In the series published by the SIOPEL group (Czauderna et al. 2002), only 15/40 patients (37%) had an underlying liver disease (13 chronic hepatitis B, 1 case of tyrosinemia, and 1 of biliary cirrhosis). On the contrary, the rate of seropositivity for HB antigens is very high in Asia because of endemic viral hepatitis in that part of the world (Ni et al. 1991). However, the introduction of neonatal hepatitis B vaccination has changed the epidemiology of this tumor. In Taiwan, it has resulted in a dramatic decrease in the incidence of HCC in children (Chang et al. 2005). Besides viral hepatitis, other risk factors for HCC in children include tyrosinemia (McKiernan 2006), Byler's disease (Jensen and Gluud 1994), metabolic diseases or Alagille syndrome (Fabre et al. 2004). In these cases, HCC may be diagnosed by systematic screening combining AFP determination and ultrasonography (Sherman 2010; Wiwanitkit 2005). These screening tests allow the detection of early tumors before the occurrence of clinical manifestations.

7.1.3 Laboratory Investigations

Liver function tests are normal in most patients with HB but may be abnormal in patients with HCC according to the underlying liver disease or to bile duct compression by the tumor.

Thrombocytosis with a platelet level exceeding 500/mL is present in 50–60% of the patients with HB at diagnosis (Pritchard et al. 2000) and is related to hyperproduction of thrombopoietin by tumor cells (Komura-Naito et al. 1997).

The main tool for the diagnosis of liver tumors in children is serum determination of AFP, which is high in more than 90% of the patients with HB and 70% of patients with HCC (Exelby et al. 1975). At the diagnosis, median AFP levels are over 10^4 ng/mL in most series of HB (von Schweinitz et al. 1997; Pritchard et al. 2000; Fuchs et al. 2002; Perilongo et al. 2004, 2009; Zsíros et al. 2010).

Elevation of this biological marker is an important argument in favor of the diagnosis of a malignant liver tumor. However, AFP elevation is not specific. Several other situations may be associated with an elevated AFP level and may lead to errors in the diagnosis in the absence of a biopsy.

At birth, the AFP level is very high and decreases throughout the first months of life (Table 7.1; Blohm et al. 1998). Consequently, in children, younger than 1 year, it may be difficult to distinguish physiological secretion of AFP from a high level due to AFP secreted by a malignant tumor. It may be helpful to have two AFP determinations several days apart. A spontaneous decline in the AFP level without any treatment is a good argument in favor of the physiological origin of the secretion of AFP.

An elevated AFP level may be associated with several other tumor types including germ cell tumors and other liver tumors such as mesenchymal hamartomas (Boman et al. 2004) and infantile hemangioendothelioma (Kim et al. 2010). Other conditions such as viral hepatitis (Alpert and Seeler 1970) or tyrosinemia (Holme and Lindstedt 1995) may also be associated with a high AFP level. In these situations, the AFP level is usually not as high as in HB. Lastly, some patients have a hereditary persistence of high AFP levels (Schefer et al. 1998).

Table 7.1 Alpha fetoprotein value references in infants (Blohm et al. 1998)

Age (days)	AFP mean (ng/mL)	AFP 95.5% interval (ng/mL)
0	41,687	9,120–190,546
1	36,391	7,943–165,959
2	31,769	6,950–144,544
3	27,733	6,026–125,893
4	24,210	5,297–109,648
5	21,135	4,624–96,605
6	18,450	4,037–84,334
7	16,107	3,524–73,621
8–14	9,333	1,480–58,887
15–21	3,631	575–22,910
22–28	1,396	316–6,310
29–45	417	30–5,754
46–60	178	16–1,995
61–90	80	6–1,045
91–120	36	3–417
121–150	20	2–216
151–180	13	1.25–129
181–720	8	0.8–87

The presence of extremely high serum AFP concentration in some patients can generate erroneously low AFP results. This effect named the "Hook effect" is a well-recognized problem that can occur in assays of most tumor markers, including AFP (Jassam et al. 2006). This finding is due to the possibility of calculation errors especially when the AFP level is very high and requires appropriate serum dilution for a reliable assessment.

In children with a normal AFP level, several diagnoses should be considered depending on their age and the clinico-radiological presentation: in infants, the rare HBs with a low AFP level (De Ioris et al. 2008), which account for only 2% of all patients enrolled in the SIOPEL 1 to 3 or rhabdoid tumors (Russo and Biegel 2009), in older children, HCC including fibrolamellar carcinomas (Katzenstein et al. 2003) and sarcomas (Bisogno et al. 2002) (Table 7.2). HBs with a normal AFP level at diagnosis are very rare and have quite different characteristics from those of the classic HB population: a young age at diagnosis, tumor multifocality, widespread extrahepatic extension, undifferentiated small cell histology, poor response to chemotherapy, and finally a worse outcome (De Ioris et al. 2008).

In patients with a fibrolamellar carcinoma, the AFP level is normal but a high serum vitamin B12 binding

Table 7.2 Liver tumors in children: diagnosis according to age and AFP level

Age	AFP level normal for age	AFP level between 10 and 10^4 ng/mL (or slightly above normal for age)	AFP > 10^4ng/mL
0–3 years	Rhabdoid tumor Biliary tree rhabdomyosarcoma Hemangioma Mesenchymal hamartoma	Hemangioma Mesenchymal hamartoma Hepatoblastoma	Hepatoblastoma
3–10 years	Biliary tree rhabdomyosarcoma Undifferentiated sarcoma of the liver Mesenchymal hamartoma Rhabdoid tumors	Mesenchymal hamartoma	Hepatoblastoma Transitional liver tumor Hepatocellular carcinoma
10–15 years	Fibrolamellar carcinoma Undifferentiated sarcoma of the liver Nodular focal hyperplasia Adenoma	Transitional liver tumors Hepatocellular carcinomas	Transitional liver tumors Hepatocellular carcinomas

capacity (transcobalamin) has been demonstrated and may be used as a tumor marker (Paradinas et al. 1982).

7.1.4 Imaging

In a child with a suspected hepatic tumor, radiologic assessment often begins with ultrasonography aimed at assessing the presence of a tumor and confirming its intrahepatic location and characteristics. Radiological assessment also aims to rule out the diagnosis of secondary liver tumors, mainly liver metastases from neuroblastomas or germ-cell tumors and hepatic lymphomas.

The majority of primary malignant hepatic tumors are solid masses with increased echogenicity. Computed tomography (CT scan) and/or magnetic resonance imaging (MRI) are mandatory to better define the site and extent of the tumor, to detect major vessel (portal and hepatic veins) involvement, and to evaluate tumor resectability. The characteristics of the mass (unifocal or multifocal), its association with extrahepatic disease, and the presence of signs of rupture should be carefully assessed.

Metastases are detected in around 20% of the cases at diagnosis, mostly in the lung. Therefore, a chest CT is mandatory at diagnosis. The other sites of metastasis (bone, brain) are very rare and have been reported mainly in infants.

In a child with a normal AFP level, some radiological features may suggest the diagnosis of sarcoma. Tumors arising in the bile duct and associated with biliary duct distension suggest the diagnosis of rhabdomysosarcoma of the biliary tree (Roebuck et al. 1998). Undifferentiated sarcoma of the liver may be associated with a large hepatic lesion that has a seemingly cystic appearance on CT and MR images and a largely solid appearance on ultrasound (Crider et al. 2009).

7.1.5 Biopsy

Even though elevated AFP in a child with unquestionable imaging of a liver tumor is very suggestive of HB or HCC, a biopsy of the tumor mass is highly recommended in order to have histological confirmation of the diagnosis in patients treated with preoperative chemotherapy. The only contraindication to a biopsy is the presence of subcapsular rupture of the tumor.

The method preferred is percutaneous ultrasound-guided needle biopsy. The aim of the biopsy is to obtain sufficient tissue to enable an accurate diagnosis, while avoiding complications. The biopsy should be performed via a short depth of healthy hepatic parenchyma in order to minimize the risk of tumor seeding. The most important potential immediate complication is hemorrhage. In the SIOPEL 1 and 2 studies, no life-threatening biopsy complications were recorded among 96 cases in which a biopsy was performed. Complications were reported in 7% of cases (7/96) and were generally minor: bleeding from the biopsy site in 4 patients, abdominal pain in 2, and a wound infection in a patient with an open biopsy.

In patients with a high AFP level, the main aim of the biopsy is to make the differential diagnosis between HB and hepatocarcinoma. This differential diagnosis may be difficult in patients without underlying liver disease and in such cases the diagnosis of a transitional liver tumor has been proposed (Prokurat et al. 2002b). In patients with a normal AFP level, the main diagnoses to be discussed are primary liver sarcoma, malignant rhabdoid tumor, and fibrolamellar carcinomas. The definition of a rhabdoid tumor classically relies on a characteristic morphology and loss of hSNF5/INI1 tumor suppressor gene expression (Russo and Biegel 2009). In cases lacking the typical histological features, the loss of expression of the INI1 gene product is an essential diagnostic tool.

7.2 Benign Tumors

7.2.1 Vascular Tumors

Hemangioma is the most frequent benign liver tumor in children and commonly occurs during the first 6 months of life. Most hemangiomas are asymptomatic and are discovered serendipitously (Prokurat et al. 2002a). They may be associated with cutaneous hemangiomas. Infantile hemangioendothelioma is a subtype of hemangioma occurring in infants, which may be complicated by cardiac failure and/or coagulopathy with thrombocytopenia (Kasabach–Meritt syndrome). CT scan reveals the typical feature of peripheral contrast enhancement with subsequent filling of the lesion and the liver.

7.2.2 Mesenchymal Hamartomas

Mesenchymal hamartomas are rare tumors often revealed by abdominal distension during the first 2 years of life. Some patients may be diagnosed before birth by an antenatal ultrasound. The vast majority involve the right side of the liver and are almost always solitary lesions. The radiological appearance is characterized by a well-circumscribed multilocular cystic mass with solid septae. They may be associated with a high AFP level, which may mimic HB (Boman et al. 2004). A biopsy is recommended in cases with a solid component in order to rule out a malignant tumor.

7.2.3 Focal Nodular Hyperplasia

Focal nodular hyperplasia is rarely diagnosed in children. Most cases of focal nodular hyperplasia are discovered serendipitously (Fabre et al. 2004). Contrast enhancement on CT scan or MRI is characterized by an early intense contrast-enhanced homogeneous lesion that becomes isodense with the normal liver on delayed images. A characteristic central scar is pathognomonic but is present in only 50% of the cases (Okada et al. 2006).

7.2.4 Adenoma

Adenomas are rare in children and most often asymptomatic. They may be associated with glycogen storage disease or androgen therapy (Fabre et al. 2004). They can also demonstrate early enhancement but have a tendency to bleed and thus appear more heterogeneous than focal nodular hyperplasia.

7.3 Conclusion

The diagnosis of liver tumors can be suspected in the majority of the cases based on the child's age, clinical information, biological data (in particular the AFP level), and radiological characteristics. However, a biopsy is now considered mandatory before any chemotherapy in children with a liver tumor.

References

Alpert ME, Seeler RA (1970) Alpha fetoprotein in embryonal hepatoblastoma. J Pediatr 77(6):1058–1060

Bisogno G, Pilz T et al (2002) Undifferentiated sarcoma of the liver in childhood: a curable disease. Cancer 94(1):252–257

Blohm ME, Vesterling-Horner D et al (1998) Alpha 1-fetoprotein (AFP) reference values in infants up to 2 years of age. Pediatr Hematol Oncol 15(2):135–142

Boman F, Bossard C et al (2004) Mesenchymal hamartomas of the liver may be associated with increased serum alpha foetoprotein concentrations and mimic hepatoblastomas. Eur J Pediatr Surg 14(1):63–66

Chan KL, Fan ST et al (2002) Management of spontaneously ruptured hepatoblastoma in infancy. Med Pediatr Oncol 38(2):137–138

Chang MH, Chen TH et al (2005) Prevention of hepatocellular carcinoma by universal vaccination against hepatitis B virus: the effect and problems. Clin Cancer Res 11(21): 7953–7957

Crider MH, Hoggard E et al (2009) Undifferentiated (embryonal) sarcoma of the liver. Radiographics 29(6):1665–1668

Czauderna P (2002) Adult type vs. childhood hepatocellular carcinoma – are they the same or different lesions? Biology, natural history, prognosis, and treatment. Med Pediatr Oncol 39(5):519–523

Czauderna P, Mackinlay G et al (2002) Hepatocellular carcinoma in children: results of the first prospective study of the International Society of Pediatric Oncology group. J Clin Oncol 20(12):2798–2804

De Ioris M, Brugieres L et al (2008) Hepatoblastoma with a low serum alpha-fetoprotein level at diagnosis: the SIOPEL group experience. Eur J Cancer 44(4):545–550

Exelby PR, Filler RM et al (1975) Liver tumors in children in the particular reference to hepatoblastoma and hepatocellular carcinoma: American Academy of Pediatrics Surgical Section Survey – 1974. J Pediatr Surg 10(3):329–337

Fabre M, Yilmaz F et al (2004) Hepatic tumors in childhood: experience on 245 tumors and review of literature. Ann Pathol 24(6):536–555

Fuchs J, Rydzynski J et al (2002) Pretreatment prognostic factors and treatment results in children with hepatoblastoma: a report from the German Cooperative Pediatric Liver Tumor Study HB 94. Cancer 95(1):172–182

Holme E, Lindstedt S (1995) Diagnosis and management of tyrosinemia type I. Curr Opin Pediatr 7(6):726–732

Horton JD, Lee S et al (2009) Survival trends in children with hepatoblastoma. Pediatr Surg Int 25(5):407–412

Jassam N, Jones CM et al (2006) The hook effect: a need for constant vigilance. Ann Clin Biochem 43(Pt 4):314–317

Jensen K, Gluud C (1994) The Mallory body: morphological, clinical and experimental studies (Part 1 of a literature survey). Hepatology 20(4 Pt 1):1061–1077

Katzenstein HM, Krailo MD et al (2002) Hepatocellular carcinoma in children and adolescents: results from the Pediatric Oncology Group and the Children's Cancer Group intergroup study. J Clin Oncol 20(12):2789–2797

Katzenstein HM, Krailo MD et al (2003) Fibrolamellar hepatocellular carcinoma in children and adolescents. Cancer 97(8):2006–2012

Kim TJ, Lee YS et al (2010) Infantile hemangioendothelioma with elevated serum alpha fetoprotein: report of 2 cases with immunohistochemical analysis. Hum Pathol 41(5):763–767

Komura-Naito E, Matsumura T et al (1997) Thrombopoietin in patients with hepatoblastoma. Blood 90(7):2849–2850

Lack EE, Neave C et al (1982) Hepatoblastoma. A clinical and pathologic study of 54 cases. Am J Surg Pathol 6(8): 693–705

McKiernan PJ (2006) Nitisinone in the treatment of hereditary tyrosinaemia type 1. Drugs 66(6):743–750

Navarro C, Corretger JM et al (1985) Paraneoplasic precocious puberty. Report of a new case with hepatoblastoma and review of the literature. Cancer 56(7):1725–1729

Ni YH, Chang MH et al (1991) Hepatocellular carcinoma in childhood. Clinical manifestations and prognosis. Cancer 68(8):1737–1741

Okada T, Sasaki F et al (2006) Management and algorithm for focal nodular hyperplasia of the liver in children. Eur J Pediatr Surg 16(4):235–240

Paradinas FJ, Melia WM et al (1982) High serum vitamin B12 binding capacity as a marker of the fibrolamellar variant of hepatocellular carcinoma. Br Med J (Clin Res Ed) 285(6345): 840–842

Perilongo G, Shafford E et al (2004) Risk-adapted treatment for childhood hepatoblastoma. Final report of the second study of the International Society of Paediatric Oncology – SIOPEL 2. Eur J Cancer 40(3):411–421

Perilongo G, Maibach R et al (2009) Cisplatin versus cisplatin plus doxorubicin for standard-risk hepatoblastoma. N Engl J Med 361(17):1662–1670

Pritchard J, Brown J et al (2000) Cisplatin, doxorubicin, and delayed surgery for childhood hepatoblastoma: a successful approach – results of the first prospective study of the International Society of Pediatric Oncology. J Clin Oncol 18(22):3819–3828

Prokurat A, Kluge P et al (2002a) Hemangioma of the liver in children: proliferating vascular tumor or congenital vascular malformation? Med Pediatr Oncol 39(5):524–529

Prokurat A, Kluge P et al (2002b) Transitional liver cell tumors (TLCT) in older children and adolescents: a novel group of aggressive hepatic tumors expressing beta-catenin. Med Pediatr Oncol 39(5):510–518

Roebuck DJ, Yang WT et al (1998) Hepatobiliary rhabdomyosarcoma in children: diagnostic radiology. Pediatr Radiol 28(2):101–108

Russo P, Biegel JA (2009) SMARCB1/INI1 alterations and hepatoblastoma: another extrarenal rhabdoid tumor revealed? Pediatr Blood Cancer 52(3):312–313

Sanz N, de Mingo L et al (1997) Rhabdomyosarcoma of the biliary tree. Pediatr Surg Int 12(2/3):200–201

Schefer H, Mattmann S et al (1998) Hereditary persistence of alpha-fetoprotein. Case report and review of the literature. Ann Oncol 9(6):667–672

Sherman M (2010) Hepatocellular carcinoma: epidemiology, surveillance, and diagnosis. Semin Liver Dis 30(1):3–16

von Schweinitz D, Byrd DJ et al (1997) Efficiency and toxicity of ifosfamide, cisplatin and doxorubicin in the treatment of childhood hepatoblastoma. Study Committee of the Cooperative Paediatric Liver Tumour Study HB89 of the German Society for Paediatric Oncology and Haematology. Eur J Cancer 33(8):1243–1249

Weinberg AG, Finegold MJ (1983) Primary hepatic tumors of childhood. Hum Pathol 14(6):512–537

Wiwanitkit V (2005) Hepatitis virus B is not a risk factor in hepatoblastoma patients. Asian Pac J Cancer Prev 6(2):213–214

Zsíros J, Maibach R et al (2010). Successful treatment of childhood high risk hepatoblastoma with dose intensive multiagent chemotherapy and surgery – final results of the SIOPEL-3HR study of the international childhood Liver tumors strategy group (SIOPEL) J Clin Oncol 28(15):2584–2590

Imaging and Staging of Pediatric Liver Tumors

8

Derek J. Roebuck

Contents

D.J. Roebuck
Department of Radiology, Great Ormond Street Hospital, NHS Trust and Institute of Child Health, Great Ormond Street, London, WC1N 3JH, United Kingdom
e-mail: roebud@gosh.nhs.uk

8.1 Imaging Techniques

Technology has advanced rapidly and continues to evolve, so any imaging guidelines must be regarded as temporary. The roles of imaging are listed in Table 8.1.

Nearly all children with malignant primary liver tumors present with an abdominal mass. A few patients have different presentations, such as abdominal bleeding.

Imaging of children with suspected liver tumors is best performed by radiologists with an interest and experience in pediatric oncology. Magnetic resonance imaging (MRI) and, to a lesser extent, computed tomography (CT) may require sedation or anesthesia in younger children. Centers familiar with pediatric oncology imaging have protocols for this, and practice varies widely between institutions. High quality studies must be obtained, because staging (and therefore treatment) is often dependent on subtle imaging findings.

8.1.1 Ultrasound (US)

This is almost always the best first technique for evaluation of a suspected abdominal mass. It should be used in all patients, because it is widely available, harmless, and can show abnormalities not detectable with other techniques.

In most liver tumors, the hepatic origin of the mass can be confirmed without difficulty (Fig. 8.1). When there is uncertainty, the pattern of movement of the mass with respiration may be diagnostic (Roebuck 2008). Assessment of the blood supply of the tumor with color Doppler US may also be helpful (Roebuck 2008).

A. Zimmermann et al. (eds.), *Pediatric Liver Tumors*, Pediatric Oncology,
DOI: 10.1007/978-3-642-14504-9_8, © Springer-Verlag Berlin Heidelberg 2011

Table 8.1 Imaging in children with suspected primary liver tumors

Confirmation of hepatic origin of the lesion
Characterization of the lesion
Differential diagnosis Is biopsy required? If so, what is the best technique for biopsy?
Staging Local disease (extent in the liver) Regional disease Metastatic disease

US is particularly useful for evaluation of the vascular anatomy of the liver and may be the best single technique for the detection of minor venous invasion (Roebuck et al. 2006; Sato et al. 2000; Ohtsuka et al. 1997). Because it is well tolerated by children and does not require sedation or ionizing radiation, US can be repeated as often as necessary, and a second examination may be helpful to resolve any uncertainties that remain after other imaging has been completed (Roebuck et al. 2006).

The overall extent and size of the tumor and the deeper parts of the portal and hepatic venous systems

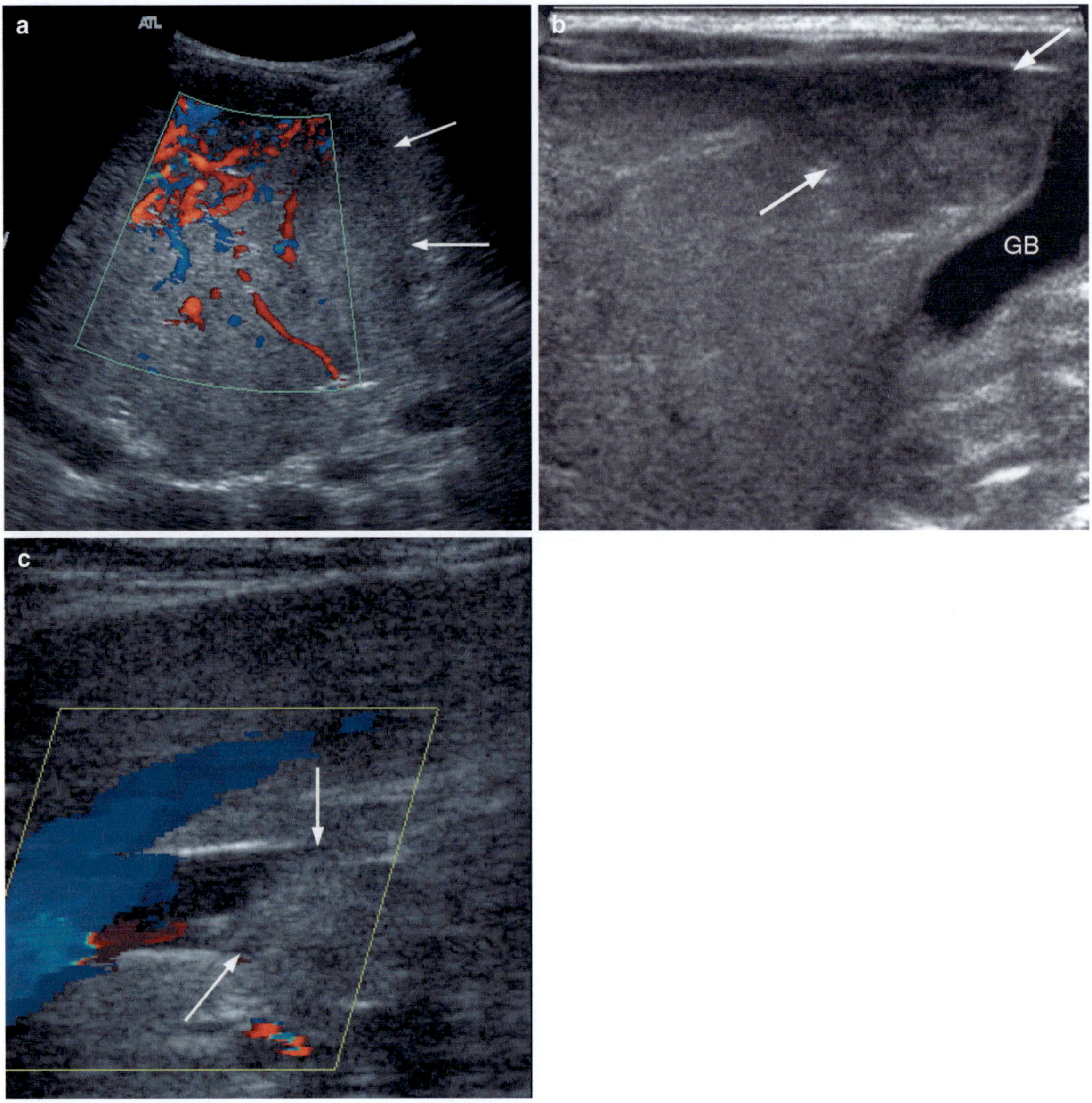

are best assessed using a relatively low frequency sector or curvilinear array transducer (Fig. 8.1a; Roebuck et al. 2006). The vessels can often be visualized at higher resolution with a high frequency (>7 MHz) linear array transducer, which is also the best way to identify and measure small tumor nodules (Fig. 8.1b and c; Roebuck et al. 2006).

8.1.2 Computed tomography (CT)

CT is essential for evaluation of the lungs (Fig. 8.2), and may also be used instead of or in addition to magnetic resonance imaging for the abdomen and pelvis. Sedation or general anesthesia (GA) is sometimes required in younger children, although this is increasingly uncommon with faster scanning times (McCarville and Kao 2006).

Because metastases often occur in the lung bases, it is important to image this area well. Unfortunately, both sedation and GA commonly cause basal lung collapse (atelectasis), and this may be aggravated by the presence of a large abdominal mass. Certain techniques may overcome this problem to some extent. Collapse can be prevented by using a gas mixture rich in nitrogen at induction, and continuing to use an inspired fraction of oxygen (F_iO_2) of only 0.3–0.4 with positive end-expiratory pressure during scanning (Hedenstierna and Rothen 2000). Additional maneuvers, such as forced expansion of the lungs at high pressure for 7–8s, may also be helpful (Hedenstierna and Rothen 2000). When basal collapse is present despite these measures, CT can be repeated with the patient in the prone position if necessary (Roebuck et al. 2006).

Although the development of multidetector CT (MDCT) systems has led to an important improvement in image quality, meticulous attention to detail is still required (Fig. 8.2b and c). The exact technique used will depend on the scanner, but in general a collimation of 0.6–1.25 mm and pitch of 0.9–1.25 should be applied. A reconstruction interval of 3 mm is optimal for detection of 5-mm metastases, but this may need to be reduced when the detection of smaller lesions is important (Fig. 8.2c). Dynamic tube current adjustment and age-appropriate tube voltage should be used to minimize radiation dose (Roebuck et al. 2006).

Images are constructed from chest CT data using soft tissue and lung algorithms, and reviewed using appropriate window widths and levels. The conspicuity of lung nodules may be improved by using maximum intensity projection (MIP) sliding thin-slab reconstructions (Napel et al. 1993; Kawel et al. 2009).

Intravenous nonionic iodinated contrast is always given when the abdomen is imaged, but oral contrast is optional (Roebuck et al. 2006). An injection pump gives the best results because the timing of the scan relative to the injection of the contrast bolus is crucial (Roebuck et al. 2006). It is usual to inject 2 mL/kg of nonionic contrast (with an iodine content of 300 mg/mL) at a rate of 1.2–3 mL/s, depending on the size of the child and the intravenous cannula. Early images (20–30 s after the start of the contrast injection in most children) show the hepatic arterial supply to the liver well, and may be useful for the detection of small hypervascular lesions, for example, in hepatocellular carcinoma or metastatic disease (McCarville and Kao 2006). Images in the portal phase (about 60 s) usually maximize the conspicuity of the margins of primary tumors, and are best for assessment of portal venous involvement. The hepatic veins opacify with contrast almost simultaneously with the portal veins, so in practice both sets of vessels may be enhanced on the same image. If only one scan is performed, it should be done in the portal venous phase. In adults, images are routinely acquired in two or more phases, but this is not a popular practice in pediatric radiology because of concerns about radiation risk. In theory, the detection of tumoral calcification would be optimal on noncontrast images, but in practice these are almost never useful. The entire abdomen and pelvis should be examined, to assess for peritoneal tumor spread.

Fig. 8.1 Use of ultrasound for the evaluation of pediatric liver tumors. (**a**) A low frequency sector transducer is useful to show the overall size of the mass in this 2-year-old male with hepatocellular carcinoma. The interface between the tumor and normal liver (arrows) is not well seen, but color Doppler imaging shows the typical disorganized tumor vasculature. (**b**) A high frequency linear array transducer is better for the detection of smaller lesions. Here a small tumor (arrows) is identified in the gallbladder (GB) fossa in a female infant with PRETEXT IV F1 hepatoblastoma. (**c**) Vascular invasion (arrows) is shown with a high frequency linear array transducer and color Doppler imaging

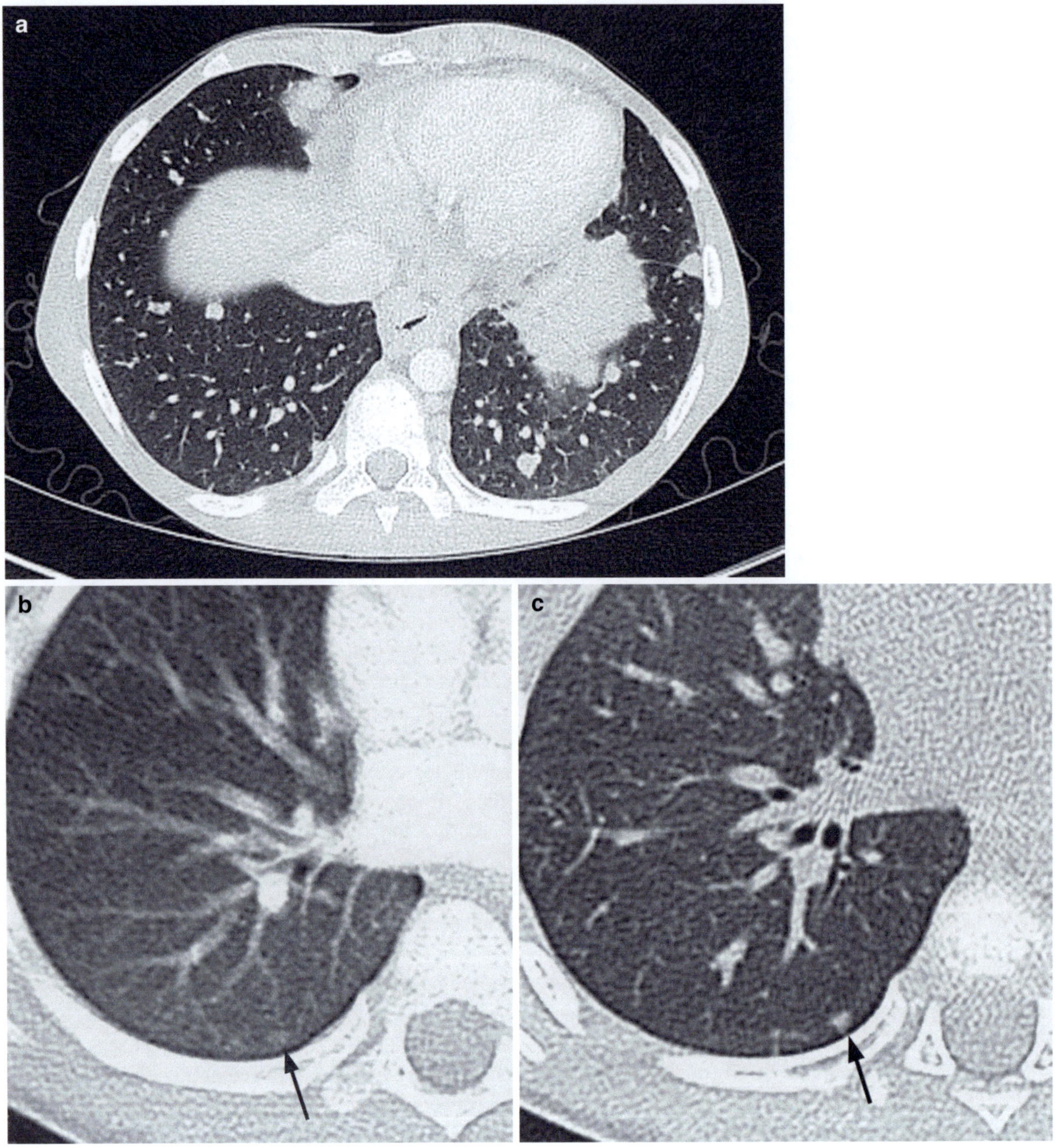

Fig. 8.2 Computed tomography of the lungs. (**a**) Typical appearances of multiple lung metastases in an 11-year-old male with fibrolamellar carcinoma. (**b**) Multidetector CT data reconstructed as 5-mm slices in a 5-year-old male. There is an almost imperceptible 3-mm lesion in the superior segment of the right lower lobe (arrow). (**c**) The same patient was rescanned in the prone position, and images were reconstructed at 1 mm slice thickness. The nodule (arrow) is much more obvious

The optimal reconstruction interval for detection of small liver lesions is a trade-off between contrast-to-noise ratio and partial volume averaging, which impair detection of lesions at smaller and larger intervals respectively. In general, a reconstruction interval of 5 mm is probably best (Soo et al. 2010).

MDCT technology generates a three-dimensional dataset with approximately isotropic voxels (i.e., the spatial resolution is the same along all three axes). These data can be manipulated on a workstation to present slices in any plane (multiplanar reconstruction, MPR) or generate 3D-like images (volume rendering techniques, VRT). MPR may be helpful, especially to assess the relationship of the tumor to vascular structures. VRT images are often very elegant (Dong et al. 2007), but are not routinely used in clinical practice. MIP images may be used to demonstrate hepatic and portal venous structures (Catalano et al. 2008), but should not be interpreted in isolation as they tend to misrepresent spatial relationships. Recent developments in segmentation software allow depiction of the true segmental liver anatomy, based on the portal venous branching pattern (Fuchs et al. 2005).

All CT studies should be reviewed using bone windows, especially in children with suspected hepatocellular carcinoma.

8.1.3 Magnetic Resonance Imaging (MRI)

The proliferation of MRI sequences means that only a selection can be performed in each patient. Although the sequences could be selected on an individual patient basis, it is more usual to use a standard protocol. Unfortunately, there are at least as many protocols as there are children's hospitals. In general, only broad guidelines are given in published recommendations (Roebuck et al. 2006; McCarville and Kao 2006; Roebuck 2009; Albuquerque et al. 2009; Siegel et al. 2008).

A flexible phased-array body coil can be used in older children, but in infants it is better to use an adult head coil (Roebuck et al. 2006; Siegel et al. 2008). Sequences obtained with breath-holding, either in cooperative older patients or under GA, give the best images (Vasanawala et al. 2010). When breath-holding is not feasible, respiratory triggering (Roebuck et al. 2006) or navigator pulses (Vasanawala et al. 2010) can be used. Both techniques prolong scan time.

It is conventional to obtain unenhanced T1-weighted images (spin echo or gradient echo) in transverse and coronal planes. Corresponding fast spin echo T2-weighted sequences are usually fat suppressed (Albuquerque et al. 2009; Siegel et al. 2008; Vasanawala 2010). Volumetric acquisition of T2-weighted images (variously known as FSE XETA, T2-SPACE, and VISTA) is also possible (Vasanawala 2010). In-phase and out-of-phase low flip angle T1-weighted gradient-echo images can identify lipid in tumors, but are not routinely used (Siegel et al. 2008). Recently, diffusion-weighted MRI (DWI) has been used to evaluate pediatric tumors (Humphries et al. 2007). Although DWI does not discriminate perfectly between benign and malignant masses, it can potentially be used to decide which part of a lesion is the best to biopsy, as regions with restricted diffusion of water molecules tend to be more cellular.

Conventional intravenous MRI contrast agents (gadolinium chelates) are used routinely. Post-contrast images are usually acquired using dynamic spoiled gradient echo (FLASH, SPGR, and T1-FFE) or balanced steady-state free precession (TrueFISP, FIESTA, b-FFE) techniques (Roebuck et al. 2006; Albuquerque et al. 2009; Siegel et al. 2008; Vasanawala 2010). Because these sequences are very rapid, they can be used to construct angiogram-like images of the arterial and venous anatomy of the liver.

Although liver specific (reticuloendothelial or hepatocellular) contrast agents are rarely used in children, there may be a role for superparamagnetic iron oxide agents in the diagnosis of focal nodular hyperplasia and the detection of small satellite lesions in children with malignant tumors.

8.1.4 Nuclear Medicine

Bone metastases are extremely rare at diagnosis in hepatoblastoma, and bone scintigraphy is not routinely performed because of the high prevalence of false-positive findings, probably related to abnormal calcium metabolism (Roebuck et al. 2006). Bone scintigraphy is, however, appropriate for staging in children with hepatocellular carcinoma.

Although positron emission tomography (PET) can, in principle, be used to detect hepatoblastoma (Figarola et al. 2005), its clinical role is yet to be defined (McCarville and Kao 2006).

8.1.5 Obsolete Imaging Techniques

Plain film radiography and sulfur colloid scintigraphy are now obsolete in the evaluation of children with liver masses. Catheter angiography is now only used as the basis of some therapeutic procedures (Chap. 13).

8.2 Approach to Differential Diagnosis

Nearly all solid liver masses in children are neoplastic, but many, especially in infancy, are benign (Table 8.2). Clinical, laboratory, and imaging information can be combined to construct a differential diagnosis for each patient. Clinical clues include relevant history (e.g., family history, known predisposing conditions) and examination findings (e.g., multiple cutaneous hemangiomas, pyrexia). Laboratory findings such as platelet count and hepatitis serology may also be helpful. The contribution of imaging at this stage is to identify lesions, such as vascular tumors and mesenchymal hamartoma, where biopsy may not be necessary to direct treatment. Imaging alone is not useful in making a precise diagnosis of malignant tumor type.

8.2.1 Benign Tumors

The most important benign neoplasms are the vascular tumors of infancy, each of which may also occur elsewhere in the body. The literature on this subject is confusing, and many authorities do not make all the clinically important distinctions. Infantile hemangioma (Fig. 8.3a) is relatively common, and almost always multifocal or diffuse. Biopsy is almost never required, and the only important differential diagnosis is metastatic neuroblastoma. MRI and CT both show a characteristic pattern of nodular, progressive, and almost complete centripetal contrast enhancement. Infantile hemangioma regresses after a period of growth in the first year of life. Unfortunately, a small number of children originally diagnosed with hemangioma subsequently go on to develop angiosarcoma, and prolonged imaging follow-up is therefore appropriate to confirm resolution.

Table 8.2 Large solid liver lesions, by age group (Modified from Roebuck [2008])

Neonates and infants
Infantile hemangioma
Rapidly involuting congenital hemangioma (RICH)
(Cystic) mesenchymal hamartoma
Hepatoblastoma
Rhabdoid tumor
Metastases (especially in neuroblastoma)
Young children (1–10 years)
Hepatoblastoma
Transitional liver cell tumor
Undifferentiated (embryonal) sarcoma
Non-Hodgkin lymphoma
Biliary rhabdomyosarcoma
Angiosarcoma
Metastases
Adolescents (10 years and older)
Transitional liver cell tumor
Fibrolamellar carcinoma
Hepatocellular carcinoma
Hepatic adenoma
Undifferentiated (embryonal) sarcoma
Epithelioid hemangioendothelioma
Non-Hodgkin lymphoma
Metastases

The second most important vascular tumor is rapidly involuting congenital hemangioma (RICH). RICH almost always presents as a solitary mass with peripheral enhancement and relatively low attenuation centrally on CT (Fig. 8.3b). It does not appear to be associated with angiosarcoma. The other benign vascular neoplasms of infancy, non-involuting congenital hemangioma and kaposiform hemangioendothelioma, rarely occur in the liver.

Mesenchymal hamartoma (Fig. 8.3c) shows a variety of imaging appearances, reflecting the highly variable mix of cystic and solid elements (Kim et al. 2007). Focal nodular hyperplasia (FNH, Fig. 8.3d) has an inconstant imaging appearance in children, and is sometimes difficult to diagnose without biopsy (Cheon et al. 1998). The use of superparamagnetic iron oxide MRI contrast agents is a promising method for the diagnosis of FNH (Okada et al. 2005).

8.2.2 Malignant Tumors

The distinction between primary and secondary liver tumors is usually not a problem in children. With the exception of neuroblastoma (Fig. 8.4a), hepatic metastatic disease from an unknown primary tumor is extremely rare.

The relatively common primary liver tumors (hepatoblastoma and hepatocellular carcinoma) have no characteristic imaging features. In each of these diseases large size and/or multifocality, calcification, and vascular invasion are all fairly common. Certain unusual appearances at CT or MRI may suggest the diagnosis of rare malignancies. Undifferentiated (embryonal) sarcoma often presents as a

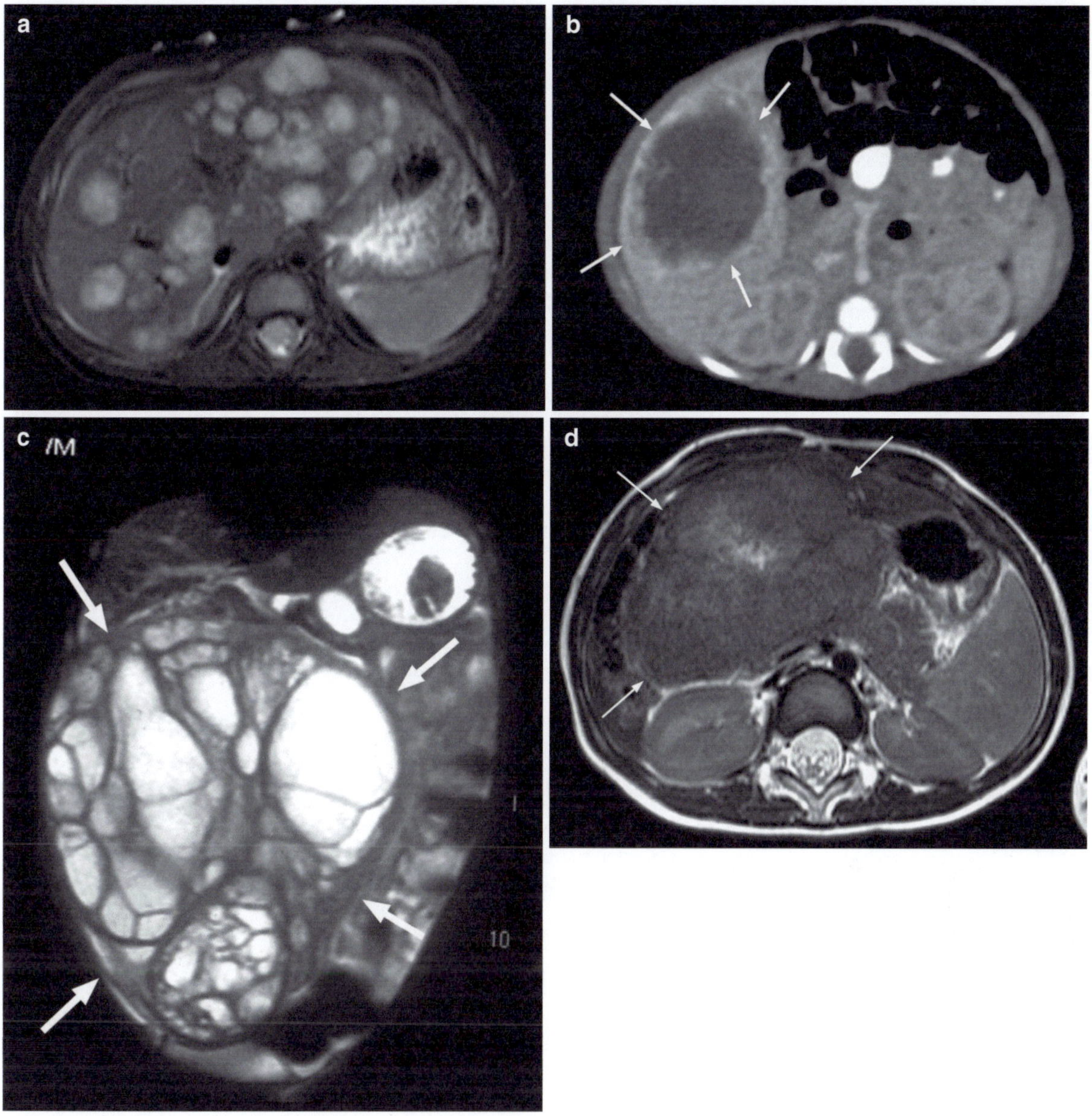

Fig. 8.3 Common benign tumors of the liver. (a) Infantile hemangioma (transverse fat-suppressed T2-weighted MRI). This lesion (histologically identical to, and often associated with, "strawberry" hemangiomas of the skin) is almost always multifocal or diffuse. This condition sometimes mimics metastatic neuroblastoma (Fig. 8.4a). (b) Rapidly-involuting congenital hemangioma (contrast-enhanced CT, delayed images). The mass (arrows) shows only peripheral enhancement; its central area shows low attenuation. (c) Mesenchymal hamartoma (T2-weighted coronal MRI). This is an example of multicystic morphology (arrows), but this lesion may be partly or even entirely solid. (d) Focal nodular hyperplasia (arrows) in a 3-year-old female (T2-weighted transverse MRI). There is a central "scar"

large, solid mass with low CT attenuation and T2-hyperintensity at MRI, similar to water (Fig. 8.4b; Buetow et al. 1997). Epithelioid hemangioendothelioma is usually multifocal. The lesions may enhance with a "target" pattern, and may be associated with local capsular retraction (Da Ines et al. 2010; Thin et al. 2009).

Fibrolamellar carcinoma (FLC) may have a central, fibrous scar, and this may be detectable by imaging. It has been proposed that, as opposed to FNH, the scar in FLC does not enhance with intravenous contrast, but this finding may not be reliable (McLarney et al. 1999).

Biliary rhabdomyosarcoma typically shows an intraductal growth pattern (Roebuck et al. 1998).

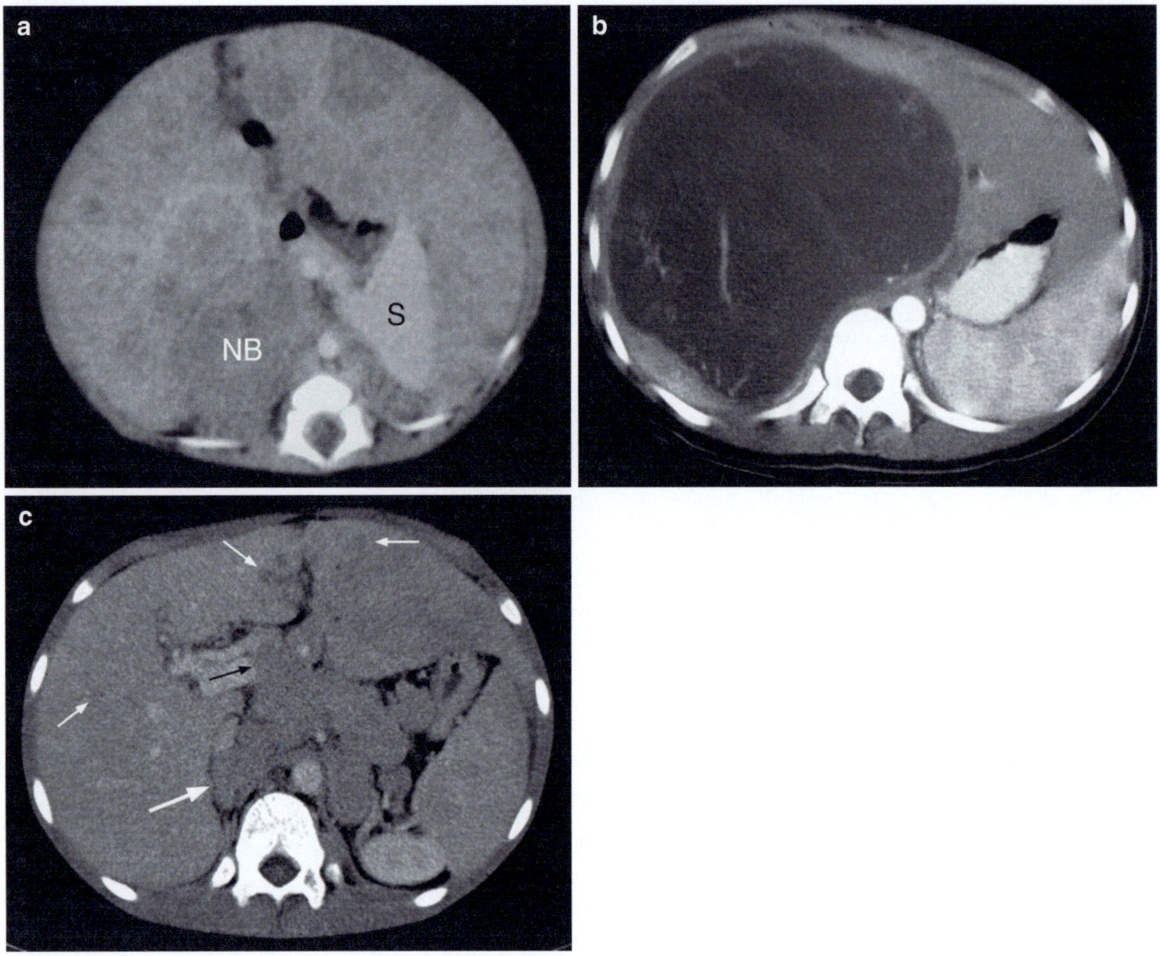

Fig. 8.4 Other malignant tumors of the liver. (a) Stage 4S (MS) neuroblastoma with diffuse liver metastases. Contrast-enhanced computed tomography shows typical appearance of gross heterogeneous hepatomegaly. Note that the left lobe has expanded to surround the spleen (S). The primary tumor was in the right adrenal (NB). This multifocal pattern resembles that seen in infantile hemangioma (Fig. 8.3a). (b) Undifferentiated (embryonal) sarcoma (contrast-enhanced CT). The very low attenuation of the mass is characteristic. (c) Multifocal (F1) fibrolamellar carcinoma in an 11-year-old male (contrast-enhanced CT). There are innumerable liver lesions (small white arrows). CT also shows lymph node metastases (N1, black arrow) and direct extension into the retroperitoneum, posterior to the inferior vena cava (large white arrow)

8.3 Staging Systems

Two major staging systems are in current use. The International Children's Liver Tumor Strategy Group (SIOPEL) uses a preoperative staging system, PRETEXT (from PRETreatment EXTent of disease, Table 8.3 and Fig. 8.5), which is based on imaging findings (Roebuck et al. 2007a). PRETEXT has also been adopted by other groups for purposes of data collection, in addition to the Children's Oncology Group's postsurgical staging system (Table 8.4; Ortega et al. 1991). The Japanese TNM classification (Morita et al. 1983) can be considered a forerunner of the PRETEXT system.

8.4 Local Staging

8.4.1 PRETEXT

The primary tumor is classified to one of four PRETEXT groups, using the upper case Roman numerals I to IV, based on its extent within the liver (Table 8.3, Figs. 8.5 to 8.9). It should be noted that this system does not perfectly represent the true segmental anatomy of the liver, based on the branching pattern of the intrahepatic branches of the portal vein, which define segments of quite variable size and extent in different

Table 8.3 PRETEXT grouping for primary liver tumors (Roebuck et al. 2007a), and current SIOPEL risk stratification for hepatoblastoma

PRETEXT I	One section is involved, and three contiguous sections are free of tumor
PRETEXT II	One or two sections are involved, and two contiguous sections are free of tumor
PRETEXT III	Two or three sections are involved, and no two contiguous sections are free of tumor
PRETEXT IV	All four sections are involved
High risk hepatoblastoma (any of the following features)	
PRETEXT IV	
E1, E1a, E2, or E2a	
H1 (tumor rupture at diagnosis)	
M1	
N1 or N2	
P2 or P2a	
V3 or V3a	
Serum alpha-fetoprotein <100 μg/L	
Standard risk hepatoblastoma	
All other patients	

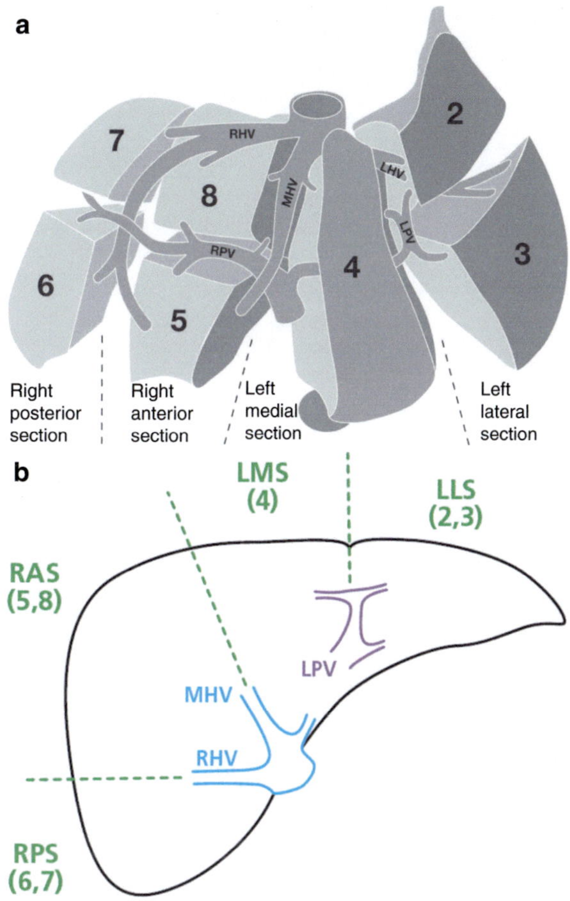

Fig. 8.5 PRETEXT staging of the extent of the primary liver tumor. (**a**) "Exploded" frontal view showing the segmental anatomy of the liver. The hepatic and portal veins define the sections of the liver (numbered here 2–8). Segment 1, which lies between the right portal vein (RPV) and the inferior vena cava, is obscured in this view. The left hepatic vein (LHV) runs between segments 2 and 3 and is not used in PRETEXT staging. (**b**) Schematic transverse section of the liver, showing the planes of the major venous structures used to determine the PRETEXT number (dashed lines). The right hepatic (RHV) and middle hepatic (MHV) veins indicate the borders between the right anterior section (RAS) and the right posterior (RPS) and left medial (LMS) sections. The umbilical portion of the left portal vein (LPV) separates the LMS from the left lateral section (LLS). Note that the LPV actually lies caudal to the confluence of the hepatic veins, and is not seen in the same transverse image in clinical practice. The segment numbers of each section are given in parenthesis. Reproduced with permission from: Roebuck DJ, Aronson D, Clapuyt P, et al. (2007) 2005 PRETEXT: a revised staging system for primary malignant liver tumours of childhood developed by the SIOPEL group. Pediatr Radiol 37:123-132

individuals. Broadly speaking, the PRETEXT groups approximate the difficulty of surgical resection, if vascular and other forms of local extension are ignored.

8.4.1.1 PRETEXT I (Fig. 8.6)

By definition, PRETEXT I tumors involve only the right posterior section (segments 6 and/or 7) or left lateral section (segments 2 and/or 3), and are therefore almost always resectable at diagnosis (Fig. 8.6a). Very small PRETEXT I tumors are sometimes detected by screening, for example, in children with Beckwith–Wiedemann syndrome, or as an incidental finding (Fig. 8.6b; Roebuck 2008). Larger lesions are more common, however (Fig. 8.6c).

8.4.1.2 PRETEXT II (Fig. 8.7)

PRETEXT II tumors are almost always unifocal and restricted to either the right or left lobe (Fig. 8.7a and b). In theory, multifocal tumors involving only the left lateral and right posterior sections would also qualify. Originally, there was no classification for tumors involving only the caudate lobe (segment 1). This was

Table 8.4 Children's Oncology Group postsurgical staging system (Ortega et al. 1991), and current risk stratification for hepatoblastoma (AHEP0731)

Stage I	No metastatic disease, tumor completely resected
Stage II	No metastatic disease, microscopic residual disease after resection of tumor, or tumor rupture (including tumor spill at the time of surgery)
Stage III	No distant metastases, tumor unresectable or resected with gross residual disease, or lymph node metastases
Stage IV	Distant metastases, irrespective of local extent of tumor
Low risk hepatoblastoma	
Stage I PFH	
Stage I non-PFH non-SCUD	
Stage II non-SCUD	
Intermediate risk hepatoblastoma	
Stage I SCUD	
Stage II SCUD	
Stage III	
High risk hepatoblastoma	
Stage IV	
AFP < 100 μg/L	
PFH	Pure fetal histology
SCUD	Small cell undifferentiated histology
AFP	Alpha-fetoprotein

corrected in the revised PRETEXT system (Roebuck et al. 2007a), and now caudate lobe involvement makes a tumor PRETEXT II as a minimum (Fig. 8.7c), and is also classified as **C1**.

8.4.1.3 PRETEXT III (Fig. 8.8)

The most important single task in local staging in hepatoblastoma is to distinguish PRETEXT III tumors from PRETEXT IV. This is easier for right-sided tumors, which are separated from the left lateral section (segments 2 and 3) by the fissure for the ligamentum teres and the left portal vein. These structures are usually easy to identify on transverse and coronal images. When the tumor is left-sided, the crucial structure is the right hepatic vein, which is often harder to identify, and which must be distinguished from accessory veins, which drain into the retrohepatic inferior vena cava (IVC).

8.4.1.4 PRETEXT IV (Fig. 8.9)

PRETEXT IV tumors involve all four sections of the liver, and are therefore (with extremely rare exceptions based on unconventional operations) unresectable at diagnosis without the use of transplantation. Results from SIOPEL studies suggest that many children with large unifocal PRETEXT IV hepatoblastoma (Fig. 8.9a) have undergone trisectionectomy following preoperative chemotherapy. It is not clear whether some of these patients were incorrectly staged at diagnosis. Multifocal hepatoblastoma is often PRETEXT IV (Fig. 8.9b), and again occasional patients have been successfully treated without transplantation. Despite these observations, all PRETEXT IV patients should be referred for assessment by a transplant center at diagnosis.

8.4.2 Imaging of Segmental and Vascular Anatomy

The vascular anatomy of the liver is the key to evaluation of the segmental extent of the tumor (Fig. 8.5), and imaging is not complete until all the relevant information has been obtained.

The anatomy of the (main) portal vein (MPV) is almost always predictable. It bifurcates at the porta hepatis into two large branches: the left portal vein (LPV) and the right portal vein (RPV). Trifurcation of the MPV is an uncommon variant.

The anatomy of the hepatic veins is much more variable (Catalano et al. 2008). The standard pattern, in which three major vessels, the left (LHV), middle (MHV), and right (RHV) hepatic veins, converge on the superior end of the IVC is seen in a minority of individuals (Catalano et al. 2008). The most common variants are to have a short common trunk of the LHV and MHV, and/or multiple MHVs. A useful clue for identifying the MHV is that it tends to lie in the same oblique plane as the gallbladder fossa. Accessory RHVs are common but are not important for PRETEXT grouping.

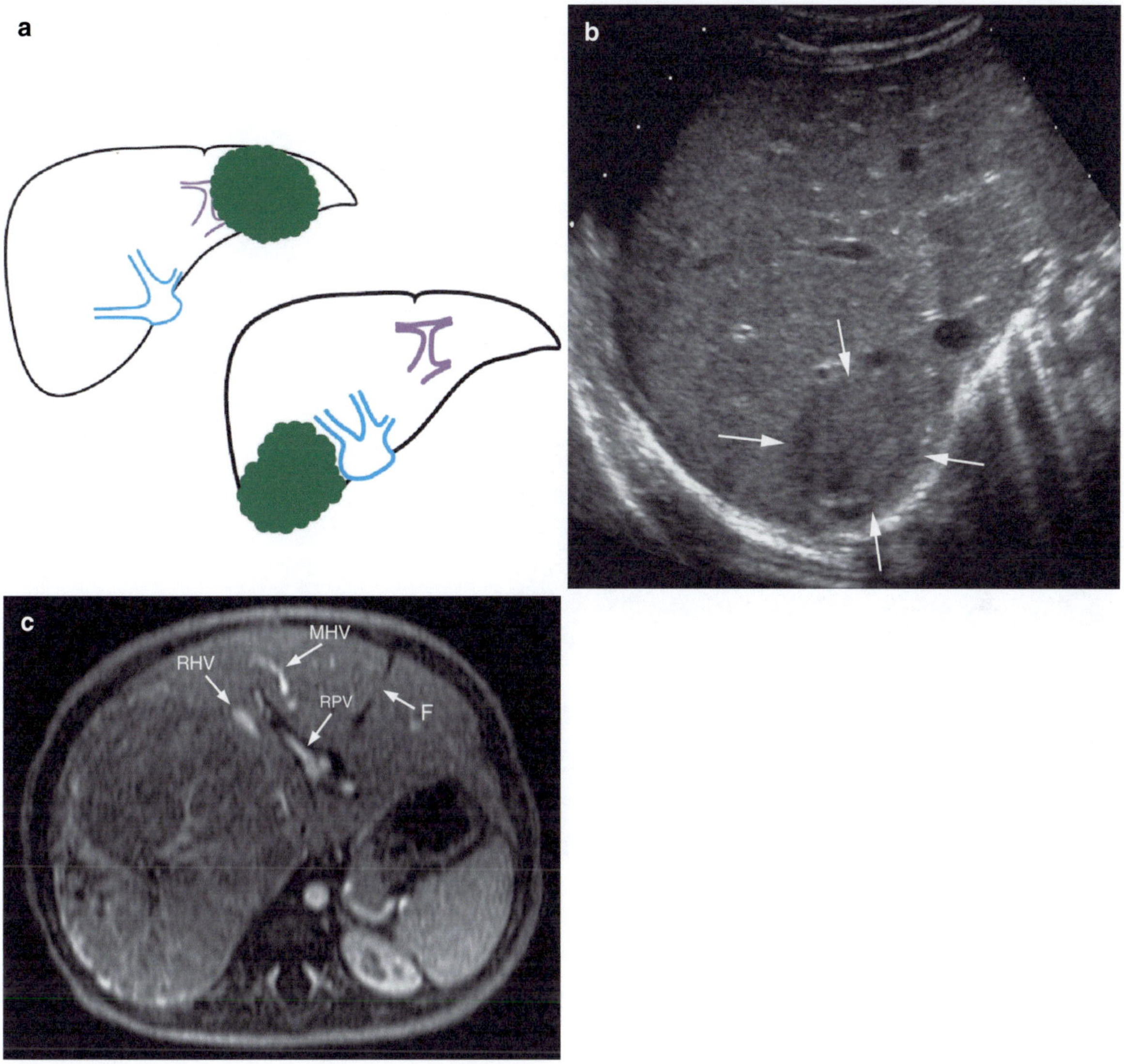

Fig. 8.6 PRETEXT I. (**a**) The two possible patterns of PRETEXT I tumor. Reproduced with permission from: Roebuck DJ, Aronson D, Clapuyt P, et al. (2007) 2005 PRETEXT: a revised staging system for primary malignant liver tumours of childhood developed by the SIOPEL group. Pediatr Radiol 37:123-132. (**b**) Ultrasound shows a small PRETEXT I tumor (arrows), an incidental finding in a 4-month-old male with Beckwith-Wiedemann syndrome. (**c**) Contrast-enhanced MRI shows a large PRETEXT I tumor, which arises from segments 6 and 7, and displaces the right hepatic vein (RHV) anteriorly and to the left (arrow). The fissure for the ligamentum teres (F) lies in the plane of the umbilical segment of the left portal vein, separating segments 2 and 3 from segment 4. MHV = middle hepatic vein, RPV = right portal vein

8.4.3 Multifocal Tumor (F)

It seems likely that the distinction between multifocal (and perhaps diffuse) tumors and unifocal lesions is clinically useful (Roebuck et al. 2007a). The presence of more than one intrahepatic nodule, regardless of size or PRETEXT group, is classified as **F1** (Figs. 8.1b, 8.4c, and 8.9b), and unifocal lesions as **F0**.

8.5 Vascular Involvement (P, V)

Involvement of both the portal venous system and the systemic veins (hepatic veins and/or inferior vena cava) is common in hepatoblastoma and hepatocellular carcinoma. The 2005 PRETEXT revision defines the word "involvement" quite clearly (Fig. 8.10; Roebuck et al. 2007a). The first type of involvement is *invasion*

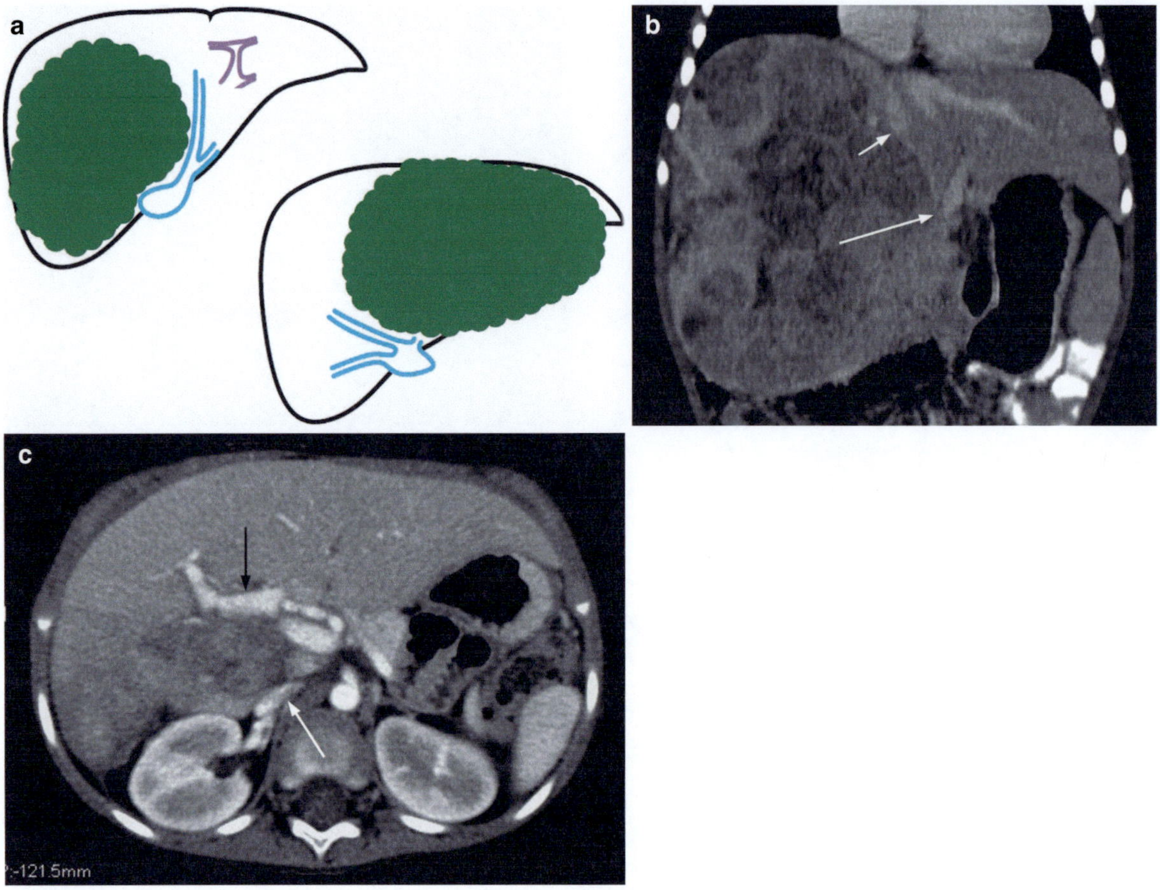

Fig. 8.7 PRETEXT II. (**a**) The most common patterns of PRETEXT II tumors. Other configurations are possible but uncommon. Reproduced with permission from: Roebuck DJ, Aronson D, Clapuyt P, et al. (2007) 2005 PRETEXT: a revised staging system for primary malignant liver tumours of childhood developed by the SIOPEL group. Pediatr Radiol 37:123-132. (**b**) Coronal contrast-enhanced CT image, showing a large PRETEXT II tumor displacing the middle hepatic vein (arrows) to the left. (**c**) Tumor involving the caudate lobe (C1), between the right portal vein (black arrow) and the inferior vena cava (white arrow). Caudate lobe involvement is by definition at least PRETEXT II.

of the lumen of the vein (Figs. 8.1c and 8.11b). The second is complete *encasement* of the vein, with or without obstruction of its lumen (Fig. 8.11a). It is reasonable to assume that a vein is encased if no vessel is seen in its expected location (allowing for possible displacement by the tumor). On CT studies, this only applies if the images were obtained after the appropriate time delay for that type of vessel following contrast injection (see above). Although both of these forms of involvement are likely to be indicators of a relatively poor prognosis, invasion may be worse than encasement. A tumor that abuts a vein without completely encircling it does not involve the vein according to this definition (Roebuck et al. 2007a).

Involvement of either the LPV or the RPV, or one of their major branches, is classified as **P1** (Fig. 8.11). When there is involvement of both branches and/or the MPV, the patient is categorized as **P2**.

Involvement of one or two of the hepatic veins, or their major tributaries, is classified as **V1** or **V2**, respectively (Fig. 8.12). The term **V3** is used when there is involvement of all three hepatic veins and/or the IVC. IVC compression is very commonly seen in children with large tumors, often accompanied by enlargement of veins of the azygos system. This finding by itself is not considered involvement.

In each case, invasion of the vein (as opposed to encasement), is indicated by the suffix **–a**.

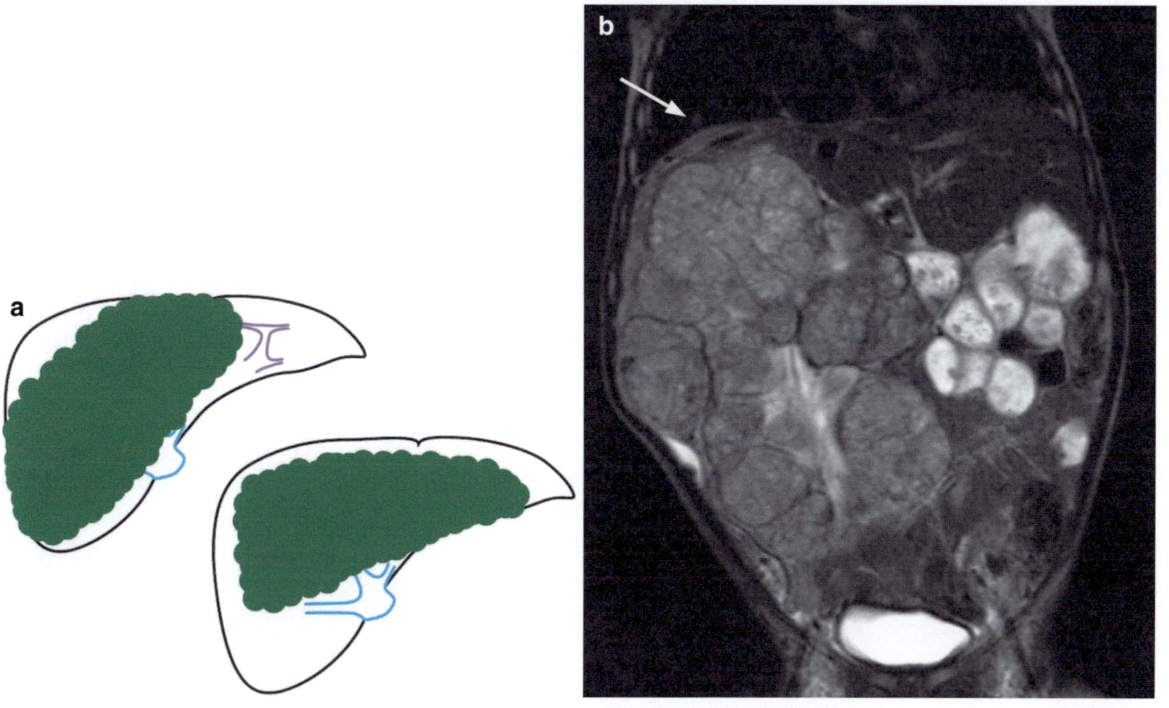

Fig. 8.8 PRETEXT III. (**a**) The most common patterns of PRETEXT III tumors. Other configurations are possible but uncommon. Reproduced with permission from: Roebuck DJ, Aronson D, Clapuyt P, et al. (2007) 2005 PRETEXT: a revised staging system for primary malignant liver tumours of childhood developed by the SIOPEL group. Pediatr Radiol 37: 123-132. (**b**) Coronal T2-weighted MRI shows a PRETEXT III tumor, apparently arising from the right lobe and involving segment 4. There is a lung metastasis (M1p, arrow)

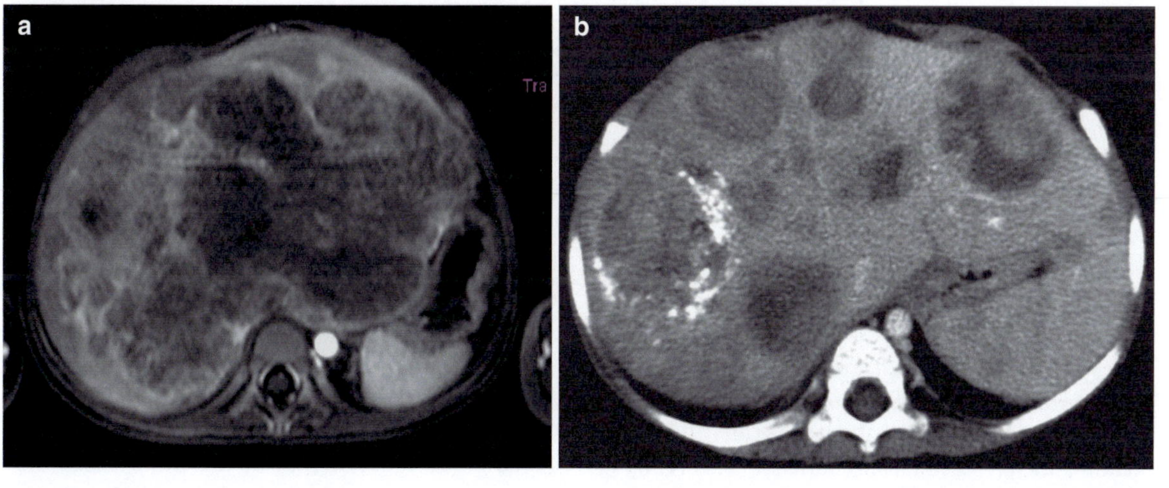

Fig. 8.9 PRETEXT IV. (**a**) Contrast-enhanced MRI shows a huge unifocal tumor involving all four sections of the liver (PRETEXT IV F0). (**b**) Contrast-enhanced CT shows multifocal tumor involving all four sections of the liver (PRETEXT IV F1)

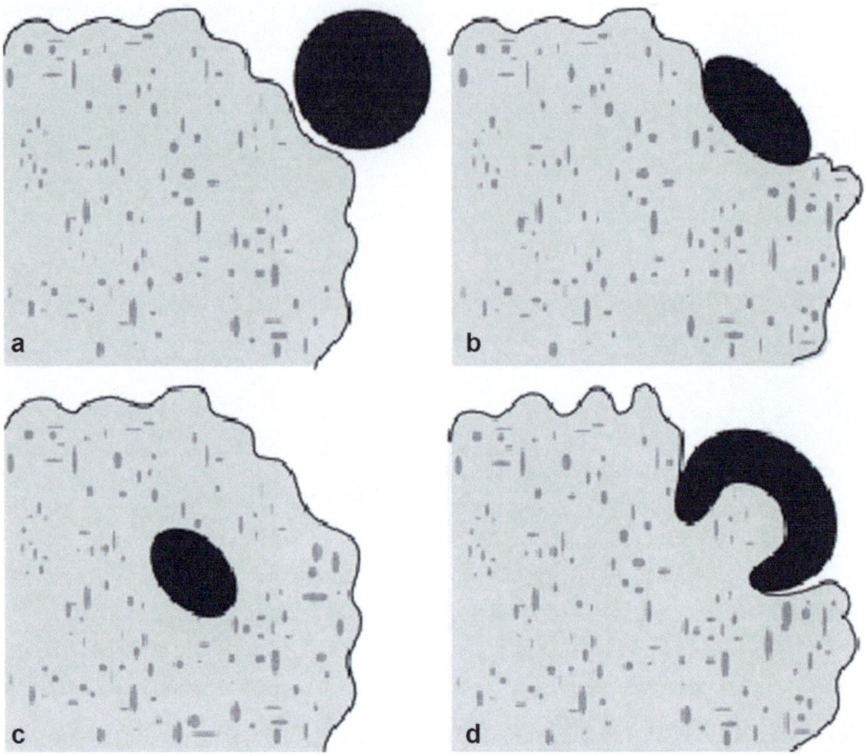

Fig. 8.10 Venous involvement, either portal or systemic, according to the PRETEXT system. A tumor which approaches (**a**) or abuts (**b**) a vessel does not involve it. Involvement is defined as either encasement (**c**) or invasion (**d**). Reproduced with permission from: Roebuck DJ, Olsen Ø, Pariente D (2006) Radiological staging in children with hepatoblastoma. Pediatr Radiol 36:176-182

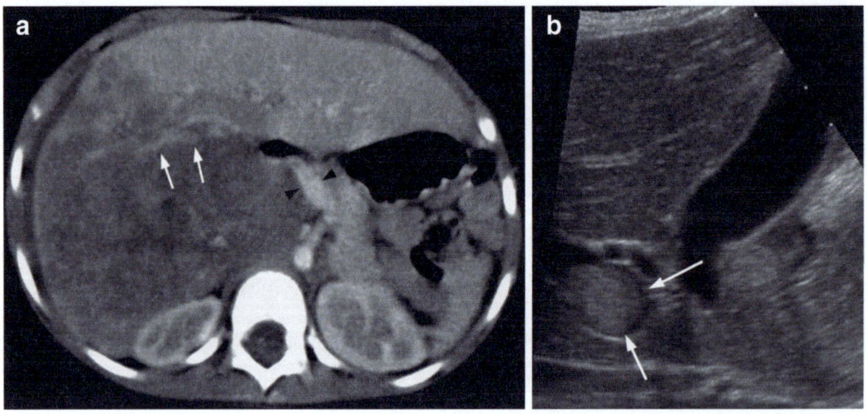

Fig. 8.11 Involvement of the portal venous system (P). (**a**) P1. The right portal vein (white arrows) is encased by tumor. The (main) portal vein (black arrowheads) and left portal vein (not shown) are not involved. (**b**) P2a. Venous invasion. Ultrasound shows tumor growing within the (main) portal vein (arrows)

8.6 Extrahepatic Spread in the Abdomen (E, H)

The PRETEXT system classifies direct extension of tumor from the liver and peritoneal spread of disease as **E1**, **E1a**, **E2**, or **E2a** (Roebuck et al. 2007a). In addition, the presence (**H1**) or absence (**H0**) of tumor rupture at diagnosis is also recorded. Although there is no proof that **E1**, **E2**, or **H1** are adverse prognostic factors, they are both currently regarded as defining features of high-risk hepatoblastoma by SIOPEL.

A primary liver tumor may invade the abdominal wall, the diaphragm, or adjacent organs such as the pancreas or colon (Roebuck et al. 2007b). Although advances in CT and MRI have made this form of spread easier to detect, it remains quite uncommon in hepatoblastoma (Roebuck et al. 2007b). Direct extension of tumor is classified as **E1**. Biopsy

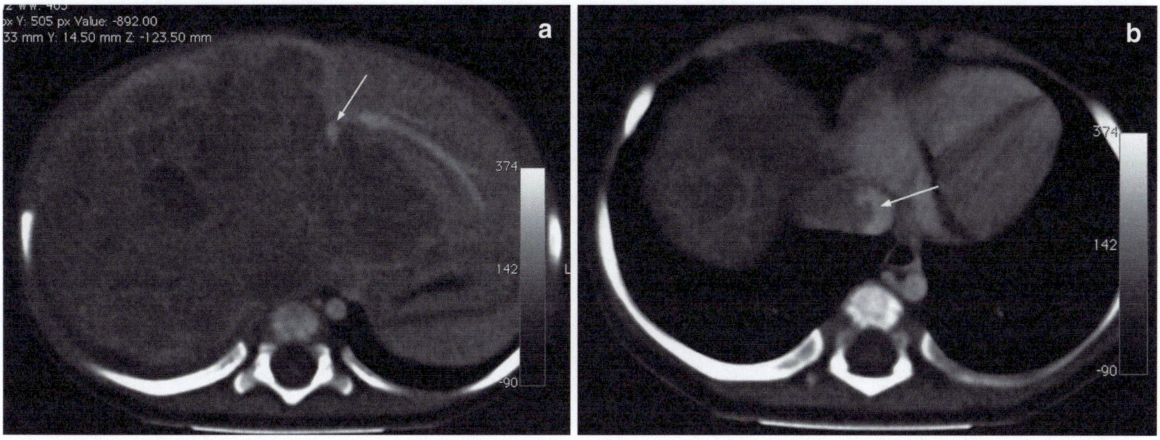

Fig. 8.12 Involvement of the inferior vena cava (IVC) and/or hepatic veins (V). (**a**) V2. Transverse contrast-enhanced CT image shows encasement of the middle hepatic vein (arrow). The right hepatic vein is completely obliterated. (**b**) V3a. Transverse contrast-enhanced CT image shows that tumor has extended to involve the suprahepatic IVC (arrows)

confirmation is not required if the imaging features are unequivocal (Roebuck et al. 2007a). The presence of an exophytic or pedunculated growth pattern alone has probably no adverse effect on prognosis, and is not sufficient for **E1**. Although the 2005 PRETEXT revision does not specifically address this issue, invasion of the gallbladder alone should not be regarded as **E1**.

Peritoneal spread (in the form of separate tumor nodules) is often detectable by CT, MRI, and, particularly in the presence of ascites, US (Fig. 8.13; Roebuck et al. 2007b). This form of spread is classified as **E2**, regardless of the size of the lesion.

It is not known whether the presence of ascites alone is an independent risk factor in children with primary liver tumors. In order to facilitate future data analysis, the suffix **–a** is added to the classification (i.e., **E0a**, **E1a**, or **E2a**) when ascites is present.

Tumor rupture (as shown by the presence of hemoperitoneum) is classified as **H1** (Fig. 8.14a). This requires either a combination of clinical, laboratory, and imaging findings (e.g., presentation with sudden abdominal pain, possibly after trauma, hypotension, or low hematocrit, and echogenic peritoneal fluid on US) or aspiration of blood at paracentesis. Tumor rupture is not uncommon in hepatoblastoma and hepatocellular carcinoma (Ishak and Glunz 1967; Iida et al. 2004; Chan et al. 2002), and may require urgent surgery or embolization. Localized (e.g., subcapsular) hemorrhage and biopsy-related bleeding are not sufficient for **H1** (Fig. 8.14b).

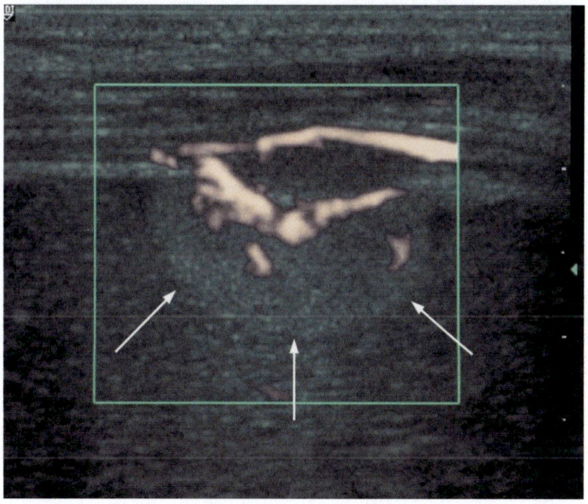

Fig. 8.13 Peritoneal tumor nodule without ascites (E2). Ultrasound shows a tiny echogenic peritoneal nodule (arrows), overlying the liver, which has recruited blood supply from the abdominal wall. This is currently the only feasible imaging technique which can distinguish between a peripheral liver nodule (F1) and a peritoneal metastasis (E2)

8.7 Metastatic Disease (M, N)

The 2005 revision separates distant metastases into two separate categories, as is common in adult tumors using the TNM system. Presumed hematogenous metastases are classified as **M1**. In hepatoblastoma, almost all metastases at diagnosis are found in the lungs (**M1p**, Fig. 8.2), but in hepatocellular carcinoma lesions are

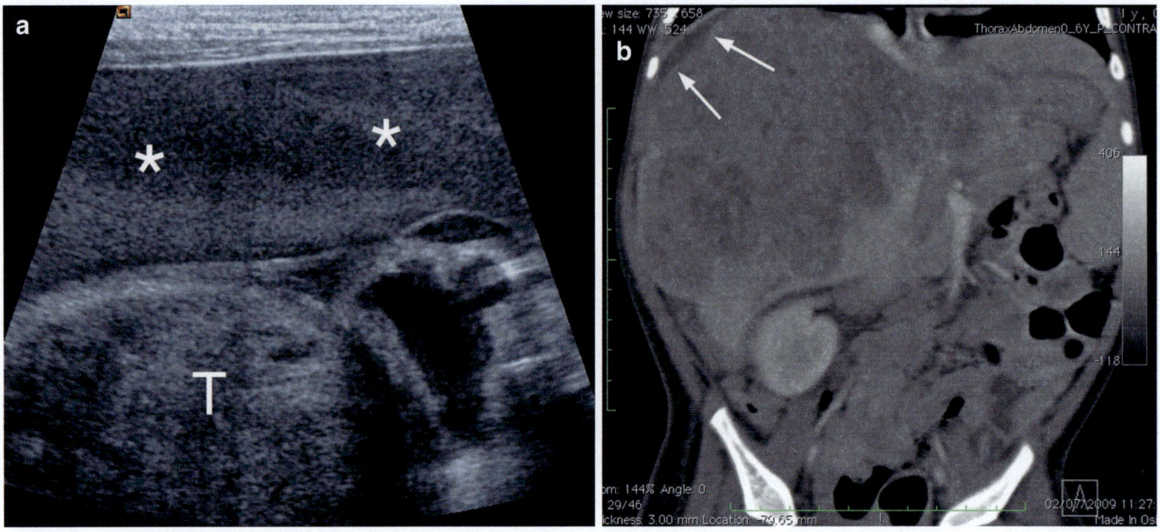

Fig. 8.14 Tumor rupture at diagnosis (H). (**a**) H1. Abdominal ultrasound shows fresh intraperitoneal blood, shown as a layer of mixed echogenicity fluid (asterisks), anterior to the tumor (T). (**b**) H0. Coronal contrast-enhanced CT image shows an isolated, possibly subcapsular, fluid collection (arrows)

sometimes found in the skeleton (**M1s**, Fig. 8.15), central nervous system (**M1c**), bone marrow (**M1m**), or other sites (**M1x**). Biopsy proof is not required in the presence of convincing imaging findings.

Although multidetector CT technology is now widely available, high-quality imaging of all of the lungs is sometimes not possible for various reasons, despite best techniques for anesthesia or sedation (see above). Even with ideal imaging, the diagnosis of pulmonary metastases in children is fraught with difficulties (McCarville et al. 2006), and most of the available information comes from children with nonhepatic primary tumors (Absalon et al. 2008). Various benign lesions may simulate solitary or multiple metastases. The most common of these are granulomas, which may be seen after bacterial, fungal, or viral infections (e.g., tuberculosis, histoplasmosis, and varicella). There is a significant geographical variation in the frequency of postinfective lung nodules (McCarville et al. 2006). Hamartomas and intrapulmonary lymph nodes may also simulate metastases. Various factors, including basal distribution, subpleural location, smooth margins (McCarville et al. 2006), and size and number of lesions (McCarville et al. 2006) have been proposed as signs that lung lesions are likely to be due to metastatic disease, but these are unreliable (McCarville et al. 2006). Interobserver variability in prediction of malignancy is quite high, but there is some evidence that radiologists who practice predominantly in pediatric oncology may perform better than general pediatric radiologists (McCarville et al. 2006).

The PRETEXT system takes a pragmatic approach to this problem. Rather than insisting on biopsy in all patients who have lung lesions compatible with metastases, it classifies them as **M1p** and leaves the decision about risk stratification (e.g., on the basis of the size and/or number of lesions) to individual treatment protocols. For example, the SIOPEL 4 protocol required not just **M1p**, but the presence of at least one lung lesion >10 mm, or "several" (interpreted as >1) lesions, at least one of which was >5 mm, for a patient to qualify as having high-risk hepatoblastoma.

Lymph node metastases are uncommon in hepatoblastoma (Morita et al. 1983), and even when they are present it is not clear that they are a significant prognostic factor (Reyes et al. 2000). Benign enlargement may also occur. For these reasons, the PRETEXT system requires biopsy proof. In the future, it may be possible to detect malignant nodes using imaging techniques such as positron emission tomography or diffusion-weighted MRI. Currently, the best approach may be to biopsy very large nodes (>15 mm in short axis) in children with hepatoblastoma. In hepatocellular carcinoma and fibrolamellar carcinoma, where lymph nodes metastases are much more common (Fig. 8.4c), biopsy confirmation is not required if the short axis diameter is >15 mm (Roebuck et al. 2007a).

Abdominal lymph node metastases are coded as **N1** (Fig. 8.4c) and distant nodal metastases as **N2**.

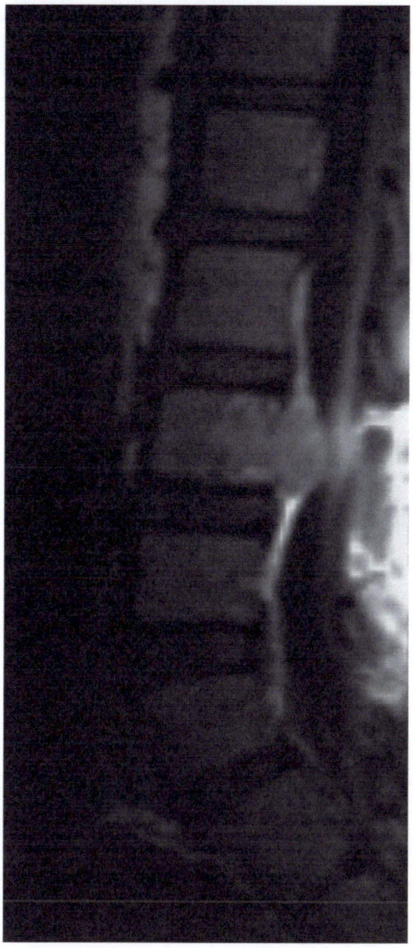

Fig. 8.15 Bony metastasis in hepatocellular carcinoma (M1s). Sagittal contrast-enhanced T1-weighted MRI shows a metastasis which arises from the body of L3 and extends into the spinal canal

References

Absalon MJ, McCarville MB, Liu T et al (2008) Pulmonary nodules discovered during the initial evaluation of pediatric patients with bone and soft-tissue sarcoma. Pediatr Blood Cancer 50:1147–1153

Albuquerque PA, Morales Ramos DA, Faingold R (2009) Magnetic resonance imaging of the liver and biliary tree in children. Curr Probl Diagn Radiol 38:126–134

Buetow PC, Buck JL, Pantongrag-Brown L et al (1997) Undifferentiated (embryonal) sarcoma of the liver: pathologic basis of imaging findings in 28 cases. Radiology 203:779–783

Catalano OA, Singh AH, Uppot RN et al (2008) Vascular and biliary variants in the liver: implications for liver surgery. Radiographics 28:359–378

Chan KL, Fan ST, Tam PK et al (2002) Management of spontaneously ruptured hepatoblastoma in infancy. Med Pediatr Oncol 38:137–138

Cheon JE, Kim WS, Kim IO et al (1998) Radiological features of focal nodular hyperplasia of the liver in children. Pediatr Radiol 28:878–883

Da Ines D, Petitcolin V, Joubert-Zakeyh J, Demeocq F, Garcier JM (2010) Epithelioid hemangioendothelioma of the liver with metastatic coeliac lymph nodes in an 11-year-old boy. Pediatr Radiol 40(7):1293-1296

Dong Q, Xu W, Jiang B et al (2007) Clinical applications of computerized tomography 3-D reconstruction imaging for diagnosis and surgery in children with large liver tumors or tumors at the hepatic hilum. Pediatr Surg Int 23:1045–1050

Figarola MS, McQuiston SA, Wilson F et al (2005) Recurrent hepatoblastoma with localization by PET-CT. Pediatr Radiol 35:1254–1258

Fuchs J, Warmann SW, Szavay P et al (2005) Three-dimensional visualization and virtual simulation of resections in pediatric solid tumors. J Pediatr Surg 40:364–370

Hedenstierna G, Rothen HU (2000) Atelectasis formation during anesthesia: causes and measures to prevent it. J Clin Monit Comput 16:329–335

Humphries PD, Sebire NJ, Siegel MJ et al (2007) Tumors in pediatric patients at diffusion-weighted MR imaging: apparent diffusion coefficient and tumor cellularity. Radiology 245:848–854

Iida T, Suenaga M, Takeuchi Y et al (2004) Successful resection of a ruptured hepatoblastoma prior to chemotherapy: report of a case. Surg Today 34:710–714

Ishak KG, Glunz PR (1967) Hepatoblastoma and hepatocarcinoma in infancy and childhood. Report of 47 cases. Cancer 20:396–422

Kawel N, Seifert B, Luetolf M et al (2009) Effect of slab thickness on the CT detection of pulmonary nodules: use of sliding thin-slab maximum intensity projection and volume rendering. AJR Am J Roentgenol 192:1324–1329

Kim SH, Kim WS, Cheon JE et al (2007) Radiological spectrum of hepatic mesenchymal hamartoma in children. Korean J Radiol 8:498–505

McCarville MB, Kao SC (2006) Imaging recommendations for malignant liver neoplasms in children. Pediatr Blood Cancer 46:2–7

McCarville MB, Lederman HM, Santana VM et al (2006) Distinguishing benign from malignant pulmonary nodules with helical chest CT in children with malignant solid tumors. Radiology 239:514–520

McLarney JK, Rucker PT, Bender GN et al (1999) Fibrolamellar carcinoma of the liver: radiologic-pathologic correlation. Radiographics 19:453–471

Morita K, Okabe I, Uchino J et al (1983) The proposed Japanese TNM classification of primary liver carcinoma in infants and children. Jpn J Clin Oncol 13:361–369

Napel S, Rubin GD, Jeffrey RB Jr (1993) STS-MIP: a new reconstruction technique for CT of the chest. J Comput Assist Tomogr 17:832–838

Ohtsuka Y, Takahashi H, Ohnuma N et al (1997) Detection of tumor thrombus in children using color Doppler ultrasonography. J Pediatr Surg 32:1507–1510

Okada T, Sasaki F, Kamiyama T et al (2005) Focal nodular hyperplasia of the liver: usefulness of superparamagnetic iron oxide-enhanced magnetic resonance imaging. J Pediatr Surg 40:E21–25

Ortega JA, Krailo MD, Haas JE et al (1991) Effective treatment of unresectable or metastatic hepatoblastoma with cisplatin and continuous infusion doxorubicin chemotherapy: a report from the Childrens Cancer Study Group. J Clin Oncol 9:2167–2176

Reyes JD, Carr B, Dvorchik I et al (2000) Liver transplantation and chemotherapy for hepatoblastoma and hepatocellular cancer in childhood and adolescence. J Pediatr 136: 795–804

Roebuck D (2008) Focal liver lesion in children. Pediatr Radiol 38(Suppl 3):S518–522

Roebuck DJ (2009) Assessment of malignant liver tumors in children. Cancer Imaging 9(Spec No A):S98–S103

Roebuck DJ, Yang WT, Lam WW et al (1998) Hepatobiliary rhabdomyosarcoma in children: diagnostic radiology. Pediatr Radiol 28:101–108

Roebuck DJ, Olsen O, Pariente D (2006) Radiological staging in children with hepatoblastoma. Pediatr Radiol 36:176–182

Roebuck DJ, Aronson D, Clapuyt P et al (2007a) 2005 PRETEXT: a revised staging system for primary malignant liver tumours of childhood developed by the SIOPEL group. Pediatr Radiol 37:123–132, quiz 249–150

Roebuck DJ, Sebire NJ, Pariente D (2007b) Assessment of extrahepatic abdominal extension in primary malignant liver tumours of childhood. Pediatr Radiol 37:1096–1100

Sato M, Ishida H, Konno K et al (2000) Liver tumors in children and young patients: sonographic and color Doppler findings. Abdom Imaging 25:596–601

Siegel MJ, Chung EM, Conran RM (2008) Pediatric liver: focal masses. Magn Reson Imaging Clin N Am 16:437–452

Soo G, Lau KK, Yik T et al (2010) Optimal reconstructed section thickness for the detection of liver lesions with multidetector CT. Clin Radiol 65:193–197

Thin LW, Wong DD, De Boer BW, Ferguson JM, Adams L, Macquillan G, Delriviere L, Mitchell A, Jeffrey GP (2010) Hepatic epithelioid haemangioendothelioma: challenges in diagnosis and management. Intern Med J (in press)

Vasanawala SS (2010) MRI of the liver – how to do it. Pediatr Radiol 40:431–437

Vasanawala SS, Iwadate Y, Church DG et al (2010) Navigated abdominal T1-W MRI permits free-breathing image acquisition with less motion artifact. Pediatr Radiol 40:340–344

Pathology of Pediatric Liver Tumors

9

Arthur Zimmermann and Dolores Lopez-Terrada

Contents

A. Zimmermann (✉)
Institute of Pathology of the University, Murtenstrasse 31, CH-3010 Berne, Switzerland
e-mail: zimmerma@patho.unibe.ch

D. Lopez-Terrada
Department of Pathology, Texas Children's Hospital, 1 Baylor Plaza, Suite 286A, 77030 Houston, Texas, USA
e-mail: Dhterrad@texaschildrens.org

9.1 Hepatoblastoma and Related Tumors

9.1.1 Introduction

Hepatoblastoma is a term proposed by Willis for all embryonal tumors containing hepatic epithelial parenchyma more or less resembling fetal or embryonal tissue (Willis 1962). Early reports reviewed by Ishak and Glunz (1967) employed several terms to denote hepatoblastoma, including primary hepatoma or carcinoma of the liver in infancy and childhood, mixed tumors of the liver, and hepatic embryonic tumors. As the prognosis of these lesions was dismal those days, it was not thought important to classify the tumors differently. Subsequently, this changed considerably, leading to the concept of hepatoblastoma that we have today (reviews: Dehner 1978; Weinberg and Finegold 1983; Stocker 2001; Zimmermann 2005; Meyers 2007; Finegold et al. 2008). Hepatoblastoma is predominantly a disorder of the liver in small children and infants (see the chapter on epidemiology), but may occur in adults up to the age of 80 years.

9.1.2 Classification of Hepatoblastoma

Willis (1962) had classified hepatoblastoma into three types: (1) embryonic hepatoma, containing only embryonic liver tissue; (2) mixed tumors containing both epithelial and mesenchymal components; and (3) rhabdomyoblastic mixed tumors. In the same period, Edmondson still had epithelial hepatoblastomas under the category primary carcinoma of the liver, and the

A. Zimmermann et al. (eds.), *Pediatric Liver Tumors*, Pediatric Oncology,
DOI: 10.1007/978-3-642-14504-9_9, © Springer-Verlag Berlin Heidelberg 2011

Table 9.1 SIOPEL classification of hepatoblastomas

Hepatoblastoma, wholly epithelial type
Fetal subtype
Mixed embryonal/fetal subtype
Macrotrabecular subtype
Small cell undifferentiated subtype
Hepatoblastoma, mixed epithelial, and mesenchymal type
Without teratoid features
With teratoid features
Hepatoblastoma, not otherwise specified (NOS)

other lesions were mixed tumors (Edmondson 1956). Later, a so-called "pure hepatoblastoma" was added to this classification, denoting mixed tumors without osteoid (Neimann et al. 1963), while the osteoid-containing variant was identified as a separate entity (Milman and Grayzel 1951); this is currently obsolete. A major breakthrough was the proposition by Ishak and Glunz, who divided the tumors into an epithelial type and a mixed epithelial mesenchymal type, further breaking down the epithelial tumors into those with fetal or embryonal cells (Ishak and Glunz 1967), a refined and improved modification of the classification previously advocated by Willis. The criteria for modern classifications of hepatoblastoma have recently been reviewed (Rowland 2002), and a more expanded classification of the *hepatoblastoma tumor family* has been proposed (Zimmermann 2005). Table 9.1 shows the hepatoblastoma classification currently employed by SIOPEL.

About 55% of hepatoblastomas are epithelial (30% fetal, 20% fetal-embryonal, 3% macrotrabecular, 2% small cell undifferentiated), and 45% are mixed epithelial and mesenchymal, but when all types are considered, around 85% contain both fetal and embryonal components in variable proportions. There is no relationship between the age of the child and the predominant cell type in hepatoblastoma.

9.1.3 Macroscopy

Hepatoblastomas are more commonly solitary than multifocal, mostly expanding masses of roughly spherical shape (Ishak and Glunz 1967). Focal calcifications may be seen macroscopically; radiologically, coarse calcifications are present in hepatoblastoma in 50% of the cases, but many of them are in fact mineralized foci of osteoid (Dachman et al. 1987). Some tumors present with prominent feeding arteries and enlarged or engorged veins. Such tumors are hypervascular multifocal hepatoblastomas at imaging and may be confounded with hemangioendothelioma (Ingram et al. 2000; Lu and Greer 2007).

The gross and histologic work-up of hepatoblastomas has been formulated in a College of American Pathologists protocol (Finegold et al. 2007). A detailed description of the gross features delivers informations that are important for the confirmation of staging and for prognostication. Several parameters of growth patterns have been shown to be predictors of failed conservative treatment (FCT), such as multifocality, portal vein involvement, hepatic vein involvment, and vena cava involvement (Von Schweinitz et al. 1994; Davies et al. 2004; D'Antiga et al. 2007). Gross examination must include the precise assessment of radicality, what is sometimes difficult owing to the complexity of resection surfaces, especially in the fixed state of specimens. For the evaluation of surgical resection margins (Dicken et al. 2004) and the assessment of microscopic residual disease, it is recommended that surgeons and pathologists find a way to identify critical margin areas and the vascular and biliary trees, for example, by use of colored sutures or inking. In newborns with congenital hepatoblastoma, macroscopy must include the examination of the placenta, because hepatoblastoma can metastasize to this organ (Robinson and Bolande 1985; Doss et al. 1998).

9.1.4 Histopathology of Hepatoblastomas

Based on the histomorphologic features that had led to the current classifications, the specific features of the types and subtypes of hepatoblastoma have been worked out (Edmondson 1956; Ishak and Glunz 1967; Lack et al. 1982; Weinberg and Finegold 1983; Dehner and Manivel 1988; Haas et al. 1989; Conran et al. 1992). In the following overview, the types and subtypes follow the SIOPEL classification.

9.1.4.1 Fetal Hepatoblastoma: The Differentiated Phenotype with a Favorable Histology

The morphology of fetal-type cells has already been specified in detail in 1967 (Ishak and Glunz 1967). They are smaller than normal adult hepatocytes but larger than normal fetal hepatocytes, with a well-defined outline, and present a cytoplasm that varies from eosinophil and is slightly granular to clear (Fig. 9.1a and b), resulting in a characteristic dark-and-clear cell pattern, or a pattern of light and dark lobules. The pale or clear aspect of the cytoplasm is sometimes striking (Fig. 9.1d) and is caused by accumulation of glycogen and lipids. Marked lipid accumulation induces vacuolization of the cell, commonly seen after chemotherapy. Bile production can be noted, sometimes with dense bile deposits in canalicular-like structures. The nuclei are round to slightly ovoid, with a rather fine chromatin structure and one small acidophilic nucleolus. Fetal cells are arranged in cords, nests, or nodules, without a prominent stroma (except around feeding vessels or in certain tumor variants with a lobular growth pattern and hamartoma-like features) and with a rather poorly developed network of reticular tissue (Ishak and Glunz 1967). In compact areas, sinusoids may be absent, resulting in a cellular mosaic pattern (Haas et al. 1989). Extramedullary hematopoiesis is a typical feature (Fig. 9.1c), whereby erythroblasts predominate, but megakaryocytes are also in evidence. These foci are intrasinusoidal and are not seen in the adjacent normal liver tissue.

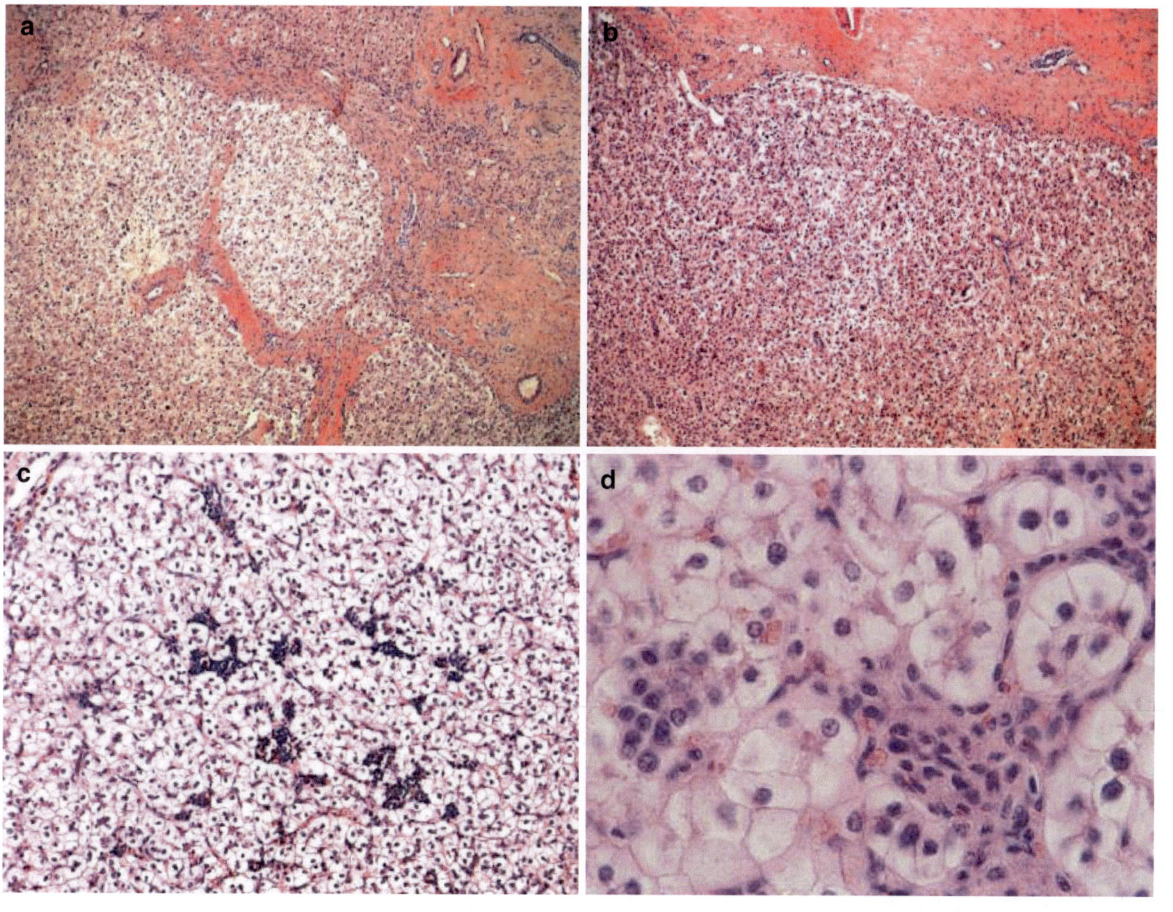

Fig. 9.1 (**a**) Fetal hepatoblastoma. The cells form solid formations and nodules, and exhibit a clear cytoplasm (hematoxylin and eosin stain). (**b**) In this fetal hepatoblastoma, both clear and dark cells are noted (hematoxylin and eosin stain). (**c**) Several hematopoietic clusters are seen in this fetal hepatoblastoma (hematoxylin and eosin stain). (**d**) Clear cells of a fetal hepatoblastoma at higher magnification (hematoxylin and eosin stain)

In the well-differentiated variety of fetal hepatoblastoma, there is little mitotic activity (two or less than two mitotic figures per ten high-power [×40 objective] fields; pure fetal histology). A subset of fetal hepatoblastoma shows significant mitotic activity (>2 mitotic figures in ten high-power fields). This variant is called mitotically active fetal or crowded fetal hepatoblastoma, because cytoplasmic glycogen storage is less and hence the proportion of a sample occupied by nuclei is increased.

9.1.4.2 Embryonal Histology: A Common Partner of Fetal Tissue Components

The embryonal pattern almost always occurs in combination with fetal components (purely embryonal hepatoblastomas are exceptional observations Borman et al. 1961). Embryonal hepatoblastoma cells are less differentiated than fetal cells, poorly cohesive, elongated, and have a high nuclear cytoplasmic ratio and a sparse, compact basophilic or amphophilic, poorly outlined cytoplasm (Fig. 9.2a). Bile production is not seen. The nuclei are oval rather than round and show a coarser chromatin, with prominent parachromatin and one enlarged amphophilic or acidophilic nucleolus. Mitoses are more frequent than in the fetal subtype. Transitions between fetal cells and embryonal cells are common, and sometimes embryonal tissue is seen at the periphery of otherwise fetal tissue areas (Fig. 9.2b). The growth pattern of embryonal areas is complex and includes solid sheets or plates of variable thickness, incomplete or complete tubuloacinar profiles

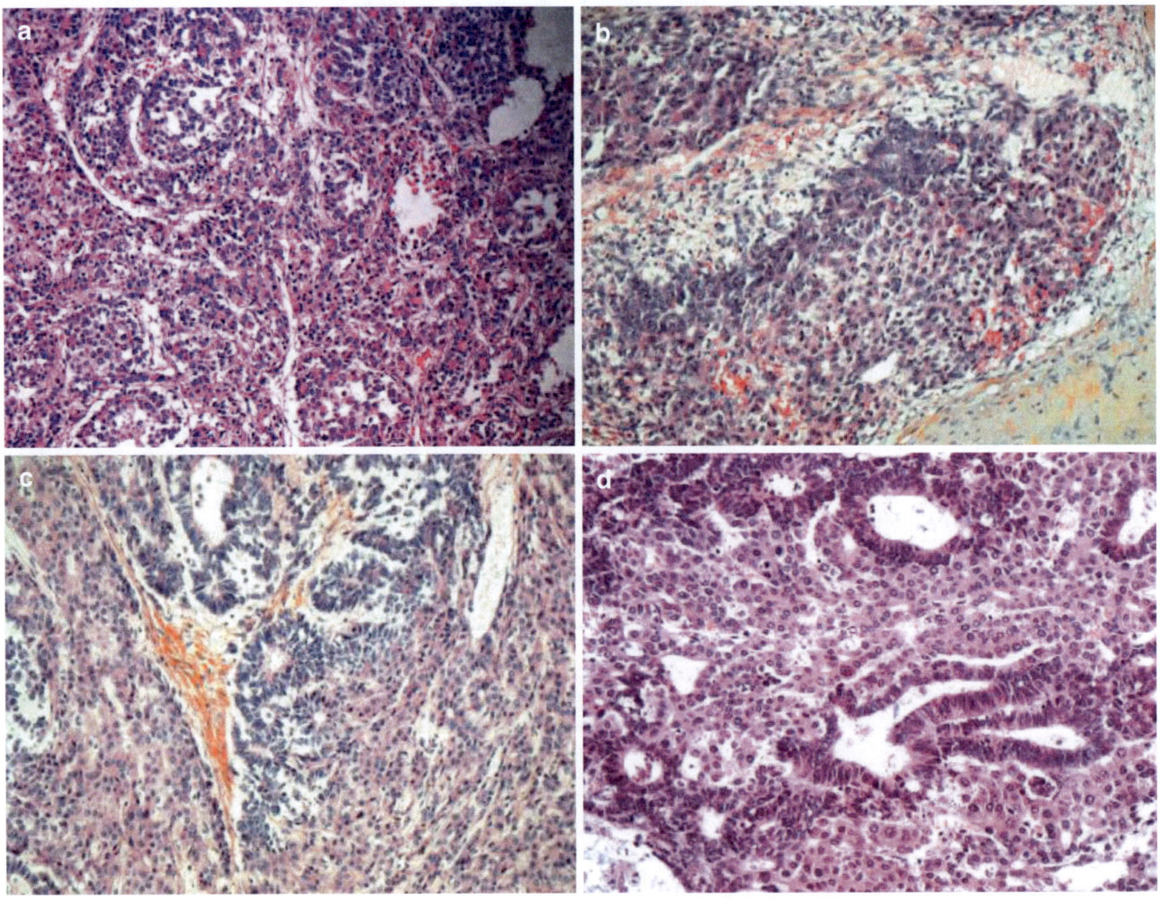

Fig. 9.2 (**a**) Embryonal components of a mixed epithelial hepatoblastoma (hematoxylin and eosin stain). (**b**) In this embryonal/fetal hepatoblastoma, embryonal components are located to the periphery of fetal parts (hematoxylin and eosin stain). (**c**) Embryonal area of a hepatoblastoma with acinar formations (hematoxylin and eosin stain). (**d**) In this embryonal area, immature tubular structures are present (hematoxylin and eosin stain)

(Fig. 9.2c), and rosette-like configurations (pseudorosettes) resembling primitive bile ducts of the embryonic liver prior to the sixth week of gestation (Gonzalez-Crussi et al. 1982; Fig. 9.2d). Micropapillary structures may occur and sometimes form a dominant pattern. The vascular network differs from that of fetal-type tumors, in that a fine capillary network and larger vascular channels are present, sometimes forming dilated channels with incomplete endothelial lining (vascular lakes lined by tumor cells; Ishak and Glunz 1967) or pelioid areas. In contrast to fetal tumors, extramedullary hematopoiesis is very rarely observed in embryonal areas. Embryonal tumor tissue exhibits necroses and apoptotic bodies, most marked in chemotherapy-treated tumors.

9.1.4.3 Macrotrabecular Hepatoblastoma: A Distinct Growth Pattern

Gonzalez Crussi and coworkers have described hepatoblastoma areas having a macrotrabecular growth pattern in otherwise typical tumors. Macrotrabecules are 10–20 or more cells thick, resulting in a typical pattern (Fig. 9.3a and b). The cells in the macrotrabecular parts may be fetal, embryonal, or indistinguishable from those of adult-type hepatocellular carcinoma (Gonzalez-Crussi et al. 1982). The macrotrabecular phenotype occurs as a pure form, but may also be mixed with other histologies. It has been proposed that a hepatoblastoma with only an isolated macrotrabecular focus should not be classified as a macrotrabecular subtype (Conran et al. 1992), but the cut-off criteria have not yet been defined.

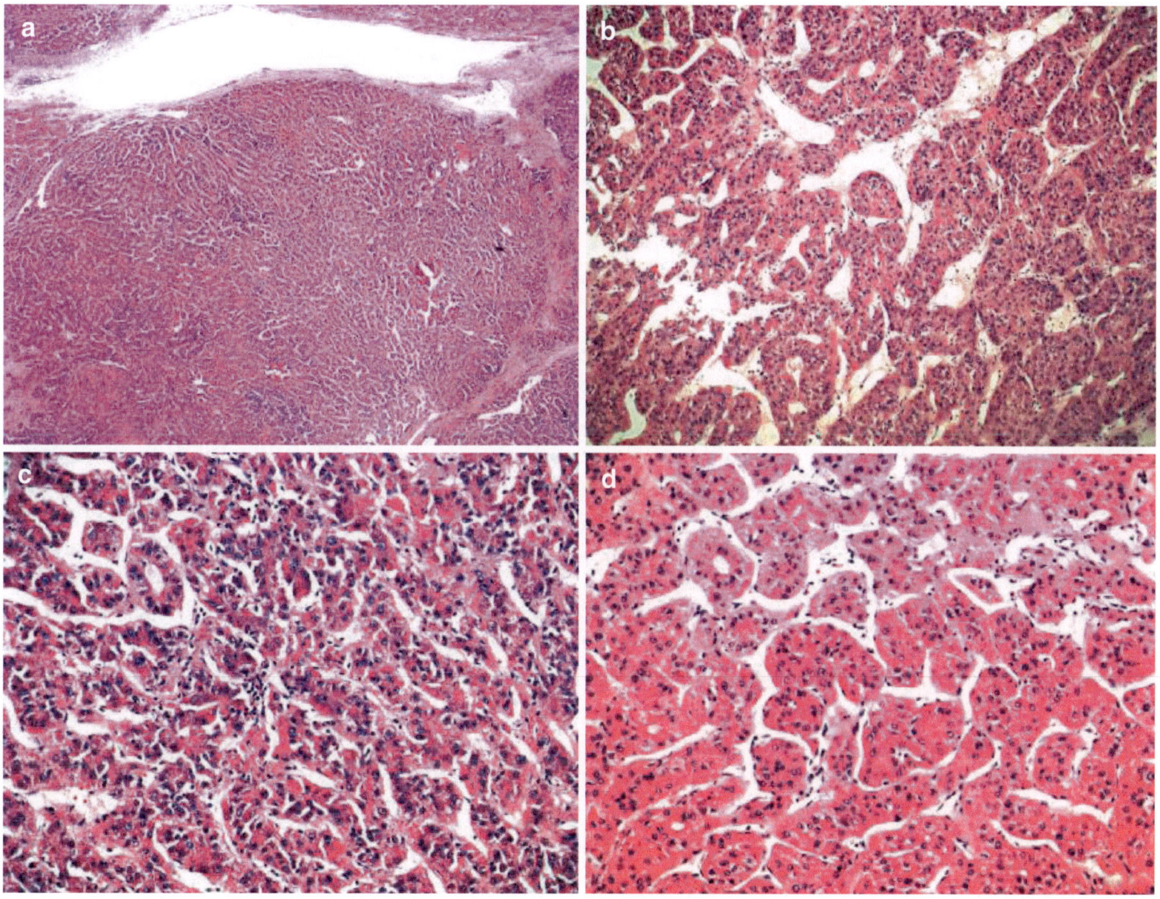

Fig. 9.3 (**a**) Macrotrabecular hepatoblastoma at low magnification. Note the resemblance to hepatocellular carcinoma (hematoxylin and eosin stain). (**b**) The large cell plates (macrotrabecules) are clearly seen in this tumor (Hematoxylin and eosin stain). (**c**) Macrotrabecular hepatoblastoma consisting of embryonal and fetal cells (MT-2; hematoxylin and eosin stain). (**d**) Macrotrabecular hepatoblastoma consisting of hepatocyte-like cells (MT-1; hematoxylin and eosin stain)

Previously, macrotrabecular hepatoblastoma was characterized by a repetitive arrangement of fetal or embryonal cells in macrotrabecules (Haas et al. 1989), but these authors noted that occasionally the tumor cell size may resemble the cells of hepatocellular carcinoma. It has therefore been proposed to divide macrotrabecular hepatoblastomas into two categories (Zimmermann 2005): MT-1 composed of hepatocyte/HCC-like cells (Fig. 9.3d), and MT-2 composed of fetal and/or embryonal cells (Fig. 9.3c).

With regard to the biology of macrotrabecular hepatoblastomas, only two therapy studies have specifically referred to this variant. In the first study of 168 patients with hepatoblastoma, 18 patients had macrotrabecular tumors, and their estimated 24-month survival probability was 50% in comparison with 92%, 63%, and 0% for the purely fetal, embryonal, and small cell undifferentiated histologies, respectively (Haas et al. 1989). In a later second investigation that also identified the macrotrabecular variant, the histology of any type or subtype of hepatoblastoma did not have a significant prognostic effect (Conran et al. 1992). In summary, there are presently too few observations on this subtype to be certain whether it is prognostically unfavorable or not, but it is believed that the MT1 phenotype is a high-risk histology.

9.1.4.4 Undifferentiated Epithelial Hepatoblastomas

This rare subgroup of wholly epithelial hepatoblastomas is characterized by poorly differentiated or undifferentiated (anaplastic) cells cytologically resembling those of other "blue cellular tumors." So far, undifferentiated hepatoblastoma is defined as an aggressive (high-risk) neoplasm composed of small cells, mostly with a diffuse growth pattern (hepatoblastoma, small cell undifferentiated; HB-SCUD). However, this group of tumors is heterogeneous and contains, apart from HB-SCUD, neoplasms with focal expression of anaplasia, tumors with undifferentiated cells of intermediate or large cells rather than small cells, and a subset of lesions, which seem to be related to malignant rhabdoid tumors.

Small Cell Undifferentiated Hepatoblastoma (HB-SCUD)

This neoplasm was originally termed, "anaplastic type," and described as a lesion having small cells resembling those of neuroblastoma (Kasai and Watanabe 1970). However, small undifferentiated round and spindle-shaped cells have been described in hepatoblastoma earlier (Misugi et al. 1967). Haas et al. proposed to replace "anaplasia" by "small cell undifferentiated" (SCUD) (Haas et al. 1989). The small cell cytologic and histologic patterns have since been reported several times, but mostly in small numbers only (Sinniah et al. 1974; Lack et al. 1982; Weinberg and Finegold 1983; Haas et al. 1989; Gonzalez-Crussi 1991; Hansen et al. 1992; Stocker 1994). When the small cell feature is present in a significant proportion of a hepatoblastoma (75%) or as the sole cell type, this tumor subtype is typically found in infants younger than 1 year. The SCUD phenotype can be combined with any other hepatoblastoma types and subtypes. HB-SCUD is a rapidly growing and highly aggressive subtype of hepatoblastoma, with an estimated 2-year patient survival rate probably not exceeding 0% (Haas et al. 1989). Few studies have, however, systematically analyzed the clinical behavior of HB-SCUD, also related to the rarity of this lesion. In a study of completely resected hepatoblastoma, the 38% recurrence rate in tumors with a SCUD histology compared unfavorably with the overall estimated event-free survival rate of 91% for the entire group (Ortega et al. 2000). HB-SCUD is, therefore, one of the phenotypes in the hepatoblastoma family of tumors with an "unfavorable histology."

Histologically, the typical growth pattern of HB-SCUD is diffuse (Fig. 9.4a) or spotty (Fig. 9.4b), with small cells being ovoid, stellate, or spindle-shaped with slight eosinophilia or amphophilia of the poorly developed cytoplasm. The nuclei exhibit a dense chromatin and variably prominent nucleoli (Fig. 9.4c). In silver stains, delicate reticulin fibers surround small to large clusters or sheets of tumor cells, without a distinct pattern.The stroma is usually scanty or lacking. The tumor tends to invade the adjacent liver substance, often with a prominent intravascular growth (Fig. 9.4d), and the neoplastic tissue may engulf preexisting bile ducts and ductules (Haas et al. 1989; Fig. 9.4e). Necrosis may be extensive (Fig. 9.4f). Immunohistochemically, the tumor cells are reactive for vimentin, pankeratin, and cytokeratins 8 (Fig. 9.5a). The proliferative activity is sometimes markedly increased (Fig. 9.5b).Typically, the tumor cells do not usually stain for AFP (with few exceptions; Abenoza et al. 1987), and in fact part of tumors with normal or only slightly elevated serum

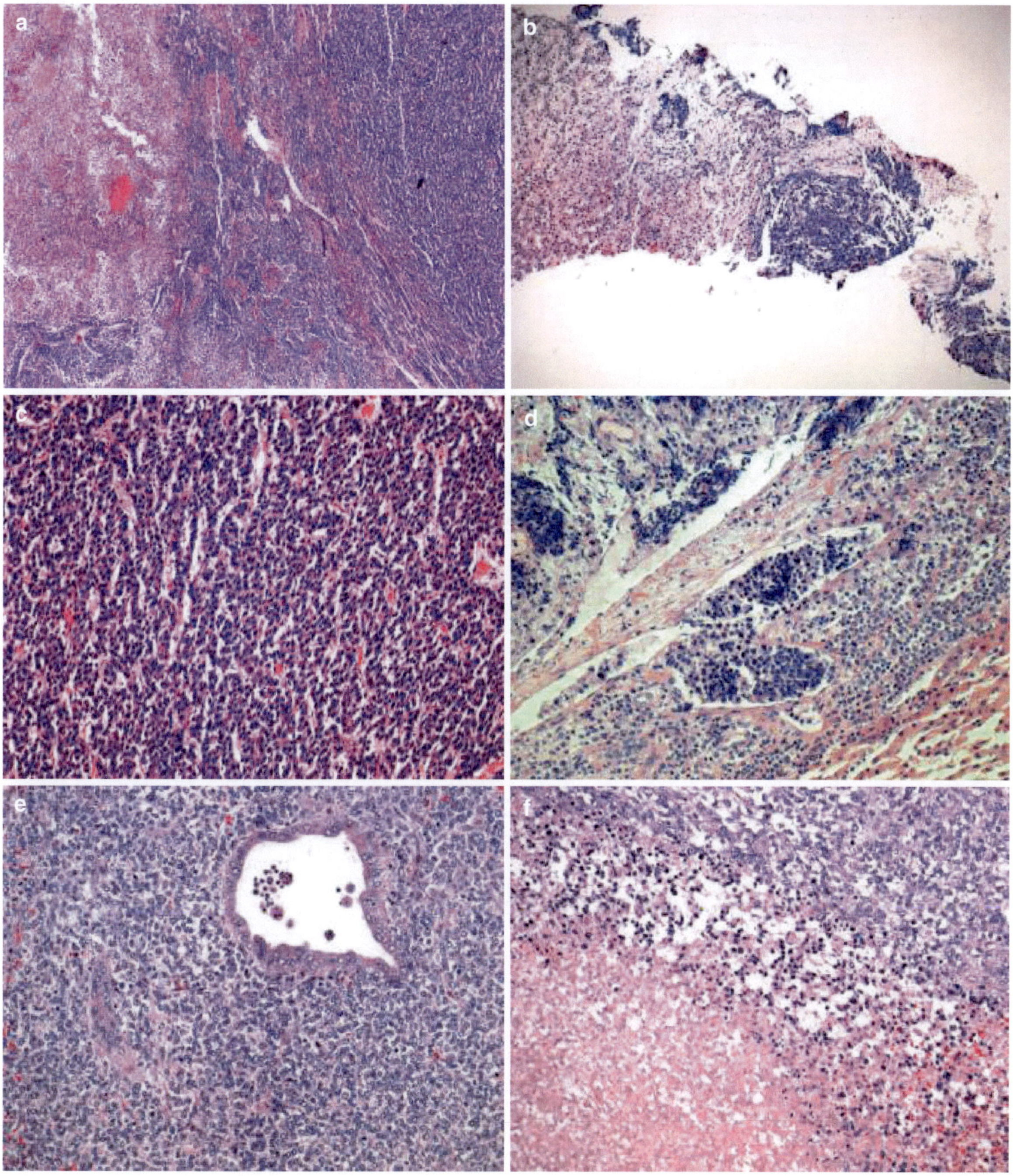

Fig. 9.4 (**a**) Small cell undifferentiated hepatoblastoma, diffuse growth pattern (hematoxylin and eosin stain). (**b**) Small cell undifferentiated hepatoblastoma, spotty growth pattern (ematoxylin and eosin stain). (**c**) Cellular phenotype of small cell undifferentiated hepatoblastoma (hematoxylin and eosin stain). (**d**) Vascular invasion of small cell undifferentiated hepatoblastoma (hematoxylin and eosin stain). (**e**) In this small cell undifferentiated hepatoblastoma, tumor cells have infiltrated the tissue surrounding a bile duct (hematoxylin and eosin stain). (**f**) This tumor has undergone partial necrosis, visualized as an eosinophilic mass with ghost cells (*lower half of figure*) and a zone of damaged cells (hematoxylin and eosin stain)

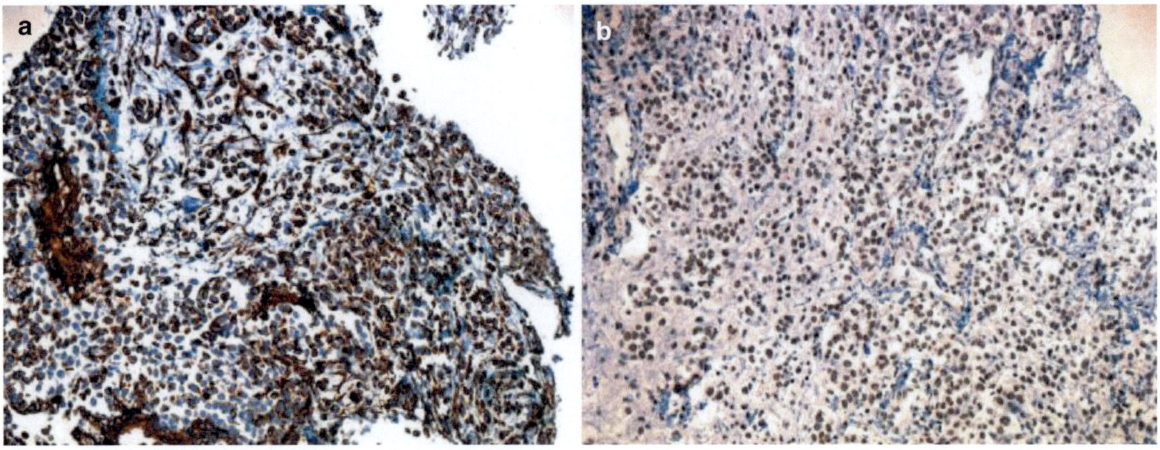

Fig. 9.5 (**a**) Cytokeratin 8 expression in cells of small cell undifferentiated hepatoblastoma (brown reaction product; CK8 immunostain). (**b**) Small cell undifferentiated hepatoblastomas may show high proliferative activity (proliferation marker/Ki-67 immunostain).

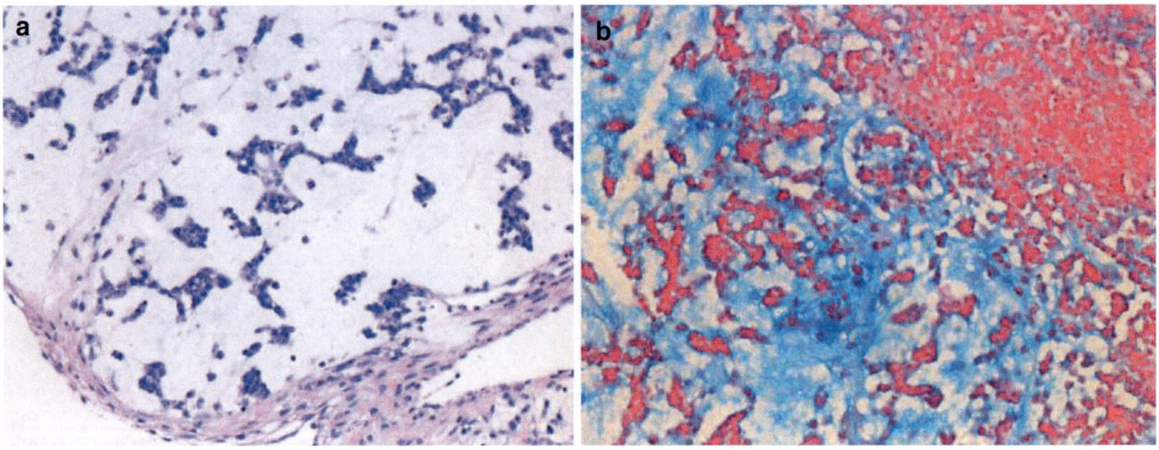

Fig. 9.6 (**a**) Myxoid variant of small cell undifferentiated hepatoblastoma. Note the prominent myxoid (*whitish-blue*) intercellular matrix (hematoxylin and eosin stain). (**b**) The myxoid matrix is rich in glycosaminoglycans (maxtrix in *blue*, tumor cells in *red*; alcaline Alcian blue stain)

AFP and aggressive biology are HB-SCUD (De Ioris et al. 2008). Rare variants of HB-SCUD exhibit a myxoid stroma with large amounts of glycosaminoglycans (Fig. 9.6a and b), sometimes with mucoid microcysts ("mucoid anaplastic hepatoblastoma"; Joshi et al. 1984).

The SCUD phenotype may be focal and associated with fetal- and/or embryonal-type tumor cells; this phenomenon has previously been noted in descriptions of hepatoblastomas (Gonzalez-Crussi et al. 1982). Even incomplete, that is, nondiffuse expression of the SCUD phenotype has been shown to be unfavorable (Douglass et al. 1993; Haas et al. 2001). In a CCG report of 33 patients with Stage I hepatoblastoma, 3/18 patients whose completely resected hepatoblastomas were believed to be of pure fetal histology later developed pulmonary metastases. The histology review showed that all three tumors contained scattered microscopic foci of SCUD histology (Feusner et al. 1993; Haas et al. 2001).

Other Phenotypes of Undifferentiated Hepatoblastoma

Rare cases of undifferentiated hepatoblastomas do not express a small cell phenotype, but are composed of intermediate-sized cells or even large cells (hepatoblastoma, intermediate cell undifferentiated, HB-ICUD; hepatoblastoma, large cell undifferentiated, HB-LCUD; Zimmermann 2005). Medium-sized cells in undifferentiated hepatoblastoma have previously been noted (Lack et al. 1982) and earlier observations of large cells occurring in hepatoblastomas have been described (Weinberg and Finegold 1983). Large cell features associated with aggressive course are also recognized for other blastomas, including large cell medulloblastoma and large cell neuroblastoma. Some large cell hepatoblastomas are CD99-positive, in the absence of any other PNET features (Zimmermann 2005), but CD99 positivity has also been found in other hepatoblastomas (Ramsay et al. 2008).

Undifferentiated Hepatoblastoma with Rhabdoid Features and Malignant Rhabdoid Tumor

At least part of HB-SCUD seems to have a relationship to malignant rhabdoid tumors (MRT), which also occur in the liver (Parham et al. 1994; Scheimberg et al. 1996; Garcés-Inigo et al. 2009). MRT is histologically characterized by sheets of large polygonal cells with abundant cytoplasm and vesicular nuclei with a central prominent nucleolus. Part of the cells discloses the feature of so-called rhabdoid cells (Fig. 9.7a). The rhabdoid cell, which is a hallmark of MRT (although not present in each tumor), has an eosinophilic or amphophilic cytoplasm containing a spheroid perinuclear inclusion body that consists of intermediate filament whorls, and which is immunoreactive for both, epithelial and mesenchymal markers (mainly cytokeratins 8 and 18, and vimentin; Fig. 9.7b). A large subset, if not the majority, of MRTs are characterized by a recurrent deletion of region 11.2 of the long arm of chromosome 22 (22q11.2) and show truncating frameshift or nonsense mutations of INI1, immunohistochemically detectable by the loss of BAF47 reactivity.

In the liver of infants and small children, polyphenotypic tumors may develop, which are difficult to

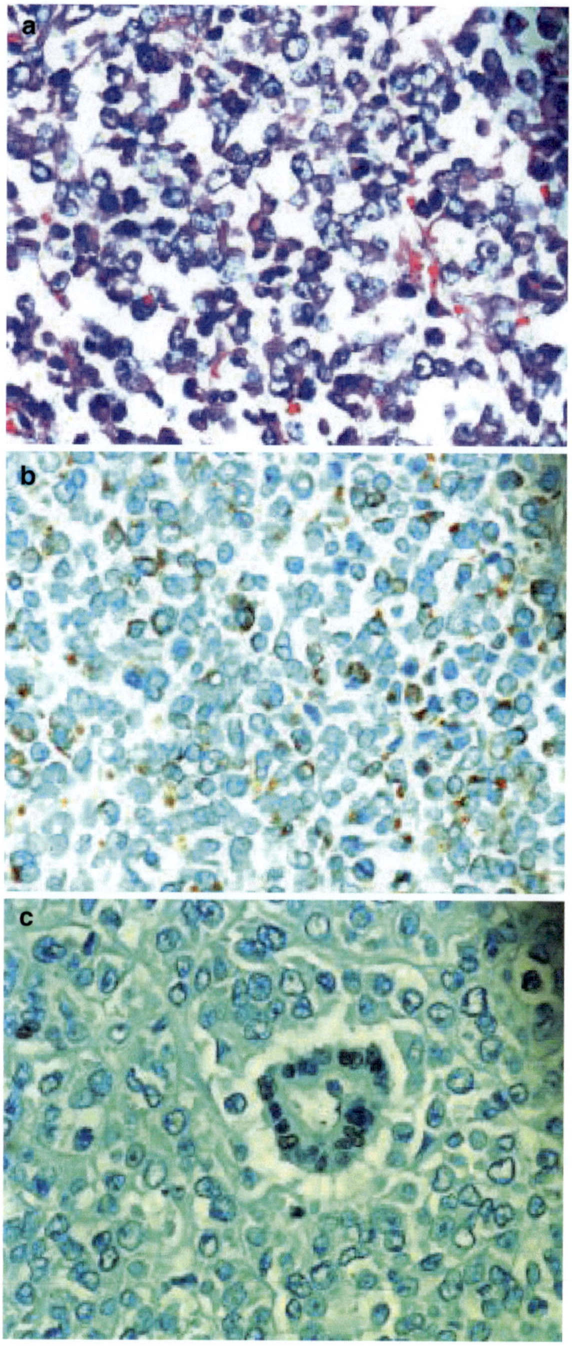

Fig. 9.7 (**a**) Malignant rhabdoid tumor of the liver. Some of the cells display so-called rhabdoid features (hematoxylin and eosin stain). (**b**) Part of the rhabdoid cells show excentric intermediate filament staining (vimentin immunostain). (**c**) Small cell undifferentiated hepatoblastoma with rhabdoid features. Note that the nuclei of a normal bile duct (*center*) stain for INI1, whereas the tumor cells do not (BAF47 immunostain)

allocate to either MRT or undifferentiated hepatoblastoma, because they may share features with both tumor types (Wagner et al. 2007; Russo and Biegel 2009). This constellation has been confirmed in a recent study of 11 patients with hepatoblastomas showing normal or minimally increased serum AFP and a SCUD histology. Ten of these patients died of disease progression, and immunostaining revealed that tumors from six of six patients tested were INI1 negative, suggesting that at least some HB-SCUD cases may actually represent a form of MRTs (Trobaugh-Lotrario et al. 2009). This subset of INI1-negative SCUD tumors may be termed, rhabdoid-like tumors or HB-SCUD with rhabdoid features (Fig. 9.7c). Apart from their diagnostic and clinical relevance, these observations may provide clues for a deeper understanding of pathogenic pathways involved in undifferentiated hepatoblastoma. This issue is further discussed in Chap. 3.

9.1.4.5 Grading of Epithelial Types of Hepatoblastoma

So far, grading of hepatoblastomas or at least of their epithelial components is based on the concept of favorable versus unfavorable histology and still requires more studies. Hepatoblastomas with favorable histology are, in principle, purely fetal, well-differentiated neoplasms with minimal recognizable mitotic activity (see above). The typical unfavorable histology comprises a small cell undifferentiated phenotype with or without associated rhabdoid features, and the malignant rhabdoid tumor itself. The remaining tumor types and subtypes are, provisionally, classified as having "less favorable histopathologies," that is, somewhere in between favorable and unfavorable. Probably, the deeper analysis of large studies will clarify this situation.

9.1.4.6 Mixed Epithelial and Mesenchymal Hepatoblastomas

This type of hepatoblastoma was described in detail in 1967 by use of the terms, epithelial and mesenchymal type or mixed hepatoblastoma (19 out of 35 analyzed hepatoblastomas; Ishak and Glunz 1967). This form of hepatoblastoma is characterized by a complex mixture of epithelial lineages and an immature-looking mesenchyme making part of the tumor itself rather than representing a stromal reaction. Later it was recognized that some of these tumors may contain heterologous components resembling those found in a teratoma. This is the reason why new classifications distinguish mixed hepatoblastomas with or without teratoid features.

Mixed Epithelial and Mesenchymal Hepatoblastoma Without Teratoid Features

This is the more common variant. Typically, the epithelial component is either fetal or mixed fetal-embryonal. In addition to the connective tissue following the vascular tree or forming septa there are areas of a primitive, sometimes hypercellular mesenchyme intimately admixed with the tumor epithelia. The cells forming this mesenchyme are spindle-shaped (sometimes fibroblastoid) or stellate, with delicate processes and elongated, inconspicuous nuclei. The cytoplasm is scanty. The extracellular matrix contains reticulin fibers and sometimes a myxoid alcianophilic substance. Foci of osteoid with or without mineralization are often seen (Fig. 9.8a). The cells within this tumor osteoid are indistinguishable from osteoblasts, but also stain for epithelial markers in addition to vimentin (cytokeratins). Bone formation may occur in metastases of hepatoblastomas, sometimes indistinguishable from osteosarcoma (Weinberg and Finegold 1983). Cartilage tissue seems to occur in mixed hepatoblastoma (review: Pang 1961), but true (hyaline) cartilaginous tissue is probably not common; it was not noted by Ishak and Glunz (1967) and was observed in the large SIOPEL pathology review only once. Mixed tumors may contain foci of squamous epithelia with formation of concentric pearls. They can express keratohylaine granules, sometimes with marked keratinization and a foreign body reaction with giant cells (Ishak and Glunz 1967).

Mixed Epithelial and Mesenchymal Hepatoblastoma with Teratoid Features

These are mixed hepatoblastomas, which reveal multiple lines of cell and tissue differentiation in addition to

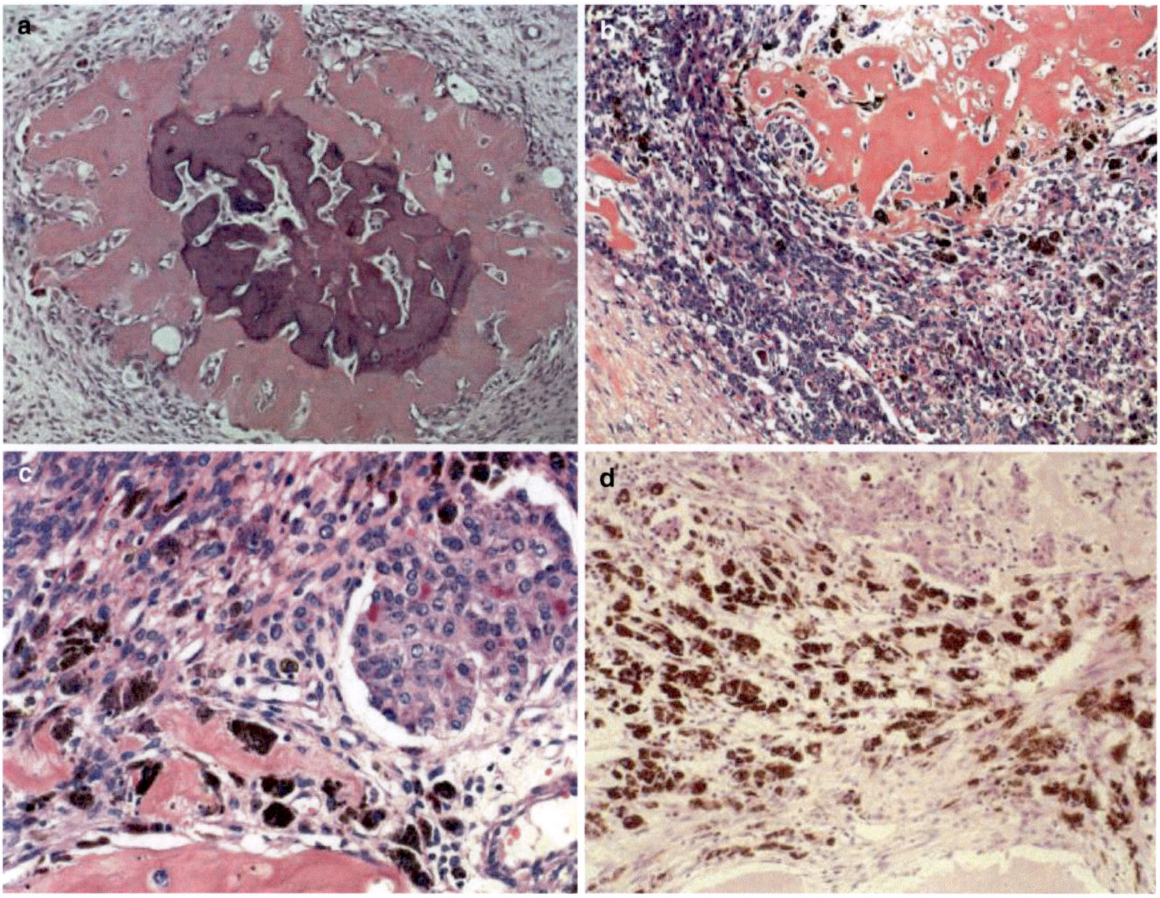

Fig. 9.8 (**a**) Osteoid formation in mixed epithelial and mesenchymal hepatoblastoma (hematoxylin and eosin stain). (**b**) In this mixed epithelial and mesenchymal hepatoblastoma, cells in epithelium and in osteoid contain melanin (*brown*), a feature of the teratoid variant (hematoxylin and eosin stain). (**c**) Melanin formation at higher magnification (hematoxylin and eosin stain). (**d**) Tumor necrosis in melanotic teratoid hepatoblastoma causes accumulation of melanin in macrophages (phagocytosis of melanosomes; hematoxylin and eosin stain)

immature mesenchyme, myoid cell lineages, and osteoid tissue. These so-called teratoid lines include intestinal or mucinous epithelium, melanin-containing cells, endocrine elements, immature striated muscle cells, and glioneural tissue (Watanabe et al. 1975; Manivel et al. 1986; Abenoza et al. 1987; Conran et al. 1992; Kim et al. 2001). It is noteworthy that the first pediatric osteoid-containing liver tumor was described in 1898 under the term, teratoma hepatis (Misick 1898), but the term, teratoid hepatoblastoma, was coined in 1986 (Manivel et al. 1986) and is now frequently replaced by the term proposed by the SIOPEL classification, that is, mixed epithelial and mesenchymal hepatoblastoma with teratoid features. This subtype of hepatoblastoma has no connection with teratomas, which are germ cell tumors, but there are very rare instances where teratoid hepatoblastoma occurs together with true hepatic teratoma (Conrad et al. 1993) or with yolk sac tumor (Cross and Variend 1992).

Teratoid hepatoblastomas exhibit the same epithelial components as other hepatoblastomas and they often also contain osteoid, sometimes in an excessive manner (Schlecht et al. 1996). "Teratoid" epithelia come as mucinous or goblet cell formations resembling intestinal or bronchial linings and neuroepithelium. Smooth and striated muscle cells may occur, but are rare. Glioneural components are characterized by a fibrillary glial matrix immunostaining for glial fibrillary acidic protein. Well-differentiated ganglionic cells may be seen. Melanin-containing cells are sometimes prominent (melanotic hepatoblastoma; Fig. 9.8b and c); they contain densely packed melanosomes and are immunoreactive for the marker, HMB45. Melanin-containing granules are also present in neoplastic epithelial cells and are sometimes observed in osteoblast-like cells located within osteoid (Fig. 9.8b) and in macrophages (Fig. 9.8d). Endocrine/neuroendocrine differentiation can occur in teratoid hepatoblastoma (Ruck and Kaiserling 1993). In contrast to other hepatoblastoma types and subtypes, teratoid components are negative for glypican 3 expression (Zynger et al. 2008). Neuroendocrine components and melanin-containing cells seem to be more resistant to chemotherapy than epithelial lineages (Forouhar et al. 1984), but it is not known whether this has an impact for prognosis.

9.1.5 Immunohistochemistry of Hepatoblastomas

The immunohistochemical assessment of hepatoblastomas is a somewhat problematic issue, because these neoplasms display variable immunophenotypes, can express antigens seen in other pediatric malignancies, and hence do not possess a distinct immunohistochemical profile (Ramsay et al. 2008).

Hepatoblastomas express the cytokeratins of hepatocyte lineages, that is, cytokeratins 8 and 18 (Abenoza et al. 1987; Van Eyken et al. 1990; Ramsay et al. 2008). Also the osteoblastoid/osteocytoid cells located within osteoid of mixed hepatoblastomas express cytokeratins 7, 8, and 18 (Van Eyken et al. 1990). The higher differentiation status of fetal-type cells, with production of a canalicular domain, is shown by positivity for polyclonal CEA (Fasano et al. 1998), and by a difference of claudin expression in comparison with embryonal-type tissue (Halasz et al. 2006). Alpha-fetoprotein (AFP) is long known to be expressed in about half of hepatoblastomas (Abenoza et al. 1987; Ramsay et al. 2008), but is consistently lacking in HB-SCUD. In a systemtic study, AFP was detected in about half of the cases of hepatoblastoma (Ramsay et al. 2008).

As outlined elsewhere, hepatoblastomas and related tumors exhibit abnormalities of the Wnt/beta-catenin signaling pathway (Buendia 2002; Yamaoka et al. 2006; Lopez-Terrada et al. 2009a; Fig. 9.9a–c). Subsequent to mutations in the beta-catenin (CTNNB1) gene, beta-catenin bypassing the proteasomal degradation pathway is translocated to the nucleus, where it

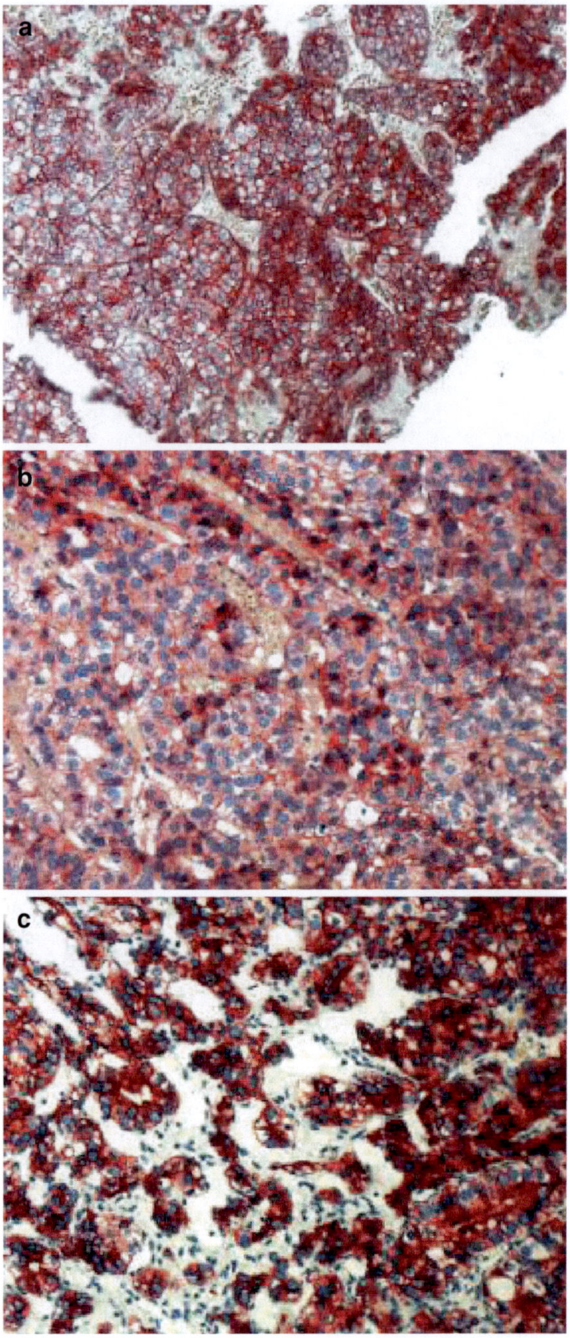

Fig. 9.9 (**a**) Fetal hepatoblastoma with membranous expression of beta-catenin (in *red*; beta-catenin immunostain). (**b**) This hepatoblastoma in part shows cytoplasmic beta-catenin expression (beta-catenin immunostain). (**c**) In addition to cytoplasmic expression, this tumor displays nuclear reactivity for beta-catenin, indicating beta-catenin gene mutation (beta-catenin immunostain)

can be detected by immunohistochemistry, mainly in less differentiated cells (Wei et al. 2000; Yamaoka et al. 2006), a phenomenon which is an important prognostic marker in hepatoblastoma (Park et al. 2001) and is associated with overexpression of cyclin D1 and fibronectin and poorly differentiated histology in hepatoblastoma (Takayasu et al. 2001).

Hepatoblastomas can express glypican 3 (GPC3; mutated in the Simpson-Golabi-Behmel tissue overgrowth syndrome), one of the six known members of a heparin sulfate proteoglycan anchored to the cell membrane and detected in hepatic stem cells and being one of the most overexpressed genes in hepatoblastoma by microarray analysis (Luo et al. 2006). In a study of 65 hepatoblastomas, all cases had cytoplasmic immunoreactivity for GPC3 with greater than 90% of cases showing strong and diffuse positivity. GPC3 was present in epithelial lineages (including the small cell undifferentiated subtype), but not in mesenchymal or teratoid components (Zynger et al. 2008).

A subset of hepatoblastomas expresses human choriogonadotropins (hCG) in the tumor cells, clinically causing virilization and precocious puberty (Behrle et al. 1963; review: Nakagawara et al. 1982). Expression of hCG may be associated with concomitant secretion of AFP (Nakagawara et al. 1985). These two markers showed a discordant behavior of the plasma levels during chemotherapy and radiotherapy in two patients (Hung et al. 1963; Braunstein et al. 1972) and a concordant behavior in one (Kumar et al. 1978). Interestingly, one study uncovered that all out of seven hCG-producing hepatoblastomas showed hCG expression in multinucleated syncytiotrophoblast-like giant cells accompanied by round and clear cells with squamous metaplasia, suggesting a choriocarcinoma lineage (Watanabe et al. 1987). Another hormone that may exceptionally be produced by hepatoblastoma is renin, associated with hyperreninemia and hypertension (Moritake et al. 2000).

9.1.6 Growth Patterns, Proliferation, and Differentiation Characteristics in Hepatoblastomas

Hepatoblastomas show various growth patterns. One which is crucial for outcome is angioinvasion that may extensively involve tumor-associated vessels (Fig. 9.10a), small vessels in portal tracks (Fig. 9.10b), and larger veins, including the portal vein (Fig. 9.10c) and branches thereof (Fig. 9.10d). Apart from components of the invasive machinery, these growth patterns require distinct proliferation features. There is a significant association between the histologic type, DNA content, and proliferation, in that fetal tissue is diploid, embryonal tissue is aneuploid, and the proliferative index is higher in embryonal cells than in fetal cells (Rugge et al. 1998; Zerbini et al. 1998; Tsai et al. 2009). The proliferation is commonly lowest in the fetal phenotype (Rugge et al. 1998; Tsai et al. 2009). The proliferative activity of hepatoblastomas has been found to be lower in low stage tumors than in stages III and IV, and was higher in metastases than in primary tumors (Ara et al. 1997).

Among cell cycle regulators, cyclins and cyclin-dependent kinase inhibitors (CDKNs) are in part deregulated in hepatoblastomas (Gray et al. 2000). Cyclin D1 acts as a switch at the G1-S checkpoint, and a polymorphism of codon 242 of the cyclin D1 gene affects the age of onset of hepatoblastoma (Pakakasama et al. 2004). It has been found that CDKN2A, CDKN2B, and CDKN2C genes are structurally unmodified in these tumors, whereas CDKN2A, normally silenced in the liver, and CDKN2C are expressed in hepatoblastoma, and cyclin D exhibits a shift in expression (Iolascon et al. 1998). Expression of the cyclin-dependent kinase inhibitor, p27(KIP1) is generally decreased in more aggressive tumors and this has also been found to play a role in hepatoblastoma. P27(KIP1) is not mutated in hepatoblastoma but shows increased transcriptional activity (Hartmann et al. 2000). Well-differentiated low-proliferative fetal tumors markedly express p27, embryonal patterns show a variable expression (less in proliferative areas), and most small cell hepatoblastomas do not express p27 (Brotto and Finegold 2002). Continuous growth of hepatoblastomas is also mediated by high expression of spindle checkpoint kinases, specifically Polo-like kinase 1 (PLK1), being a poor-prognosis indicator (Yamada et al. 2004). The Wnt/beta-catenin signaling pathway, which plays a role in the pathogenesis of hepatoblastoma, affects proliferation and growth, in that stabilized beta-catenin promotes hepatocyte proliferation and inhibits TNFalpha-induced apoptosis (Shang et al. 2004), and is associated with overexpression of cyclin D1 in hepatoblastomas (Takayasu et al. 2001).

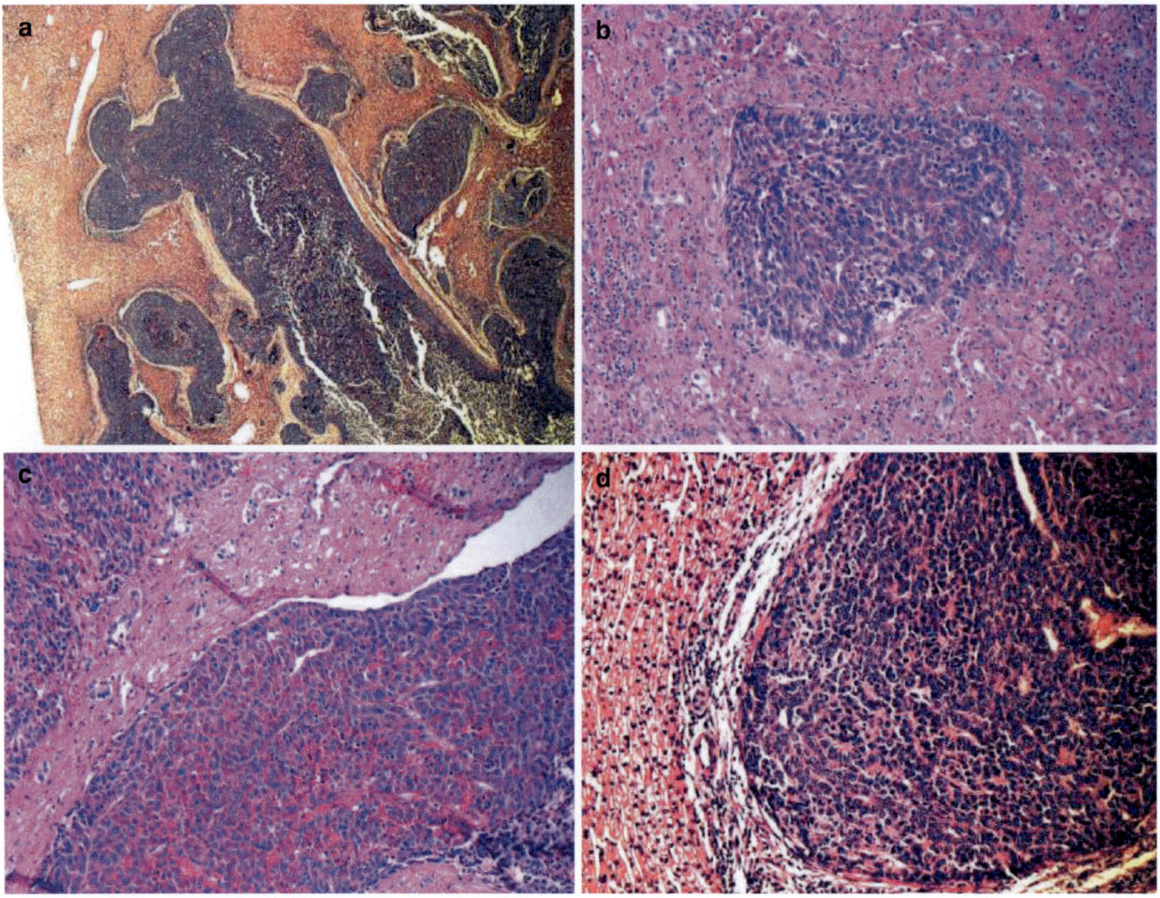

Fig. 9.10 (**a**) This hepatoblastoma exhibits massive angioinvasion with formation of tumor plugs (hematoxylin and eosin stain). (**b**) Hepatoblastoma angioinvasion in small portal tract vessels (hematoxylin and eosin stain). (**c**) Invasion of the portal vein, with formation of a tumor thrombus. The wall of the vein (*pink*) is seen to the left and above the center (hematoxylin and eosin stain). (**d**) Obturation of a small portal vein branch by hepatoblastoma (hematoxylin and eosin stain)

Growth regulation of hepatoblastomas involves the insulin-like growth factor-II (IGF2) signaling pathway (Li et al. 1995; Rainier et al. 1995; Yun et al. 1998; Tomizawa and Saisho 2006). IGF2 is a maternally imprinted gene and encodes a fetal peptide hormone that regulates cell proliferation, differentiation, and cell migration. IGF2 acts via binding to the type 1 IGF tyrosine kinase receptor (IGF-1R). IGF2 is expressed in hepatoblastomas and this expression is inversely correlated with the degree of differentiation, lacking in fetal-type cells and being high in embryonal-type cells (Akmal et al. 1995).The allelic expression of IGF2 is regulated by the methylation status of a distinct site (CTCF) in the H19 gene differentially methylated region (DMR) that represents the parental origin of the IGF2 allele: in normal tissues, the maternal allele is unmethylated, whereas the paternal CTCF site is methylated. The maternally expressed H19 gene belongs to an imprinted cluster on chromosome 11p15 and encodes a noncoding mRNA, which controls the expression of the neighboring, paternally transcribed IGF2 gene. Hepatoblastomas show monoallelic expression of H19 (Ross et al. 2000). Loss of imprinting of IGF2 in hepatoblastomas correlates with hypermethylation of the H19 region (Honda et al. 2008), and there is a high frequency of inactivation of H19 in sporadic hepatoblastomas (Fukuzawa et al. 1999). In hepatoblastoma, the IGF2/IGF-IR pathway is interacting with PLAG1, a developmentally regulated zinc finger transcription factor, which positively regulates IGF2 (Van Dyck et al. 2007), and which is overexpressed in hepatoblastomas (Zatkova et al. 2004).

9.1.7 Chemotherapy Effects in Hepatoblastomas

Hepatoblastomas treated by chemotherapy undergo complex changes that may mimic or obscure viable tumor persistence, rendering interpretation of post-chemotherapy resection specimens sometimes difficult (Lowichik et al. 2000).

The main chemotherapy-induced tumor changes comprise necrosis, apoptosis, and inflammatory/immune reactions directed against decaying tumor, fibrosis, vascular changes, and cellular alterations of residual (viable) tumor. Macroscopically, treated tumors appear contracted and nodular, more sharply delineated than native lesions (Fig. 9.11a). Histologically, most of the former tumor usually consists of a fibrous tissue. Often these fibrotic areas are present in the form of nodular hypocellular structures containing blood vessels and old hemorrhage (Fig. 9.11b). It is assumed that the shape of these structures reflects the previous vascular tree of the tumor. Chemotherapy-induced necrosis presents as an eosinophilic and slightly granular mass (Fig. 9.11c), which is sharply demarcated from the adjacent liver by granulation and fibrous tissue containing macrophages and lymphocytes, and sometimes foreign body giant cells. Focal

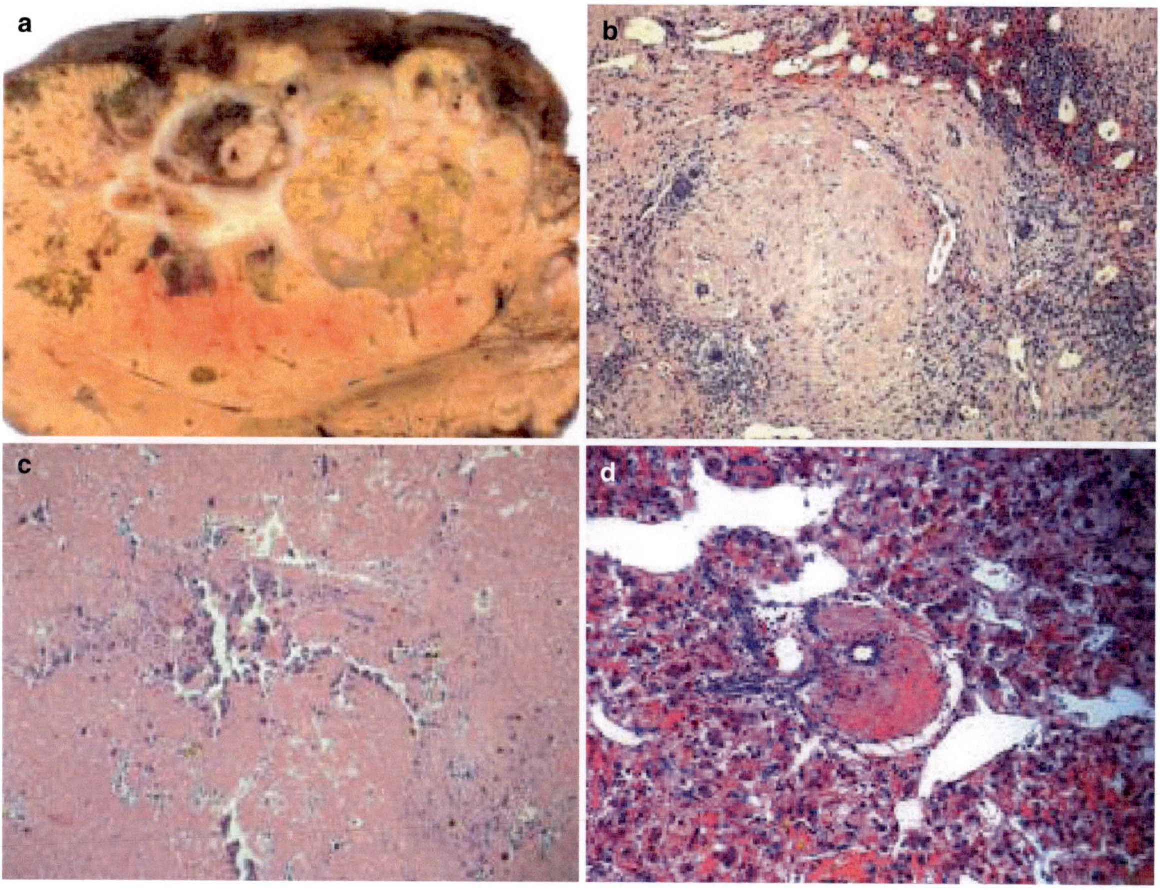

Fig. 9.11 (**a**) Macroscopic features of resected hepatoblastoma post-chemotherapy (cut surface). The tumor appears contracted, consists of yellowish nodules, and reveals white areas of fibrosis/scarring. (**b**) Nodular areas of fibrosis and perifocal liver atrophy after chemotherapy (hematoxylin and eosin stain). (**c**) Hepatoblastoma with post-chemotherapy necrosis (hematoxylin and eosin stain). (**d**) Chemotherapy-induced vascular change with marked thickening of the vessel wall and vascular stenosis (*center*; hematoxylin and eosin stain). (**e**) Marked fatty change of fetal hepatoblastoma after chemotherapy (hematoxylin and eosin stain). (**f**) Prominent cellular and nuclear atypia in hepatoblastoma after chemotherapy (hematoxylin and eosin stain). (**g**) Post-chemotherapy hepatoblastoma rich in osteoid. The nature of the small epithelial focus to the left of the red osteoid (residual tumor vs. atrophic liver) is difficult to assess (hematoxylin and eosin stain). (**h**) Several foci of squamous epithelium after chemotherapy of hepatoblastoma (hematoxylin and eosin stain)

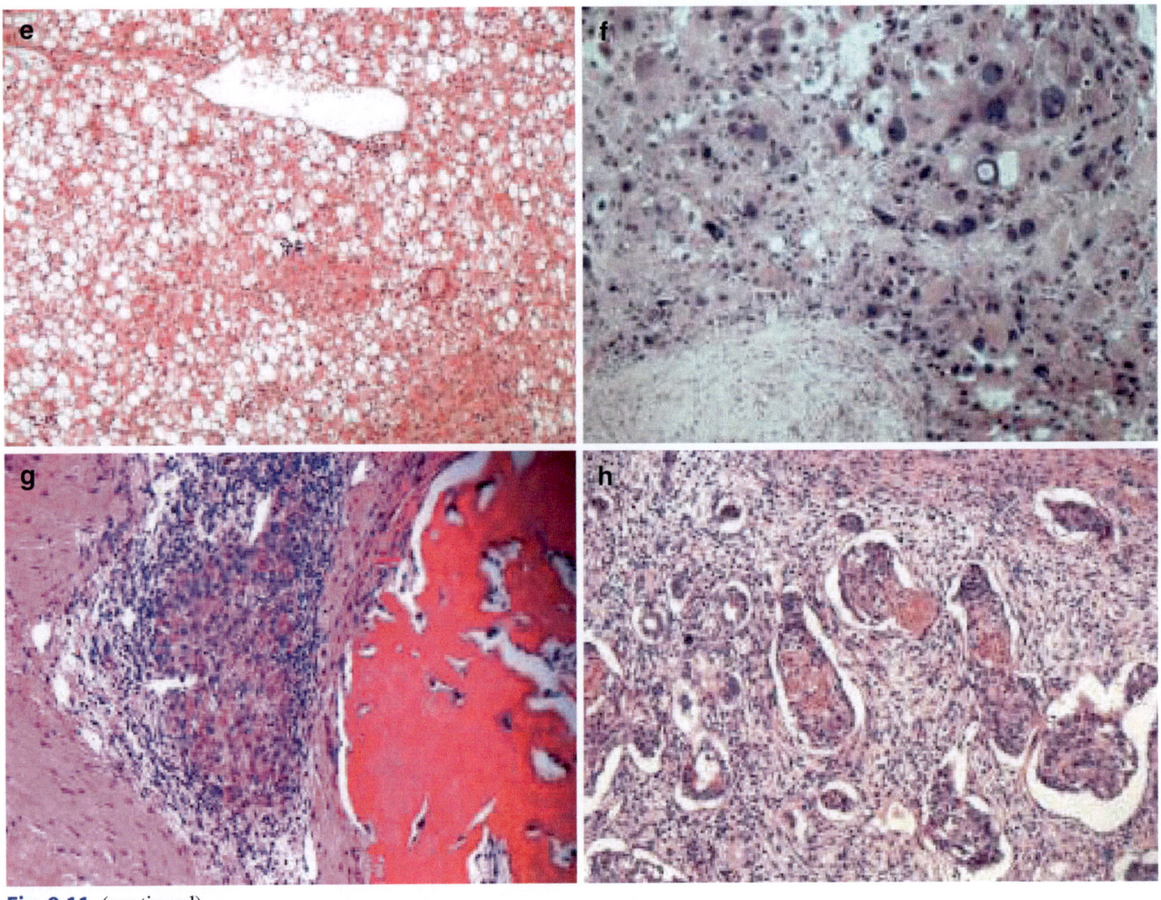

Fig. 9.11 (continued)

calcifications/mineralizations may be seen.In a study of 17 hepatoblastomas treated with preoperative chemotherapy, there was no obvious correlation between the extent of necrosis and the number of courses of chemotherapy (Saxena et al. 1993). In some cases, necroses contain clusters of epithelial-like cells that are very difficult to identify in regard to their nature, so that the question as to residual viable tumor should be answered with great caution. Chemotherapy induces marked vascular changes, characterized by thickening of the vessel wall and vascular stenosis (Fig. 9.11d). Fetal hepatoblastoma may undergo marked steatosis subsequent to chemotherapy (Fig. 9.11e). Therapy-associated cellular and nuclear anomalies of viable tumor may render the classification of the residual tumor impossible (Fig. 9.11f). A notable feature in tumors treated with chemotherapy is the extensive presence of osteoid (Fig. 9.11g). In a comparative study, osteoid was present in 36% of untreated cases, occupying less than 5% of the surface area, compared with 82% in the treated group (Saxena et al. 1993). Whether this phenomenon reflects a distinct effect of chemotherapy (Heifetz et al. 1997) or is caused by other factors, including sampling effects, has not yet been clarified. Keratinizing squamous epithelia are a typical chemotherapy effect (Fig. 9.11h).

Several post-chemotherapy histological features apparently having an impact on outcome have been described in hepatoblastoma. They comprise vascular invasion in the tumor capsule (risk factor for subsequent metastatic disease), necrosis greater than 75% (favorable prognostic indicator), and increased proliferative activity in residual tumor (poor prognostic indicator). No reproducible effects were found for marked osteoid production, fibroblastic proliferation around necrosis, and intimal thickening, occlusion or hyalinosis of blood vessels (review: Lowichik et al. 2000).

9.1.8 Cholangioblastic Hepatoblastoma (Hepatoblastomas with Cholangioblastic Features) and "Ductal Plate Tumors"

A small subset of hepatoblastomas exhibits, mostly at the periphery of the otherwise typical hepatoblast formations, cytokeratin 19-positive bile duct cells and even duct-like profiles in a focal distribution pattern (Fig. 9.12a) (Zimmermann 2002; Libbrecht et al. 2003). As these biliary epithelial cells are remote from preexisting ductular and ductal cells of the host liver, but rather constitute part of the tumor itself, these lesions have been proposed to be termed, hepatoblastoma with cholangioblastic features or cholangioblastic hepatoblastoma (Zimmermann 2002, 2005). The cholangioblastic features may not be recognizable with ease in conventional sections, but immunostaining for cholangiocyte lineage markers will uncover the cells of interest (Fig. 9.12b). In other situations, organoid tumors reveal numerous and small nodules consisting of immature hepatoid cells, encircled by a thin rim of biliary cells and sometimes with slits resulting in a double layer of cholangiocytes mimicking an abnormal ductal plate (so-called "ductal plate tumor"; Gornicka et al. 2001; Zimmermann 2002; Fig. 9.12c). So far, cholangioblastic features have predominantly been detected in fetal-type and embryonal-hepatoblastoma, but the proportion of tumors exhibting these features and the prognostic impact of this change have not been elucidated so far.

9.1.9 Transitional Liver Cell Tumor (TLCT)

Transitional liver cell tumor (TLCT) is a recently described malignant liver cell neoplasm that chiefly occurs in older children and young adolescents (Prokurat et al. 2002). TLCTs have a rather characteristic clinical presentation, histopathology, immunohistochemistry, and treatment response. The tumors are highly aggressive and usually present as large neoplasms associated with high or very high serum AFP levels. Most of the lesions reported so far were initially diagnosed as hepatoblastoma in needle biopsies, and the histology was later reviewed owing to the very unfavorable outcome after chemotherapy designed for hepatoblastoma. Histologically, TLCT have a rather complex pattern, with hepatoblastoma-like cells, cells resembling those of HCC, and intermediate cell

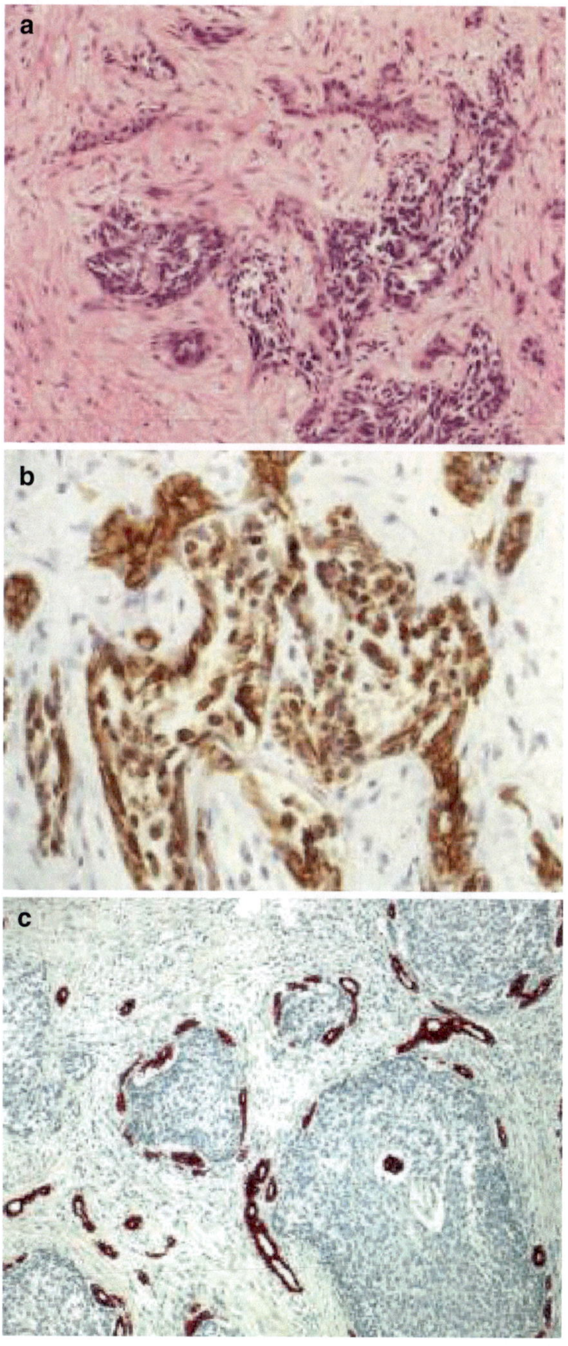

Fig. 9.12 (**a**) Hepatoblastoma with cholangioblastic features. Note the bile duct-like profiles in close association with hepatoblastoma cells (hematoxylin and eosin stain). (**b**) In this cholangioblastic hepatoblastoma, numerous cells are reactive for a bile duct cell marker (cytokeratin 19 immunostain). (**c**) Ductal plate tumor consists of small hepatoid nodules ("liverlets") associated with cholangiocellular profiles mimicking components of a ductal plate (the latter in *red*; cytokeratin 19 immunostain)

forms (Fig. 9.13a). Multinucleated giant cells are a typical feature (Fig. 9.13b). The cellular features of larger cells vary from cholangiocyte-like elements (Fig. 9.13c) to immature hepatoid cells (Fig. 9.13d). A biliary phenotype is visualized by epithelial membrane antigen (EMA) staining (Fig. 9.13e). Part of the tumors express beta-catenin, with a mixed nuclear and cytoplasmic expression pattern (Fig. 9.13f). The term, transitional, has been proposed based on the hypothesis that the relevant tumor cell might be located between a hepatoblast and a hepatocyte, but this has to be analyzed in greater depth in the future, and also with molecular methods.

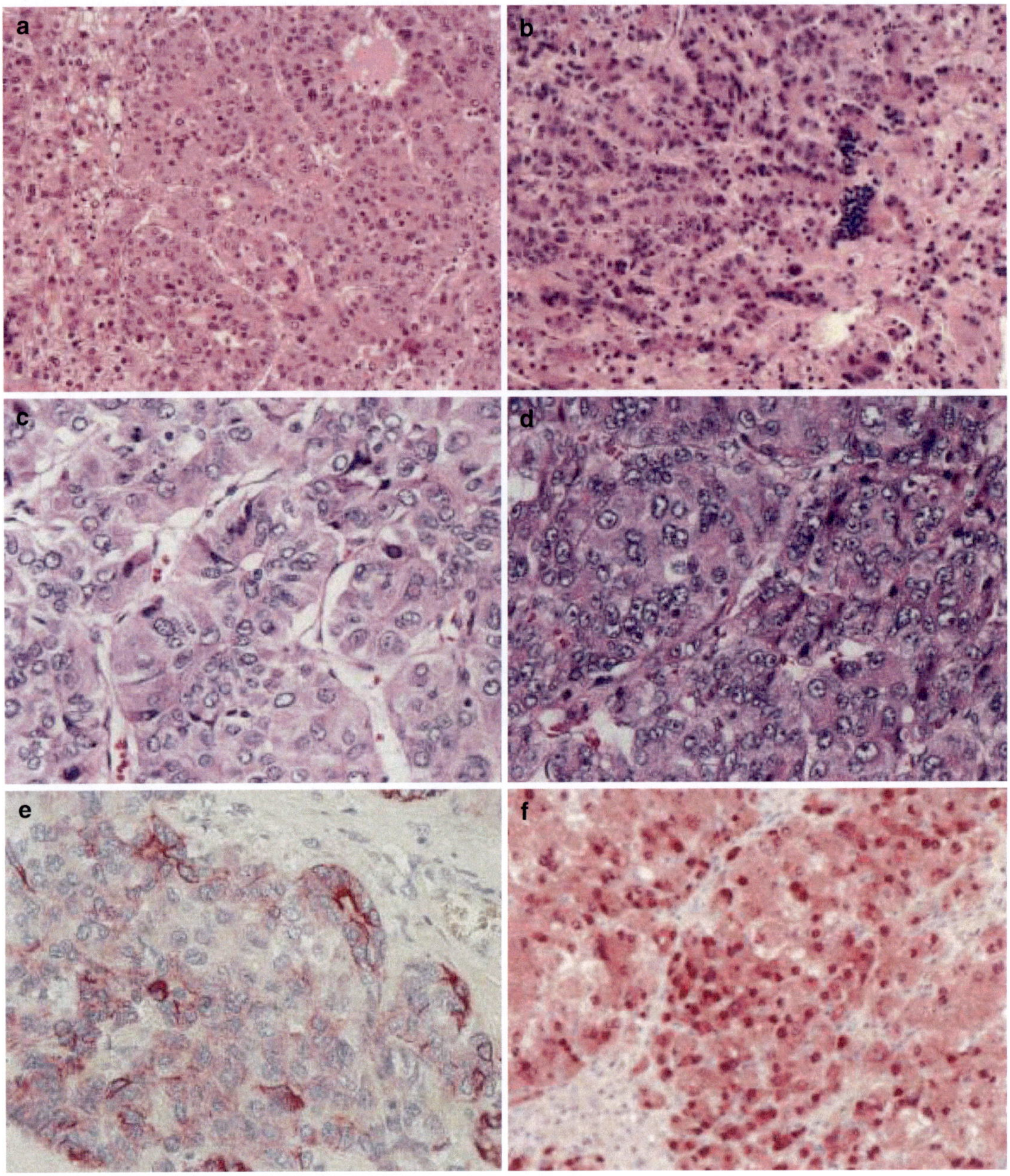

Fig. 9.13 (**a**) Transitional liver cell tumor consisting of hepatoblastoma-like cells and larger cells (hematoxylin and eosin stain). (**b**) Transitional liver cell tumors frequently show multinucleated giant cells (hematoxylin and eosin stain). (**c**) This transitional liver cell tumor exhibits cholangiocyte-like cells (hematoxylin and eosin stain). (**d**) Transitional liver cell tumor with large and poorly differentiated hepatoid cells (hematoxylin and eosin stain). (**e**) The cholangiocyte lineage in this transitional liver cell tumor is visualized by focal positivity for epithelial membrane antigen (reactivity in red; EMA immunostain). (**f**) Nuclear and cytoplasmic expression of beta-catenin in transitional liver cell tumor (reactivity in red; beta-catenin immunostain)

9.1.10 Tumors Possibly Related to the Hepatoblastoma Tumor Family

Within pathology reviews of large international prospective studies on pediatric liver tumors, most of the neoplasms are classifiable, but a minority of the lesions will not fit into known categories and may, therefore, be classified as NOS (not otherwise specified) until a precise nosological assignment is possible. In addition, there are novel tumor entities that seem to share certain features with hepatoblastomas, although the exact relation between the lesions is not yet known. According to this author's view, one of these tumors may be nested stromal epithelial tumor of the liver (Heerema-McKenney et al. 2005; Meir et al. 2009; Rod et al. 2009), also termed desmoplastic nested spindle cell tumor of the liver (Hill et al. 2005). This is a hepatic neoplasm in infants and older children and in young adolescents, associated with Cushing syndrome in some of the patients and with a variable course, one patient so far showing recurrence and extrahepatic metastasis (Brodsky et al. 2008). Histologically, nests of epithelial-like cells surrounded by spindle cells showing calcifications and osteoid are a hallmark (Fig. 9.14a and b). The epithelial cells express cytokeratin 8 (Fig. 9.14c), but not a hepatocyte marker, Hep Par1 (Fig. 9.14d). Interestingly, the nested cells

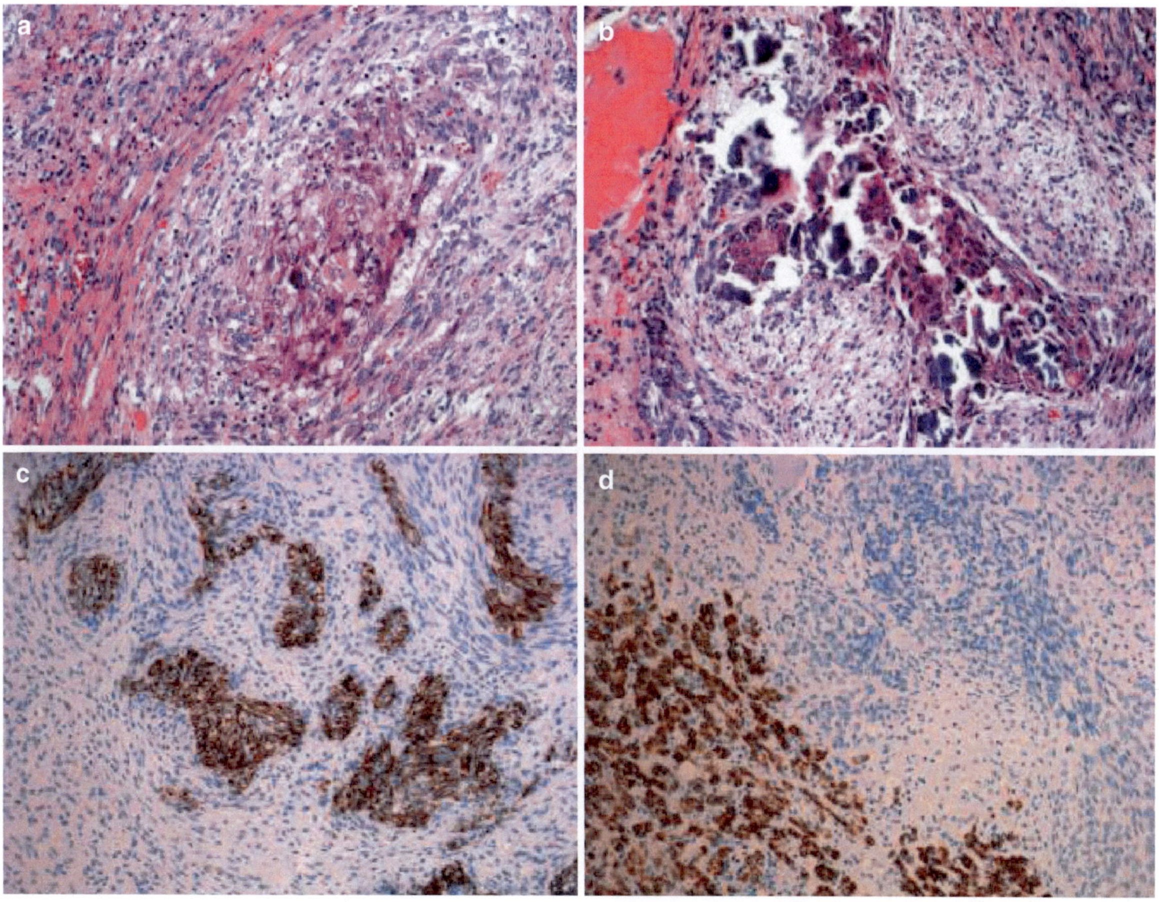

Fig. 9.14 (**a**) Epithelial cell clusters surrounded by spindle cells in nested stromal epithelial tumor of the liver (hematoxylin and eosin stain). (**b**) The nested structures may contain psammomatous calcifications and osteoid (hematoxylin and eosin stain). (**c**) Epithelia of the nested structures are positive for cytokeratin (reactivity in *brown*; cytokeratin 8 immunostain). (**d**) Normal hepatic parenchymal cells express the hepatocyte marker, Hep Par 1 (*brown; left bottom corner*), In contrast, epithelia of nested structures (to the right and top) are negative (Hep Par 1 immunostain). (**e**) Beta-catenin reactivity (in part nuclear) in nested stromal epithelial tumor (beta-catenin immunostain). (**f**) The spindle cells surrounding the epithelial clusters are positive for alpha-smooth muscle actin (*brown*; alphaSMA immunostain)

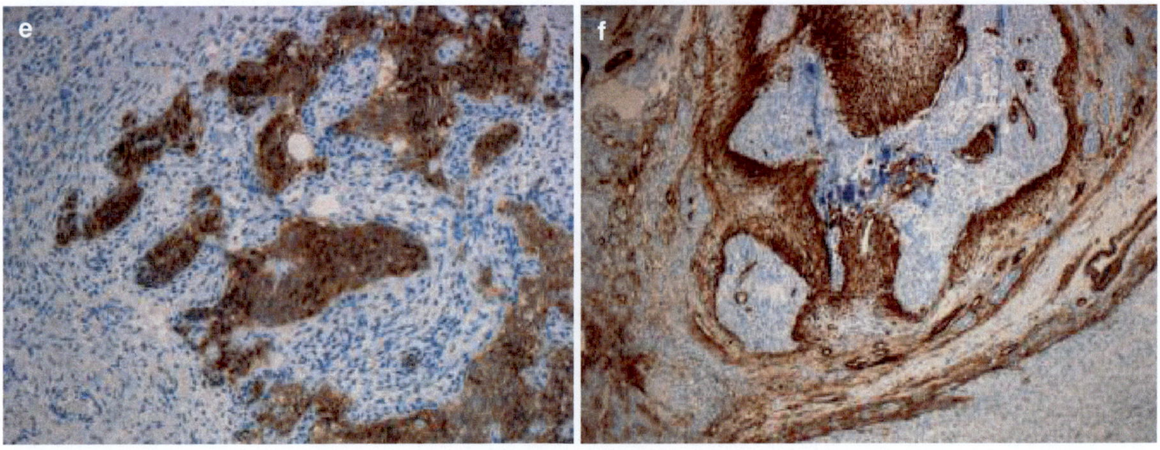

Fig. 9.14 (continued)

exhibit nuclear and cytoplasmic positivity for beta-catenin (own observations; Fig. 9.14e).The spindle cells are positive for vimentin and alpha-smooth muscle actin (myofibroblasts; Fig. 9.14f), suggesting abnormal epithelial-mesenchymal transition and resembling the morphology of a deranged liver bud. The epithelial nest cells express ACTH (Heerema-McKenney et al. 2005; Rod et al. 2009) and corticotropin-releasing hormone (Rod et al. 2009), suggesting an ectopic ACTH syndrome (EAS; Rod et al. 2009).

9.2 Pediatric Hepatocellular Carcinoma

9.2.1 Definition and Epidemiology

Hepatocellular carcinoma (HCC) is a primary malignant tumor of the liver derived from hepatocytes. HCC accounts for approximately 21% of all malignant liver tumors diagnosed in children (Weinberg and Finegold 1983; Stocker 2001), but for only a minority of pediatric solid tumors, as less than 1% of HCCs are diagnosed in patients younger than 20 years of age (Carriaga and Henson 1995). So far, it is not yet known whether pediatric HCC is the same or a disease different from adult-type HCC (Czauderna 2002). HCC is more often diagnosed in males, and mostly in children older than 10 years of age, representing the majority (87%) of malignant liver tumors diagnosed in adolescents (LaBrecque 1996; Darbari et al. 2003; SEER 2006). However, typical HCC can also occur in young children, including infants. Clinical presentation typically includes hepatomegaly and a palpable abdominal mass, often associated with abdominal pain, anorexia, abnormal liver enzymes, and AFP elevation, commonly used as a tumor marker (Ishak and Glunz 1967; Lack et al. 1983).

9.2.2 Etiology

Incidence of HCC is higher in children living in endemic hepatitis B regions (Africa and South-East Asia) (Bellani and Massimino 1993; Moore and Hesseling 1997), commonly acquired perinatally, and where incidence rates have significantly decreased due to the implementation of immunization programs (Montesano 2002; Chang 2003). Other common etiological factors associated with adult HCC, such as underlying liver disease and cirrhosis, HCV infection, chronic alcohol abuse, and exposure to aflatoxin B1, are not relevant etiologic factors for pediatric HCC. Constitutional genetic and metabolic abnormalities are more often associated with HCC diagnosed in children from countries with low HBV endemic rates (Table 9.2). HCC was reported in approximately 18% of children with hereditary tyrosinemia type 1 (fumarylacetoacetate hydrolase deficiency) (Weinberg et al. 1976; Demers et al. 2003) before therapy was available. Glycogen storage diseases, particularly type 1a, are also associated with the development of hepatic tumors in children, including HCC (Coire et al. 1987; Bianchi 1993; Siciliano et al. 2000).

Table 9.2 Genetic syndromes and other abnormalities associated with hepatocellular carcinoma in children

Disease	Associated genes	Reference
Hereditary tyrosinemia	Fumarylacetoacetate hydrolase	Weinberg et al. 1976; Demers et al. 2003
Glycogen storage diseases	–	Bianchi 1993; Siciliano et al. 2000
Familial adenomatous polyposis	*APC*	Giardello et al. 1996
Alagille syndrome	*Jagged-1*	Kaufman et al. 1987
Other familial cholestatic syndromes	*FIC1, BSEP*	Taat et al. 2004
Neurofibromatosis	*NF-1*	Ettinger and Freeman 1979
Ataxia telangiectasia	*ATM*	Weinstein et al. 1985
Fanconi anemia	*FAA, FAC,* others (20%)	Abbondanzo et al. 1986; Touraine et al. 1993
Other reported associations		
TPN	–	Vileisis et al. 1982
Osteogenesis imperfecta	*COL1A1, COL1A2 (CRTAP, LEPRE1)*	Chandra and Stocker 1992
Congenital hepatic fibrosis	Several	Manes et al. 1977
Abnormal abdominal venous drainage	–	Simson 1982; Weinberg and Finegold 1983

APC, adenomatous polyposis coli; *FIC1*, familial intrahepatic cholestasis; *BSEP*, bile salt export pump; *NF-1*, neurofibromatosis, type 1; *ATM*, ataxia telangiectasia mutated; *FAA*, Fanconi anemia complementation group A; *FAC*, Fanconi anemia complementation group C. type I; *TPN*, total parenteral nutrition

Familial adenomatous polyposis (FAP) caused by germline mutation of the *adenomatous polyposis coli (APC)* gene is typically associated with the development of hepatoblastoma in children, and has also been implicated in the pathogenesis of HCC and fibrolamellar carcinoma (Kingston et al. 1982; Giardello et al. 1996), suggesting that *APC* mutations may confer a general predisposition to tumorigenesis in the liver (Thomas et al. 2003). *APC* and beta-catenin (CTNNB1) mutations have been identified in benign precursor lesions, hepatoblastomas, and HCC (Cieply et al. 2009), and the resulting canonical Wnt pathway constitutional activation is now considerd a common oncogenic pathway in liver tumors (Zucman-Rossi et al. 2006).

HCC and cholangiocarcinomas have been observed in patients with familial cholestatic syndromes, including Alagille syndrome (Kaufman et al. 1987; Rabinovitz et al. 1989), and extrahepatic biliary atresia with both HCC and HB in children (Taat et al. 2004). HCC has also been described in cirrhotic livers of children following parenteral nutrition (Vileisis et al. 1982). Finally, pediatric liver tumors, including HCC have been reported in association with neurofibromatosis, ataxia-telangiectasia (Ettinger and Freeman 1979; Weinstein et al. 1985; Geoffroy-Perez et al. 2001; Ucar et al. 2005) and in patients with Fanconi's anemia treated with anabolic steroids, with tumor regression observed with steroids withdrawal (Abbondanzo et al. 1986; Touraine et al. 1993).

9.2.3 Pathology of Adult-Type Hepatocellular Carcinoma

9.2.3.1 Gross Presentation

Macroscopic appearance of HCC depends on the presence of underlying liver disease, size of the tumor, and intrahepatic vascular spread. The presence of cirrhosis is much less common in pediatric than in adult HCC patients. HCC can occur as a solitary, circumscribed mass in one lobe of the liver, more frequently the right, but more often involves both lobes of the liver. Tumor lesions growing without underlying cirrhosis tend to be large, nonencapsulated and exhibit an infiltrative growth pattern, with intrahepatic metastases and

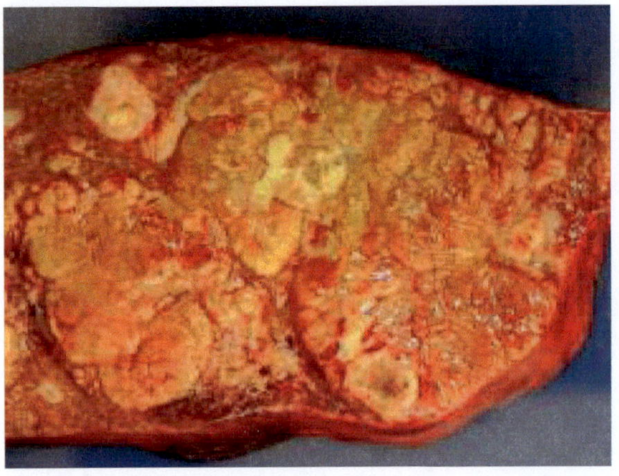

Fig. 9.15 Hepatocellular carcinoma in a 16 year-old with multiple tumor nodules, necrotic foci, and vascular invasion

numerous tumor nodules (Fig. 9.15). The cut surface is usually soft (with exception of the fibrolamellar variant) and bile-stained, different from hepatoblastoma, with areas of necrosis and hemorrhage. Four main gross growth patterns are recognized: expanding ("pushing") lesions; pedunculated ("hanging") lesions; invading lesions; and multifocal lesions (review: Zimmermann 2000). Vascular spread is common and the portal veins, hepatic veins or vena cava may be involved; however, intrahepatic metastases are usually through the portal veins (Ishak and Goodman 1999). Invasion of the biliary ducts is not common, but may cause biliary obstruction. Extrahepatic metastatic spread, often to the lungs and rarely to the brain, occurs via the hepatic veins (Katzenstein et al. 2002).

9.2.3.2 Histology of Adult-Type Hepatocellular Carcinoma

Microscopically, HCC diagnosed in children are overall similar to those in adults (Ishak and Goodman 1999; Farhi et al. 1983; Lack et al. 1983). Tumor cells variably resemble hepatocytes depending on the degree of differentiation. The nuclear/cytoplasmic ratio is elevated, and nuclei are usually prominent, irregular, and hyperchromatic. Cytoplasm is usually eosinophilic and granular, but may also appear clear, contain glycogen, fat, Mallory bodies, or ground-glass-like inclusions. Bile canaliculi are present in approximately half of the tumors. The most common architectural pattern in well and moderately well-differentiated HCC is the trabecular (plate-like) pattern, with tumor cells growing in cords separated by sinusoid-like blood spaces (Fig. 9.16a and b). A pseudoglandular and acinar pattern is commonly found admixed with the trabecular pattern. Cells can also be arranged as sheets without sinusoids (solid pattern).

According to histological grade, HCC can be classified into well-differentiated, moderately differentiated, poorly differentiated, and undifferentiated types (Hirohashi and Ishak 2000). Edmondson and Steiner (Edmondson and Steiner 1954) proposed a scale of I to IV with increasing nuclear irregularity, hyperchromatism, and nuclear/cytoplasmic ratio, associated with decreasing differentiation. Grading can also be done by nuclear features alone or in combination with microvascular invasion (Nzeako et al. 1995; Ishak and Goodman 1999). Reporting histological grade has been recommended for adult HCC resection specimens; however, the association between grade and prognosis and its clinical relevance is not entirely clear (Lai et al. 1979; Dabbs and Geisinger 2004).

Immunohistochemical stains used in combination with histomorphology, even though not helpful in most cases to distinguish HCC from hepatoblastoma or benign lesions, may be useful to differentiate HCC from other tumor types, including cholangiocarcinoma. HepPar-1 (Hepatocyte Paraffin 1), although not completely specific for hepatocytes, shows characteristic cytoplasmic granular staining in approximately 90% of HCCs. Identification of a canalicular pattern using carcinoembryotic antigen (polyclonal CEA) is also useful to differentiate HCC from other malignancies. Alpha-fetoprotein (AFP) is usually elevated in the serum of hepatoblastoma and HCC patients, and often focally present in the tumor cells. Hepatocytes express cytokeratins 8 and 18, while biliary epithelium expresses CK7, CK19, CK8, and CK18, but aberrant cytokeratin expression in HCC and cholangiocarcinoma tumor cells limits the use of these antibodies for tumor classification (Wu et al. 1996). CD34 positive immunostaining of the sinusoids can be helpful to distinguish well differentiated HCC from regenerative nodules, but not adenomas (Gouysse et al. 2004; Varma and Cohen 2004). Glypican 3 is a novel serum and histochemical marker for hepatocellular carcinoma identified by expression profiling. Glypican 3 (GPC3), a heparan sulfate proteoglycan, is expressed at a markedly elevated level in hepatocellular carcinoma and a promising marker for hepatocellular

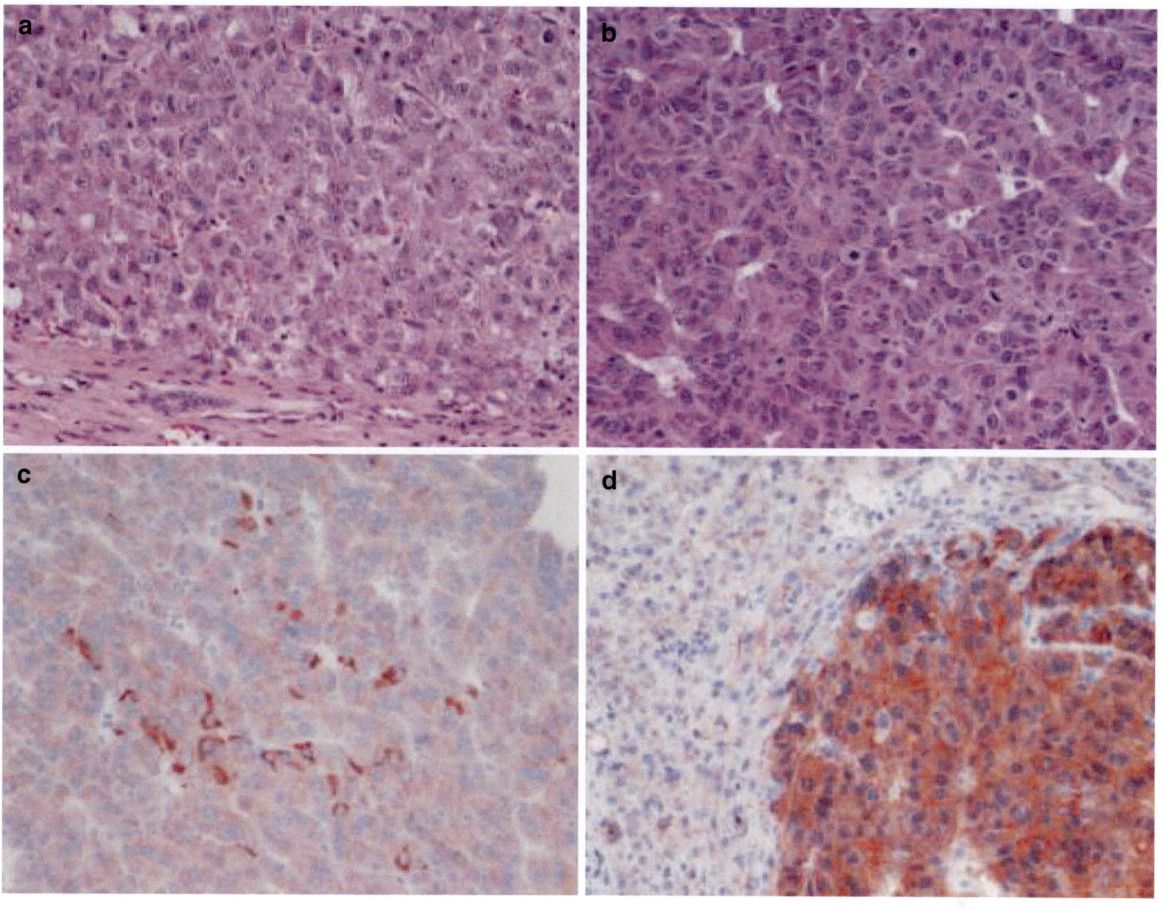

Fig. 9.16 (**a**) Moderately differentiated HCC in a patient with hereditary Tyrosinemia. (**b**) Poorly differentiated HCC in a 7 year-old, arising in a non-cirrhotic liver. Tumor cells grow in cords and macrotrabecular array, forming pseudoacini and tubules focally. Note the abundant mitoses. (**c**) Glypican staining of the same tumor showing variable cytoplasmic positivity. (**d**) β-catenin staining demonstrating strong cytoplasmic positivity in the tumor and membranous staining in the surrounding compressed liver

carcinoma in routine histological examination, and as a potential target in monoclonal antibody-based hepatocellular carcinoma therapy (Fig. 9.16c) (Capurro et al. 2003; Yamauchi et al. 2005). Beta-catenin immunostaining shows strong cytoplasmic positivity in HCC (Fig. 9.16d).

9.2.4 Fibrolamellar Hepatocellular Carcinoma

The fibrolamellar variant of HCC constitutes a distinctive clinical and histological variant of HCC that occurs almost exclusively in adolescents and young adults, accounting for almost a third of HCCs diagnosed in patients below 20 years of age (Farhi et al. 1983; Lack et al. 1983; Haas et al. 1989; El-Serag et al. 2003). The incidence of fibrolamellar HCC is similar in males and females, and characteristically presents in patients without cirrhosis, hepatitis, metabolic, or other underlying chronic liver disease. These tumors are usually slow growing, present with minimal elevation of or normal serum AFP, and are often resectable or curable by transplantation, with an overall 5 year survival that exceeds 55% in most series (Soreide et al. 1986; Pinna et al. 1997). However, and although originally thought to carry a better prognosis, this is likely due to the absence of associated cirrhosis (Kakar et al. 2005). A recent study of the Pediatric Intergroup Hepatoma Protocol INT-0098 demonstrated, unlike previous reports, that children with fibrolamellar HCC do not have a favorable prognosis and do not respond any differently to current therapeutic regimens than patients with typical HCC at similar stage (Katzenstein et al. 2003).

On gross examination they are well circumscribed, firm masses with characteristic radiating fibrous septae, resembling focal nodular hyperplasia (Fig. 9.17a). Their characteristic microscopic appearance consists of cords and nests of large neoplastic hepatocytes with granular oncocytic cytoplasm, separated by dense hyalinized collagen bands (Fig. 9.17b). Some of the cells contain so-called pale bodies.

Foci of conventional HCC and of adjacent areas of focal nodular hyperplasia have been described associated with this lesion (Saul et al. 1987; Berman et al. 1988). Staining for CK7, CEA, fibrinogen, and copper is commonly found in fibrolamellar HCC (Lefkowitch et al. 1983).

9.2.5 Differential Diagnoses

The most common differential diagnosis of pediatric HCC is hepatoblastoma and rarely other metastatic lesions, including carcinomas in older children. Cytologic atypia may be variable in pediatric HCC, as in adult HCC, but cells are in general larger than in hepatoblastoma, bile producing, with more prominent cytologic atypia and nuclear pleomorphism, and often abnormal mitoses present. Other characteristic histologic features of hepatoblastoma, such as coexistence of histologic patters, extramedullary hematopoiesis, and mesenchymal components, are not usually seen in HCC.

Hepatic adenomas occur in older children, and may be challenging to differentiate from other lesions, including well-differentiated HCC, particularly in small biopsies. Adenomas arise from non-cirrhotic livers and may be multiple, such as those seen in patients with glycogen storage disorders. In resection specimens a pushing border and, occasionally a capsule, may be identified surrounding sheets and cords of hepatocytes larger and usually paler than surrounding hepatocytes, and commonly containing cytoplasmic glycogen or fat. Immunohistochemical staining for proliferation markers such as Ki67 or endothelial markers (CD34) may be diagnostically useful (Libbrecht et al. 2001; Gouysse et al. 2004). Hepatic adenomas may sometimes be difficult to differentiate from focal nodular hyperplasia, particularly in small biopsies.

Fibrolamellar HCC can be clinically and radiographically difficult to differentiate from focal nodular hyperplasia, due to its indolent course and typical central scar. However, in most cases microscopic diagnosis can be easily made by its distinctive histologic features.

Lastly, it is worth mentioning that patients with both hepatoblastoma and HCC have been simultaneously described, and simultaneous presence of adenomas and HCC is not uncommon, particularly in patients with glycogen storage disorders (Parker et al. 1981; Coire et al. 1987).

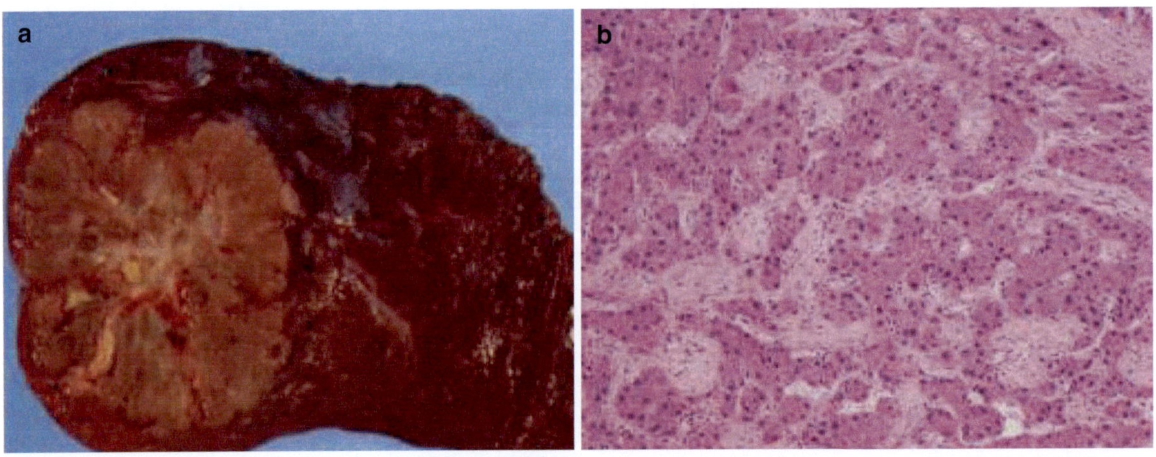

Fig. 9.17 (**a**) Well circumscribed, sclerotic appearing fibrolamellar carcinoma, with characteristic central radiating scar. (**b**) Fibrolamellar carcinoma with characteristic dense fibrous stroma separating cords and nests of neoplastic hepatocytes with abundant eosinophilic cytoplasm

9.2.6 New Knowledge on Pathogenic/Molecular Pathways

The molecular genetic alterations associated with the multistep process of hepatocarcinogenesis have been extensively studied (Bannasch 1996; Buendia 2000; Thorgeirsson and Grisham 2002, review: Zimmermann 2006; Aravalli et al. 2008). However, little knowledge is available regarding the biology of pediatric HCC, a different and heterogeneous group of tumors often occurring without underlying liver disease, and not associated with common HCC etiological factors seen in adults, with the exception of HBV infection. Hepatitis B virus is a hepatotropic DNA hepadnavirus associated with a lifetime risk of HCC for children infected at birth, of approximately 50%. Integration of HBV in the host genome has been proposed as a possible oncogenic mechanism for a proportion of patients (Matsubara and Tokino 1990; Wang et al. 1990), possibly through chromosomal instability (Bréchot 2004).

Genetic studies of mostly adult HCC have demonstrated multiple chromosomal abnormalities, predominantly losses, in contrast to HB with few characteristic chromosomal changes, commonly trisomies (Wong et al. 2000). Increased chromosomal instability has been reported in tumors associated with hepatitis B virus infection. Most common chromosomal losses are on chromosomes 17p, 13q, 9p, 6q, and 16p. LOH is common in adult HCC and frequently involves tumor suppressor genes, with deletions reported most commonly at 8p (48%), 17p (45%), 4q (38%), 1p (33%), 13q, 16q, 6q, 16p, 1q, and 9p with a frequency higher than 20% (Buendia 2002; Tornillo et al. 2002).

Alterations common to HCC and hepatoblastoma include gain of chromosomes 1q, 8q, and 17q, and loss of 4q. Another important common feature shared by the two tumor types is the frequent activation of Wnt/beta-catenin signaling by stabilizing mutations of beta-catenin (Buendia 2002) (Fig. 9.1e). Recent application of array CGH technology (Lopez-Terrada et al. 2009b) has been proposed as a genomic profiling tool applicable to surgical specimens, and useful for the differential diagnosis of HCC versus hepatoblastoma.

Genetic analysis of fibrolamellar HCC demonstrated fewer chromosomal abnormalities compared with those reported in literature for conventional hepatocellular carcinoma, with most common abnormalities on chromosomes 7 and 8. Fibrolamellar carcinomas with chromosomal changes appear to behave more aggressively than cases with normal karyotypes (Wilkens et al. 2000; Kakar et al. 2009). Epigenetic studies of a series of fibrolamellar HCCs demonstrated that genomic instability is rare in this variant when compared with viral-associated hepatocellular carcinomas (Vivekanandan et al. 2009). Signaling pathway analysis has demonstrated overexpression of genes in the RAS, MAPK, PIK3, and xenobiotic degradation pathways in this group of HCCs (Kannangai et al. 2007).

In recent years, numerous studies have aimed at identifying critical signaling pathways involved in hepatocarcinogenesis, and particularly hepatitis-associated HCC. Some of the most relevant, aberrantly activated pathways include the P53 pathway, mitogen-activated protein kinase (MAPK), Wnt/beta-catenin, epidermal growth factor (EGF), and transforming growth factor-beta (TGFbeta) pathways (Anders et al. 2003; Lee and Thorgeirsson 2005). Several gene expression profiling studies have specifically addressed differences between clinical HCC subtypes and searched for biomarkers that could serve as prognostic predictors, or therapeutic targets (Lau et al. 2000; Graveel et al. 2001; Okabe et al. 2001; Shirota et al. 2001; Delpuech et al. 2002; Lee and Thorgeirsson 2004). A recent study identified differentially expressed genes in HCC versus hepatoblastoma, and between tumors and adjacent liver (Luo et al. 2006). Other high throughput technologies (proteomics, metabolomics, micro RNA profiling) have also been applied recently to study the biology of HCC (Blanc et al. 2005; Li et al. 2005; Yang et al. 2008).

9.2.7 Conclusion

Unfortunately, most of these studies are aimed at investigating adult HCC, and it is not clear how much of what we have learned from these applies to those diagnosed in pediatric patients. Pediatric HCC is a rare, heterogeneous disease, and very little is understood today regarding how genetic predisposition, metabolic disorders, cholestasis, or even potential exposures during infancy and childhood, participate in the carcinogenesis of these rare group of tumors.

The diagnosis and clinical management of pediatric HCC still represents a tremendous challenge. Only by collaborative efforts and by incorporating new biologic parameters and traditional diagnostic algorithms, similar to other pediatric neoplasms, will it be possible to improve diagnosis, clinical stratification, and sucessfull treatment of pediatric HCC patients.

References

Abbondanzo SL, Manz HJ, Klappenbach RS et al (1986) Hepatocellular carcinoma in an 11-year-old girl with Fanconi's anemia. Report of a case and review of the literature. Am J Pediatr Hematol Oncol 8:334–337

Abenoza P, Manivel JC, Wick MR et al (1987) Hepatoblastoma: an immunohistochemical and ultrastructural study. Hum Pathol 18:1025–1035

Akmal SN, Yun K, MacLay J et al (1995) Insulin-like growth factor 2 and insulin-like factor binding protein 2 expression in hepatoblastoma. Hum Pathol 26:846–851

Anders RA, Yerian LM, Tretiakova M et al (2003) cDNA microarray analysis of macroregenerative and dysplastic nodules in end-stage hepatitis C virus-induced cirrhosis. Am J Pathol 162:991–1000

Ara T, Fukuzawa M, Oue T et al (1997) Immunohistochemical assessment of the MIB-1 labeling index in human hepatoblastoma and its prognostic relevance. J Pediatr Surg 32:1690–1694

Aravalli RN, Steer CJ, Cressman EN et al (2008) Molecular mechanisms of hepatocellular carcinoma. Hepatology 48:2047–2063

Bannasch P (1996) Pathogenesis of hepatocellular carcinoma: sequential cellular, molecular, and metabolic changes. Prog Liver Dis 14:161–197

Behrle FC, Mantz FA, Olson RL et al (1963) Virilization accompanying hepatoblastoma. Pediatrics 32:265–271

Bellani FF, Massimino M (1993) Liver tumors in childhood: epidemiology and clinics. J Surg Oncol Suppl 3:119–121

Berman MA, Burnham JA, Sheahan DG et al (1988) Fibrolamellar carcinoma of the liver: an immunohistochemical study of nineteen cases and a review of the literature. Hum Pathol 19:784–794

Bianchi L (1993) Glycogen storage disease I and hepatocellular tumours. Eur J Pediatr 152(Suppl 1):S63–S70

Blanc JF, Lalanne C, Plomion C et al (2005) Proteomic analysis of differently expressed proteins in hepatocellular carcinoma developed in patients with chronic viral hepatitis C. Proteomics 5:3778–3789

Borman JB, Harbott AJ, Morris D (1961) Hepatic lobectomy in infancy for hepatoblastoma. Br J Surg 49:11–13

Braunstein GD, Bridson WE, Glass A et al (1972) In vivo and in vitro production of human chorionic gonadotropin and alpha-fetoprotein by a virilizing hepatoblastoma. J Clin Endocrinol 35:857–862

Bréchot C (2004) Pathogenesis of hepatitis B virus-related hepatocellular carcinoma: old and new paradigms. Gastroenterology 127(Suppl 1):S56–S61

Brodsky SV, Sandoval C, Sharma N et al (2008) Recurrent nested stromal epithelial tumor of the liver with extrahepatic metastasis: case report and review of literature. Pediatr Dev Pathol 11:469–473

Brotto M, Finegold MJ (2002) Distinct patterns of p27/KIP1 gene expression in hepatoblastoma and prognostic implications with correlation before and after chemotherapy. Hum Pathol 33:198–205

Buendia MA (2000) Genetics of hepatocellular carcinoma. Semin Cancer Biol 10:185–200

Buendia MA (2002) Genetic alterations in hepatoblastoma and hepatocellular carcinoma: common and distinctive aspects. Med Pediatr Oncol 39:530–535

Capurro M, Wanless IR, Sherman M et al (2003) Glypican-3: a novel serum and histochemical marker for hepatocelular carcinoma. Gastroenterology 125:89–97

Carriaga MT, Henson DE (1995) Liver, gallbladder, exrahepatic bile ducts, and pancreas. Cancer 75(Suppl):171–190

Chandra CR, Stocker JT (1992) The liver, gallbladder and biliary tract. In: Stocker JT (ed) Pediatric pathology. JB Lippincott, Philadelphia

Chang MH (2003) Decreasing incidence of hepatocellular carcinoma among children following universal hepatitis B immunization. Liver Int 23:309–314

Cieply B, Zeng G, Proverbs-Singh T et al (2009) Unique phenotype of hepatocellular cancers with exon-3 mutations in beta-catenin gene. Hepatology 49:821–831

Coire CI, Qizilbash AH, Castelli MF et al (1987) Hepatic adenomata in type Ia glycogen storage disease. Arch Pathol Lab Med 111:166–169

Conrad RJ, Gribbin D, Walker NI et al (1993) Combined cystic teratoma and hepatoblastoma of the liver. Probable divergent differentiation of an uncommitted hepatic precursor cell. Cancer 72:2910–2913

Conran RM, Hitchcock CL, Waclawiw MA et al (1992) Hepatoblastoma: the prognostic significance of histologic type. Pediatr Pathol 12:167–183

Cross SS, Variend S (1992) Combined hepatoblastoma and yolk sac tumor of the liver. Cancer 69:1323–1326

Czauderna P (2002) Adult type vs. childhood hepatocellular carcinoma – are they the same of different lesions? Med Pediatr Oncol 39:519–523

Dabbs DJ, Geisinger KR (2004) Recommendations for the reporting of tissues removed as part of the surgical treatment of malignant liver tumors. Hum Pathol 35: 1315–1323

Dachman AH, Pakter RL, Ros PR et al (1987) Hepatoblastoma: radiologic-pathologic correlation in 50 cases. Radiology 164:15–19

D'Antiga L, Vallortigara F, Cillo U et al (2007) Features predicting unresectability in hepatoblastoma. Cancer 110: 1050–1057

Darbari A, Sabin KM, Shapiro CN et al (2003) Epidemiology of primary hepatic malignancies in U.S. children. Hepatology 38:560–566

Davies JQ, de la Hall PM, Kaschula RO et al (2004) Hepatoblastoma – evolution of management and outcome and significance of histology of the resected tumor. A 31-year experience with 40 cases. J Pediatr Surg 39: 1321–1327

Dehner LP (1978) Hepatic tumors in the pediatric age group: a distinctive clinicopathologic spectrum. Perspect Pediatr Pathol 4:217–268

Dehner LP, Manivel JC (1988) Hepatoblastoma: an analysis of the relationship between morphologic subtypes and prognosis. Am J Pediatr Hematol Oncol 10:301–307

De Ioris M, Brugieres L, Zimmermann A et al (2008) Hepatoblastoma with a low serum alpha-fetoprotein level at diagnosis: the SIOPEL group experience. Eur J Cancer 44:545–550

Delpuech O, Trabut JB, Carnot F et al (2002) Identification, using cDNA macroarray analysis, of distinct gene expression profiles associated with pathological and virological features of hepatocellular carcinoma. Oncogene 21:2926–2937

Demers SI, Russo P, Lettre F et al (2003) Frequent mutation reversion inversely correlates with clinical severity in a genetic liver disease, hereditary tyrosinemia. Hum Pathol 34:1313–1320

Dicken BJ, Bigam DL, Lees GM (2004) Association between surgical margins and long-term outcome in advanced hepatoblastoma. J Pediatr Surg 39:721–725

Doss BJ, Vicari J, Jacques SM (1998) Placental involvement in congenital hepatoblastoma. Pediatr Dev Pathol 1:538–542

Douglass EC, Reynolds M, Finegold M et al (1993) Cisplatin, vincristine, and fluorouracil therapy for hepatoblastoma: a Pediatric Oncology Group study. J Clin Oncol 11:96–99

Edmondson HA, Steiner PE (1954) Primary carcinoma of the liver: a study of 100 cases among 48,900 necropsies. Cancer 7:462–503

Edmondson HA (1956) Differential diagnosis of tumors and tumor-like lesions of liver in infancy and childhood. AMA J Dis Child 91:168–186

El-Serag HB, Davila JA, Petersen NJ et al (2003) The continuing increase in the incidence of hepatocellular carcinoma in the United States: an update. Ann Intern Med 139: 817–823

Ettinger LJ, Freeman AI (1979) Hepatoma in a child with neurofibromatosis. Am J Dis Child 133:528–531

Farhi DC, Shikes RH, Murani PJ et al (1983) Hepatocellular carcinoma in young people. Cancer 52:1516–1525

Fasano M, Theise ND, Nalesnik M et al (1998) Immunohistochemical evaluation of hepatoblastomas with use of hepatocyte-specific marker, hepatocyte paraffin 1, and the polyclonal anti-carcinoembryonic antigen. Mod Pathol 11: 934–938

Feusner JH, Krailo MD, Haas JE et al (1993) Treatment of pulmonary metastases of initial stage I hepatoblastoma in childhood. Report from the Childrens Cancer Group. Cancer 71:859–864

Finegold MJ, Lopez-Terrada DH, Bowen J et al (2007) Protocol for the examination of specimens from pediatric patients with hepatoblastoma. Arch Pathol Lab Med 131:520–529

Finegold MJ, Egler RA, Goss JA et al (2008) Liver tumors: pediatric population. Liver Trans 14:1545–1556

Forouhar FA, Quinn JJ, Cooke R et al (1984) The effect of chemotherapy on hepatoblastoma. Arch Pathol Lab Med 108:311–314

Fukuzawa R, Umezawa A, Ochi K et al (1999) High frequency of inactivation of the imprinted H19 gene in "sporadic" hepatoblastoma. Int J Cancer 82:490–497

Garcés-Inigo EF, Leung R, Sebire NJ et al (2009) Extrarenal rhabdoid tumours outside the central nervous system in infancy. Pediatr Radiol 39:817–822

Geoffroy-Perez B, Janin N, Ossian K et al (2001) Cancer risk in heterozygotes for ataxia-telangiectasia. Int J Cancer 93:288–293

Giardello FM, Petersen GM, Brensinger JD et al (1996) Hepatoblastoma and APC gene mutation in familial adenomatous polyposis. Gut 39:867–869

Gonzalez-Crussi F, Upton MP, Maurer HS (1982) Hepatoblastoma. Attempt at characterization of histologic subtypes. Am J Surg Pathol 6:599–612

Gonzalez-Crussi F (1991) Case 1 Undifferentiated small cell ("anaplastic") hepatoblastoma. Pediatr Pathol 11:155–162

Gornicka B, Ziarkiewicz-Wroblewska B, Michalowicz B et al (2001) Immature hepatic tumor of bimodal differentiation in a young adult patient: a novel lesion expressing β-catenin and mimicking a distinct phase of hepatogenesis. J Hepatol 34:955–961

Gouysse G, Franchon S, Hervieu V et al (2004) Endothelial cell differentiation in hepatocellular adenomas: implications for histopathological diagnosis. J Hepatol 41:259–266

Graveel CR, Jatkoe T, Madore SJ et al (2001) Expression profiling and identification of npvel genes in hepatocellular carcinomas. Oncogene 20:2704–2712

Gray SG, Hartmann W, Eriksson T et al (2000) Expression of genes involved with cell cycle control, cell growth and chromatin modification are altered in hepatoblastomas. Int J Mol Med 6:161–169

Haas JE, Muczynski KA, Krailo M et al (1989) Histopathology and prognosis in childhood hepatoblastoma and hepatocarcinoma. Cancer 64:1082–1095

Haas JE, Feusner JH, Finegold MJ (2001) Small cell undifferentiated histology in hepatoblastoma may be unfavorable. Cancer 92:3130–3134

Halasz J, Holczbauer A, Paska C et al (2006) Claudin-1 and claudin-2 differentiate fetal from embryonal components in human hepatoblastoma. Hum Pathol 37:555–561

Hansen K, Bagtas J, Mark HF et al (1992) Undifferentiated small cell hepatoblastoma with a unique chromosomal translocation: a case report. Pediatr Pathol 12:457–462

Hartmann W, Waha A, Koch A et al (2000) p57(KIP2) is not mutated in hepatoblastoma but shows increased transcriptional activity in a comparative analysis of the three imprinted genes p57(KIP2), IGF2, and H19. Am J Pathol 157: 1393–1403

Heerema-McKenney A, Leuschner I, Smith N et al (2005) Nested stromal epithelial tumor of the liver: six cases of a distinctive pediatric neoplasm with frequent calcifications and association with Cushing syndrome. Am J Surg Pathol 29:10–20

Heifetz SA, French M, Correa M et al (1997) Hepatoblastoma: the Indiana experience with preoperative chemotherapy for inoperable tumors; clinicopathological considerations. Pediatr Pathol Lab Med 17:857–874

Hill DA, Swanson PE, Anderson K et al (2005) Desmoplastic nested spindle cell tumor of liver: report of four cases of a proposed new entity. Am J Surg Pathol 29:1–9

Hirohashi S, Ishak KG (2000) Tumours of the liver and intrahepatic bile ducts. In: Hamilton SR, Aaltonen LA (eds) Pathology and genetics of tumours of the digestive system. IARC Press, Lyon

Honda S, Arai Y, Haruta M et al (2008) Loss of imprinting of IGF2 correlates with hypermethylation of teh H19 differentially methylated region in hepatoblastoma. Br J Cancer 99:1891–1899

Http://seer.cancer.gov Surveillance Epidemiology and End Results Web site

Hung W, Blizzard RM, Migeon CJ et al (1963) Precocious puberty in a boy with hepatoma and circulating gonadotropin. J Pediatr 63:895–903

Ingram DJ, Yerushalmi B, Connell J et al (2000) Hepatoblastoma in a neonate: a hypervascular presentation mimicking hemangioendothelioma. Pediatr Radiol 30:794–797

Iolascon A, Giordani L, Moretti A et al (1998) Analysis of CDKN2A, CDKN2B, CDKN2C, and cyclin Ds gene status in hepatoblastoma. Hepatology 27:989–995

Ishak KG, Glunz PR (1967) Hepatoblastoma and hepatocarcinoma in infancy and childhood. Cancer 20:396–422

Ishak KG, Goodman ZD (1999) Hepatocellular carcinoma. In: Ishak KG, Goodman ZD, Stocker JT (eds) Tumors of the liver and intrahepatic bile ducts. Armed Forces Institute of Pathology, Washington

Joshi VV, Kaur P, Ryan B et al (1984) Mucoid anaplastic hepatoblastoma. A case report. Cancer 54:2035–2039

Kakar S, Burgart LJ, Batts KP et al (2005) Clinicopathologic features and survival in fibrolamellar carcinoma: comparison with conventional hepatocellular carcinoma with and without cirrhosis. Mod Pathol 18:1417–1423

Kakar S, Chen X, Ho C et al (2009) Chromosomal changes in fibrolamellar hepatocellular carcinoma detected by array comparative genomic hybridization. Mod Pathol 22:134–141

Kannangai R, Vivekanandan P, Martinez-Murillo F et al (2007) Fibrolamellar carcinomas show overexpression of genes in the RAS, MAPK, PIK3, and xenobiotic degradation pathways. Hum Pathol 38:639–644

Kasai M, Watanabe I (1970) Histologic classification of liver-cell carcinoma in infancy and childhood and its clinical evaluation. Cancer 25:552–563

Katzenstein HM, Krailo MD, Malogolowkin MH et al (2002) Hepatocellular carcinoma in children and adolescents: results from the Pediatric Oncology Group and the Children's Cancer Group intergroup study. J Clin Oncol 20:2789–2797

Katzenstein HM, Krailo MD, Malogolowkin MH et al (2003) Fibrolamellar hepatocellular carcinoma in children and adolescents. Cancer 97:2006–2012

Kaufman SS, Wood RP, Shaw BW et al (1987) Hepatocarcinoma in a child with the Alagille syndrome. Am J Dis Child 141:698–700

Kim L, Park YN, Kim SE et al (2001) Teratoid hepatoblastoma: multidirectional differentiation of stem cell of the liver. Yonsei Med J 42:431–435

Kingston JE, Draper GJ, Mann JR et al (1982) Hepatoblastoma and polyposis coli. Lancet 1:457

Kumar EV, Kumar L, Pathak IC et al (1978) Clinical, hormonal and ultrastructure studies of a virilizing hepatoblastoma. Acta Paediatr Scand 67:389–392

LaBrecque D (1996) Neoplasia of the liver. Liver and biliary disease. W Wilkens, Baltimore, pp 391–438

Lack EE, Neave C, Vawter GF (1982) Hepatoblastoma. A clinical and pathologic study of 54 cases. Am J Surg Pathol 6:693–705

Lack EE, Neave C, Vawter GF et al (1983) Hepatocellular carcinoma. Review of 32 cases in childhood and adolescence. Cancer 52:1510–1515

Lai CL, Wu PC, Lam KC et al (1979) Histologic prognostic indicators in hepatocellular carcinoma. Cancer 44: 1677–1683

Lau WY, Lai PB, Leung MF et al (2000) Differential gene expression of hepatocellular carcinoma using cDNA microarray analysis. Oncol Res 12:59–69

Lee JS, Thorgeirsson SS (2004) Genome-scale profiling of gene expression in hepatocellular carcinoma: classification, survival prediction, and identification of therapeutic targets. Gastroenterology 127(Suppl 1):S51–S55

Lee JS, Thorgeirsson SS (2005) Genetic profiling of human hepatocellular carcinoma. Semin Liver Dis 25:125–132

Lefkowitch JH, Muschel R, Price JB et al (1983) Copper and copper-binding protein in fibrolamellar liver cell carcinoma. Cancer 51:97–100

Li X, Adam G, Cui H et al (1995) Expression, promoter usage and parental imprinting status of insulin-like growth factor II (IGF2) in human hepatoblastoma: uncoupling of IGF2 and H19 imprinting. Oncogene 11:221–229

Li C, Tan YX, Zhou H et al (2005) Proteomic analysis of hepatitis B virus-associated hepatocellular carcinoma: identification of potential tumors markers. Proteomics 5: 1125–1139

Libbrecht L, De Vos R, Cassiman D et al (2001) Hepatic progenitor cells in hepatocellular adenomas. Am J Surg Pathol 25:1388–1396

Libbrecht L, Desmet V, Roskams T (2003) Stages of normal and aberrant intrahepatic bile duct development in a mixed hepatoblastoma. Histopathology 42:618–620

Lopez-Terrada D, Gunaratne PH, Adesina AA et al (2009a) Histologic subtypes of hepatoblastoma are characterized by differential canonical Wnt and Notch pathway activation in DLK+ precursors. Hum Pathol 40:783–794

Lopez-Terrada D, Patel K et al (2009b) Characteristic chromosomal copy number changes are associated with subtypes of hepatoblastoma and HCC identified by array-CGH analysis. Society of Pediatric Pathology, Boston

Lowichik A, Zhou H, Pysher TJ et al (2000) Therapy associated changes in childhood tumors. Adv Anat Pathol 7:341–359

Lu M, Greer ML (2007) Hypervascular multifocal hepatoblastoma: dynamic gadolinium-enhanced MRI findings indistinguishable from infantile hemangio-endothelioma. Pediatr Radiol 37:587–591

Luo JH, Ren B, Keryanov S et al (2006) Transcriptomic and genomic analysis of human hepatocellular carcinomas and hepatoblastomas. Hepatology 44:1012–1024

Manes JL, Kissane JM, Valdes AJ et al (1977) Congenital hepatic fibrosis, liver cell carcinoma and adult polycystic kidneys. Cancer 39:2619–2623

Manivel C, Wick MR, Abenoza P et al (1986) Teratoid hepatoblastoma. The nosologic dilemma of solid embryonic neoplasms of childhood. Cancer 57:2168–2174

Matsubara K, Tokino T (1990) Integration of hepatitis B virus DNA and its implications for hepatocarcinogenesis. Mol Biol Med 7:243–260

Meir K, Maly A, Doviner V et al (2009) Nested (ossifying) stromal epithelial tumor of the liver: case report. Pediatr Dev Pathol 12:233–236

Meyers RL (2007) Tumors of the liver in children. Surg Oncol 16:195–203

Milman DH, Grayzel DM (1951) Mixed tumor of the liver; report of a case with a review of the literature. AMA Am J Dis Child 81:408–420

Misick OS (1898) A case of teratoma hepatis. J Pathol Bact 5:128–137

Misugi K, Okajima H, Misugi N et al (1967) Classification of primary malignant tumors of liver in infancy and childhood. Cancer 20:1760–1771

Montesano R (2002) Hepatitis B immunization and hepatocellular carcinoma: the Gambia Hepatitis Intervention Study. J Med Virol 67:444–446

Moore SW, Hesseling PB (1997) Hepatocellular carcinoma in children. Pediatr Surg Int 12:266–270

Moritake H, Taketomi A, Kamimura S et al (2000) Renin-producing hepatoblastoma. J Pediatr Hematol Oncol 22:78–80

Nakagawara A, Ikeda K, Hayashida Y et al (1982) Immunocytochemical identification of human chorionic gonadotropin- and alpha-fetoprotein-producing cells hepatoblastoma associated with precocious puberty. Virchows Arch A Pathol Anat Histopathol 398:45–51

Nakagawara A, Ikeda K, Tsuneyoshi M et al (1985) Hepatoblastoma producing both alpha-fetoprotein and human chorionic gonadotropin. Clinicopathologic analysis of four cases and a review of the literature. Cancer 56:1636–1642

Neimann N, Rauber G, Manciaux N (1963) Les tumeurs malignes du foie chez l'enfant. Rev Int Hepat 13:81–129

Nzeako UC, Goodman ZD, Ishak KG (1995) Comparison of tumor pathology with duration of survival of North American patients with hepatocellular carcinoma. Cancer 76:579–588

Okabe H, Satoh S, Kato T et al (2001) Genome-wide analysis of gene expression in human hepatocellular carcinomas using cDNA microarray: identification of genes involved in viral carcinogenesis and tumor progression. Cancer Res 61: 2129–2137

Ortega JA, Douglass EC, Feusner JH et al (2000) Randomized comparison of cisplatin/vincristine/fluorouracil and cisplatin/continuous infusion doxorubicin for treatment of paediatric hepatoblastoma: a report from the Children's Cancer Group and the Paediatric Oncology Group. J Clin Oncol 18:2665–2675

Pakakasama S, Chen TT, Frawley W et al (2004) CCND1 polymorphism and age on onset of hepatoblastoma. Oncogene 23:4789–4792

Pang SC (1961) Bony and cartilaginous hepatoblastoma. J Pathol Bacteriol 82:273–280

Parham DM, Weeks DA, Beckwith JB (1994) The clinicopathologic spectrum of putative extrarenal rhabdoid tumors. An analysis of 42 cases studied with immunohistochemistry or electron microscopy. Am J Surg Pathol 18:1010–1029

Park WS, Oh RR, Park JY et al (2001) Nuclear localization of beta-catenin is an important prognostic factor in hepatoblastoma. J Pathol 193:483–490

Parker P, Burr I, Slonim A et al (1981) Regression of hepatic adenomas in type Ia glycogen storage disease with dietary therapy. Gastroenterology 81:2129–2137

Pinna AD, Iwatsuki S, Lee RG et al (1997) Treatment of fibrolamellar hepatoma with subtotal hepatectomy or transplantation. Hepatology 26:877–883

Prokurat A, Kluge P, Kosciesza A et al (2002) Transitional liver cell tumors (TLCT) in older children and adolescents: a novel group of aggressive hepatic tumors expressing beta-catenin. Med Pediatr Oncol 39:510–518

Rabinovitz M, Imperial JC, Schade RR et al (1989) Hepatocellular carcinoma in Alagille's syndrome: a family study. J Pediatr Gastroenterol Nutr 8:26–30

Rainier S, Dobry CJ, Feinberg AP (1995) Loss of imprinting in hepatoblastoma. Cancer Res 55:1836–1838

Ramsay AD, Bates AW, Williams S et al (2008) Variable antigen expression in hepatoblastomas. Appl Immunohistochem Mol Morphol 16:140–147

Robinson HB, Bolande RP (1985) Case 3. Fetal hepatoblastoma with placental metastases. Pediatr Pathol 4:163–167

Rod A, Voicu M, Chiche L et al (2009) Cushing's syndrome associated with a nested stromal epithelial tumor of the liver: hormonal, immunohistochemical, and molecular studies. Eur J Endocrinol 161:805–810

Ross JA, Radloff GA, Davies SM (2000) H19 and IGF-2 allele-specific expression in hepatoblastoma. Br J Cancer 82:753–756

Rowland JM (2002) Hepatoblastoma: assessment of criteria for histologic classification. Med Pediatr Oncol 39:478–483

Ruck P, Kaiserling E (1993) Melanin-containing hepatoblastoma with endocrine differentiation. An immunohistochemical and ultrastructural study. Cancer 72:361–368

Rugge M, Sonego F, Pollice L et al (1998) Hepatoblastoma: DNA nuclear content, proliferation indices, and pathology. Liver 18:128–133

Russo P, Biegel JA (2009) SMARCB1/INI1 alterations and hepatoblastoma: another extrarenal rhabdoid tumor revealed? Pediatr Blood Cancer 52:312–313

Saul SH, Titelbaum DS, Gansler TS et al (1987) The fibrolamellar variant of hepatocellular carcinoma. Its association with focal nodular hyperplasia. Cancer 60:3049–3055

Saxena R, Leake JL, Shafford EA et al (1993) Chemotherapy effects on hepatoblastoma. A histological study. Am J Surg Pathol 17:1266–1271

Scheimberg I, Cullinane C, Kelsey A et al (1996) Primary hepatic malignant tumor with rhabdoid features. A histological, immunocytochemical, and electron microscopic study of four cases and a review of the literature. Am J Surg Pathol 20:1394–1400

Schlecht I, Riebel T, Henze G (1996) Unusually intensively ossified hepatoblastoma (teratoid type) in a 1-year-old girl (in German). Rofo 165:201–203

Shang XZ, Zhu H, Lin K et al (2004) Stabilized beta-catenin promotes hepatocyte proliferation and inhibits TNFalpha-induced apoptosis. Lab Invest 84:332–341

Shirota Y, Kaneko S, Honda M et al (2001) Identification of differentially expressed genes in hepatocellular carcinoma with cDNA microarrays. Hepatology 33:832–840

Siciliano M, De Candia E, Ballarin S et al (2000) Hepatocellular carcinoma complicating liver cirrhosis in type IIIa glycogen storage disease. J Clin Gastroenterol 31:80–82

Simson IW (1982) Membranous obstruction of the inferior vena cava and hepatocellular carcinoma in South Africa. Gastroenterology 82:171–178

Sinniah D, Campbell PE, Colebatch JH (1974) Primary hepatic cancer in childhood. Arch Dis Child 49:496

Soreide O, Czerniak A, Bradpiece H et al (1986) Characterstics of fibrolamellar hepatocellular carcinoma. A study of nine cases and a review of the literature. Am J Surg 151:518–523

Stocker JT (1994) Hepatoblastoma. Semin Diagn Pathol 11: 136–143

Stocker JT (2001) Hepatic tumors in children. Clin Liver Dis 5:259–281

Taat F, Bosman DK, Aaronson DC (2004) Hepatoblastoma in a girl with biliary atrasia: coincidence or co-incidence. Pediatr Blood Cancer 43:603–605

Takayasu H, Horie H, Hiyama E et al (2001) Frequent deletions and mutations of the beta-catenin gene are associated with overexpression of cyclin D1 and fibronectin and poorly differentiated histology in childhood hepatoblastoma. Clin Cancer Res 7:901–908

Thomas D, Pritchard J, Davidson R et al (2003) Familia hepatoblastoma and APC gene mutations: renewed call for molecular research. Eur J Cancer 39:2200–2204

Thorgeirsson SS, Grisham JW (2002) Molecular pathogenesis of human hepatocellular carcinoma. Nat Genet 31:339–346

Tomizawa M, Saisho H (2006) Signaling pathway of insulin-like growth factor-II as a target of molecular therapy for hepatoblastoma. Wordl J Gastroenterol 12:6531–6535

Tornillo L, Carafa V, Sauter G et al (2002) Chromosomal alterations in hepatocellular nodules by comparative genomic hybridization: high-grade dysplasic nodules represent early stages of hepatocellular carcinoma. Lab Invest 82:547–553

Touraine RL, Bertrand Y, Foray P et al (1993) Hepatic tumours during androgen therapy in Fanconi anemia. Eur J Pediatr 152:691–693

Trobaugh-Lotrario AD, Tomlinson GE, Finegold MJ et al (2009) Small cell undifferentiated variant of hepatoblastoma: adverse clinical and molecular features similar to rhabdoid tumors. Pediatr Blood Cancer 52:328–334

Tsai HW, Tsai HH, Kuo FY et al (2009) Computerized analyses of morphology and proliferative activity differentiate hepatoblastoma from paediatric hepatocellular carcinoma. Histopathology 54:328–336

Ucar C, Caliskan U, Troy H et al (2005) Hepatoblastoma in a child with neurofibromatosis type 1. Pediatr Blood Cancer 49:357–359

Van Dyck F, Declercq J, Braem CV et al (2007) PLAG1, the prototype of the PLAG gene family: versatility in tumour development. Int J Oncol 30:765–774

Van Eyken P, Sciot R, Callea F et al (1990) A cytokeratin-immunohistochemical study of hepatoblastoma. Hum Pathol 21:302–308

Varma V, Cohen C (2004) Immunohistochemical and molecular markers in the diagnosis of hepatocellular carcinoma. Adv Anat Pathol 11:239–249

Vileisis RA, Sorensen K, Gonzalez-Crussi F et al (1982) Liver malignancy after parenteral nutrition. J Pediatr 100:88–90

Vivekanandan P, Thomas D, Torbenson M et al (2009) Methylation regulates hepatitis B viral protein expression. J Infect Dis 199:1286–1291

Von Schweinitz D, Wischmeyer P, Leuschner I et al (1994) Clinico-pathological criteria with prognostic relevance in hepatoblastoma. Eur J Cancer 30A:1052–1058

Wagner LM, Garrett JK, Ballard ET et al (2007) Malignant rhabdoid tumor mimicking hepatoblastoma: a case report and literature review. Pediatr Dev Pathol 10:409–415

Wang J, Chenivesse X, Henglein B et al (1990) Hepatitis B virus integration in a cyclin A gene in a hepatocellular carcinoma. Nature 343:555–557

Watanabe I, Kasai M, Watanuki T et al (1975) Malignant mixed tumor of the liver: report of a case and a review of the literature. Acta Hepatogastroenterol (Stuttg) 22:158–164

Watanabe I, Yamaguchi M, Kasai M (1987) Histologic characteristics of gonadotropin-producing hepatoblastoma: a survey of seven cases from Japan. J Pediatr Surg 22:406–411

Wei Y, Fabre M, Branchereau S et al (2000) Activation of beta-catenin in epithelial and mesenchymal hepatoblastomas. Oncogene 19:498–504

Weinberg AG, Mize CE, Worthen HG et al (1976) The occurrence of hepatoma in the chronic form of hereditary tyrosinemia. J Pediatr 88:434–438

Weinberg AG, Finegold MJ (1983) Primary hepatic tumors of childhood. Hum Pathol 14:512–537

Weinstein S, Scottolini AG, Loo SY et al (1985) Ataxia telangiectasia with hepatocellular carcinoma in a 15-year-old girl and studies of her kindred. Arch Pathol Lab Med 109:1000–1004

Wilkens L, Bredt M, Flemming P et al (2000) Cytogenetic aberrations in primary and recurrent fibrolamellar hepatocellular carcinoma detected by comparative genomic hybridization. Am J Clin Pathol 114:867–874

Willis RA (1962) The Pathology of tumours of children. Charles C. Thomas, Springfield

Wong N, Lai P, Pang E et al (2000) A comprehensive karyotypic study on human hepatocellular carcinoma by spectral karyotyping. Hepatology 32:1060–1068

Wu PC, Fang JW, Lau VK et al (1996) Classification of hepatocellular carcinoma according to hepatocellular and biliary differentiation markers. Clinical and biological implications. Am J Pathol 149:1167–1175

Yamada S, Ohira M, Horie H et al (2004) Expression profiling and differential screening between hepatoblastomas and the corresponding normal livers: identification of high expression of the PLK1 oncogene as poor-prognosis indicator of hepatoblastomas. Oncogene 23:5901–5911

Yamaoka H, Ohtsu K, Sueda T et al (2006) Diagnostic and prognostic impact of beta-catenin alterations in pediatric liver tumors. Oncol Rep 15:551–556

Yamauchi N, Watanabe A, Hishinuma M et al (2005) The glypican 3 oncofetal protein is a promising diagnostic marker for hepatocellular carcinoma. Mod Pathol 18:1591–1598

Yang J, Zhou F, Xu T et al (2008) Analysis of sequence variations in 59 microRNAs in hepatocellular carcinoma. Mutat Res 638:205–209

Yun K, Jinno Y, Sohda T et al (1998) Promoter-specific insulin-like growth factor 2 gene imprinting in human fetal liver and hepatoblastoma. J Pathol 185:91–98

Zatkova A, Rouillard JM, Hartmann W et al (2004) Amplification and overexpression of the IGF2 regulator PLAG1 in hepatoblastoma. Genes Chromosomes Cancer 39:126–137

Zerbini MC, Sredni ST, Grier H et al (1998) Primary malignant epithelial tumors of the liver in children: a study of DNA content and oncogene expression. Pediatr Dev Pathol 1:270–280

Zimmermann A (2000) Tumors of the liver – pathologic aspects. In: Blumgart LH (ed) Surgery of the liver, biliary tract and pancreas, vol II, 4th edn. Saunders Elsevier, Philadelphia, pp 1085–1130, Section 13, Chapter 69

Zimmermann A (2002) Hepatoblastoma with cholangioblastic features ('cholangioblastic hepatoblastoma') and other liver tumors with bimodal differentiation in young patients. Med Pediatr Oncol 39:487–491

Zimmermann A (2005) The emerging family of hepatoblastoma tumours: from ontogenesis to oncogenesis. Eur J Cancer 41:1503–1514

Zimmermann A (2006) Malignant epithelial liver tumors in children, adolescents and adults: molecular pathways of cancerogenesis, growth, and spread. In: Lee F (ed) Liver cancer: new research. Nova Biomedical Books, New York, pp 1–41, Chapter 1

Zucman-Rossi J, Jeannot E, Nhieu JT et al (2006) Genotype-phenotype correlation in hepatocellular adenoma: new classification and relationship with HCC. Hepatology 43:515–524

Zynger DL, Gupta A, Luan C et al (2008) Expression of glypican 3 in hepatoblastoma: an immunohistochemical study of 65 cases. Hum Pathol 39:224–230

Surgical Treatment

10

Piotr Czauderna and Dietrich von Schweinitz

Contents

P. Czauderna (✉)
Department of Surgery and Urology for Children and Adolescents, Medical University of Gdansk, Ul. Nowe Ogrody 1-6, 80-803, Gdansk, Poland
e-mail: pczaud@gumed.edu.pl

D. von Schweinitz
Kinderchirurgische Klinik im Dr. von Haunerschen Kinderspital, Universität München, Lindwurmstrasse 4, D-80337, München, Germany
e-mail: dietrich.schweinitz@med.uni-muenchen.de

10.1 Introduction

Tumor resection remains the main stem of treatment and the prerequisite of cure in most cases of pediatric liver tumors. However, liver surgery still remains a challenge for many less experienced centers, even though associated mortality rates dropped significantly being between 0% and 5% nowadays in major pediatric series (Pham et al. 2007; Finegold 2002). In the SIOPEL 1 study, which involved 91 centers from 30 countries, surgical mortality rate was 4% (5/115 patients) (Pritchard et al. 2000). It is often preferred, however, when the surgery is performed in well-experienced and adequately equipped centers, while many pediatric surgical institutions may only see one case of liver tumor per 1 or 2 years.

10.2 Biopsy

Careful preoperative imaging should be performed in all patients. The three largest international study groups have different approaches to biopsy in children with suspected primary malignant liver tumors. In recent SIOPEL protocols, biopsy has become mandatory in cases of suspected hepatoblastoma, regardless of the size and apparent resectability of the tumor (Czauderna et al. 2006a). In the past the *Children's Oncology Group (COG)* and the *German Pediatric Oncology and Hematology group (GPOH)* recommended laparotomy with a view to primary resection of the tumor (Fuchs et al. 2002). This approach has become somewhat modified lately and limited mainly to tumors resectable by standard hemihepatectomies as judged by preoperative imaging (Meyers et al. 2009). In the COG protocols, all other children have a diagnostic

A. Zimmermann et al. (eds.), *Pediatric Liver Tumors*, Pediatric Oncology,
DOI: 10.1007/978-3-642-14504-9_10, © Springer-Verlag Berlin Heidelberg 2011

biopsy. The GPOH group, however, regards biopsy as unnecessary in patients aged between 6 months and 3 years of age with unequivocal clinical findings, typical imaging, and highly elevated alfa-fetoprotein (AFP) level (Katzenstein et al. 2002a). So far as patients with suspected hepatocellular carcinoma including older children are concerned, particularly those with predisposing conditions, upfront resection may be recommended, whenever possible.

Although biopsy can be probably safely omitted in the so-called typical hepatoblastoma cases, listed above, it is highly recommended in every case nowadays. First, it allows using chemotherapy safely and lawfully having tissue diagnosis. Second, hepatocellular carcinoma (HCC) can occur even in very young children, for example, in the large US Intergroup report 5 out of 28 HCCs were diagnosed in patients younger than 5 years (Finegold 2002). HCC was also reported in patients as young as 3 years (Schnater et al. 2003). In young children (below 12 months of age), physiologically elevated AFP may have a confounding effect. Additionally, in this age group, benign hepatic masses, that is, hemangiomas and hemangioendotheliomas are more common.

The aim of tumor biopsy is to obtain sufficient tissue to allow an accurate diagnosis, whilst avoiding complications. In general, tumor biopsy is a safe and diagnostically reliable procedure. Complications associated with liver biopsy are mild and relatively rare occurring in 5–10% of patients at the most (Schnater et al. 2003). The single most important and potentially immediate complication is hemorrhage. There is also the possibility of seeding tumor cells into an uninvolved segment of the liver, the abdominal wall or peritoneal cavity, although this complication is very infrequent and never found in SIOPEL studies (Schnater et al. 2003). In SIOPEL 1 and 2 studies, when open biopsy was used in the majority of cases, no life-threatening biopsy complications were recorded. In the SIOPEL 1 trial complications did occur in 6% of cases (7/122) and were generally minor: bleeding from the biopsy site in four patients (one open, three closed), abdominal pain in two (one open, one closed), and a wound infection in a child who had an open biopsy (Pritchard et al. 2000). All seven patients recovered completely with conservative management. There were no cases of tumor spillage or seeding reported.

Traditionally, open biopsy was performed by exploratory laparotomy. However, the above risks can be minimized by using a percutaneous coaxial technique or (in case of laparoscopic approach) using a protecting needle to guide *tru-cut biopsies*. This is particularly important in suspected inoperable HCC, because it is associated with the high risk of biopsy tract seeding. Additionally, with recent improvements in staging by cross-sectional liver imaging (computed tomography – CT and/or magnetic resonance imaging – MRI) and percutaneous biopsy techniques, it has become clear that diagnostic laparotomy is unnecessary and probably undesirable. The SIOPEL group consequently favors image-guided needle biopsy in children with suspected HB (Czauderna et al. 2005). *Fine needle aspiration cytology* is generally not recommended as it may provide insufficient material for diagnosis and will not allow tissue storage for biological studies.

Correction of severe coagulopathy or thrombocytopenia should be attempted prior to biopsy. Biopsies may be performed under general anesthesia in children. Real-time ultrasound (US) guidance makes liver tumor biopsy easier and safer, thus it is strongly recommended. Automated or semi-automated cutting needles (16- or 18-gauge) provide sufficiently large tumor cores. A coaxial approach seems to be the best, because it allows multiple samples to be obtained with a single tissue path (Czauderna et al. 2006a). Whenever possible, the outer needle should be passed through unaffected liver for a short distance to minimize the possibility of tumor seeding. Great care should be taken, however, to avoid crossing, and therefore possibly contaminating, segments of the liver that will not be resected at subsequent surgery. The biopsy tract may be embolized through the outer needle at the end of the procedure, either with thrombogenic plugs of gelatin foam (Czauderna et al. 2006a), or with a slurry of collagen (Hoffer 2000).

Alternatively, biopsy may be performed via *laparoscopy* or in a laparoscopic-assisted fashion (Fig. 10.1). It has the potential advantage of detecting extrahepatic tumoral deposits. The biopsy tract should be marked by a stitch or tattoo and resected during the definitive surgery, especially if the diagnosis is HCC.

The samples should be sent fresh to a histopathology laboratory. In the case of very large and necrotic tumors, it may be worthwhile to confirm adequacy and viability of the pathologic material sampled by immediate frozen section examination. Biopsy results should be interpreted in the light of clinical and radiological

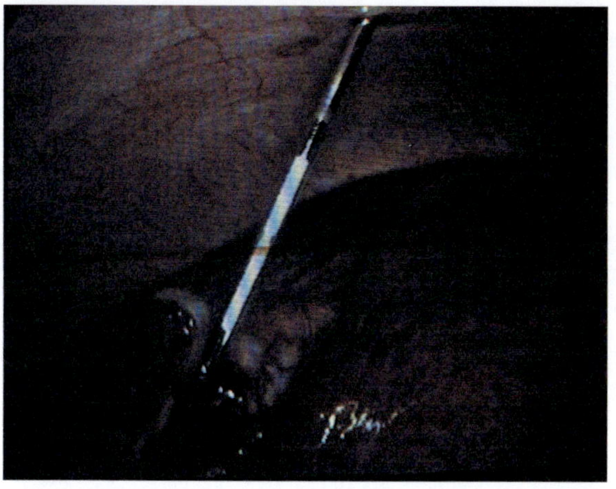

Fig. 10.1 Laparoscopic-assisted tru-cut needle liver tumor biopsy

findings, as the histological interpretation can sometimes be misleading in isolation. In addition to confirming the diagnosis, biopsy material may be stored and used for future research purposes.

10.3 Liver Resections

The ultimate goal of surgical resection in primary liver tumors is to achieve complete clearance of the tumor. In the case of hepatoblastoma, which is the most common primary malignant hepatic tumor of childhood, the approach differs between various study groups as mentioned earlier. The SIOPEL group recommends a delayed surgical approach in every case since *preoperative chemotherapy* largely facilitates resection by shrinking most tumors and even downstaging some by limiting them to fewer hepatic sections (Czauderna et al. 2005; Schnater et al. 2002). It is very unusual for a tumor to increase in size during preoperative chemotherapy: this happened in only four patients (3% of the total number) in the SIOPEL 1 study and only one of them became unresectable and later underwent a transplant and was hence completely salvaged (Czauderna et al. 2005). Contrary to past beliefs chemotherapy does not increase the number of surgical complications (Finegold 2002; Czauderna et al. 2005; Schnater et al. 2002). In fact, it makes tumors more solid, better delineated from surrounding liver parenchyma, and less prone to bleeding (Schnater et al. 2003; Czauderna et al. 2005). German data collected throughout two consecutive trials HB89 and HB94 showed that *primary hepatectomy* was associated with a significantly higher number of incomplete resections in comparison with the delayed post-chemotherapy approach: 30% (14/48) versus 19% (15/78) (Fuchs et al. 2002). In the USA, however, primary surgery is preferred, at least in tumors limited to one hepatic lobe, with a hope to avoid the potential toxicity of prolonged chemotherapy: with this approach about 40% of tumors can be resected upfront, however, another 45% can be operated successfully after preoperative chemotherapy (Finegold 2002; Meyers et al. 2009; Ortega et al. 2000).

It is well known that only complete tumor resection gives realistic hope of cure for children with malignant liver tumors, thus its planning remains crucial. This implies that all options, including *orthotopic liver transplantation* (which is the subject of a separate chapter), should be explored before declaring a tumor unresectable. This is particularly important in HCC: in the SIOPEL 1 study, the only HCC survivors were patients who underwent complete tumor removal; however, the chances for tumor recurrence in the liver is much higher in HCC than in HB being in the range of 50% (Czauderna et al. 2002). In the American Intergroup Hepatoma Study INT-0098 among 46 registered HCC patients event-free-survival at 5 years was 19% (SD=6%), while for stage I patients (completely resected at diagnosis) it was 88% (SD=12%), which underlines the importance of a complete HCC resection (Katzenstein et al. 2002b). The same applies to pediatric fibrolamellar HCC variant (Katzenstein et al. 2003). Unfortunately most of pediatric HCCs are advanced (83% in quoted American study) and never become resectable, even when some response to chemotherapy is observed (Czauderna et al. 2002; Katzenstein et al. 2002b).

The advocated *tissue margin* to achieve complete resection is somewhat controversial. Although the recommended adult minimal margin of resection is 1 cm, this is often difficult to follow in pediatric tumors; thus a close resection margin on a portal or hepatic vein should not be viewed as a contraindication to tumor resection attempt per se (Finegold et al. 2008). In fact, even a few millimeters margin may be sufficient for cure (Dicken et al. 2004). In multifocal tumors one should take into consideration a possibility of resecting completely all invaded liver sections as determined by imaging at diagnosis, if feasible, even if they had been cleared lately with preoperative chemotherapy. Otherwise small lesions, undetectable by preoperative imaging, may persist and the chance for local tumor recurrence may be higher. When there is any doubt on the completeness of resection and macroscopic residual tumor is found, the surgeon should definitely explore the possibility of immediate re-resection of the margin. In doubtful cases, taking extra frozen sections from both resection margins, including patient's one, may also be considered. It seems, however, that microscopic residuum is not associated with inferior outcome (see 9.3.3 Tumor residuum).

The final judgment of the completeness of resection is dependent on the definitive pathology report and especially on the return of postoperative AFP to normal, provided, of course, there is no persistent metastatic disease. This may take over 2 months, because the half-life of circulating AFP is about 6 days, and levels may be very high before surgery. It should be remembered that a minimal rise in AFP shortly after surgery may be a sign of liver regeneration.

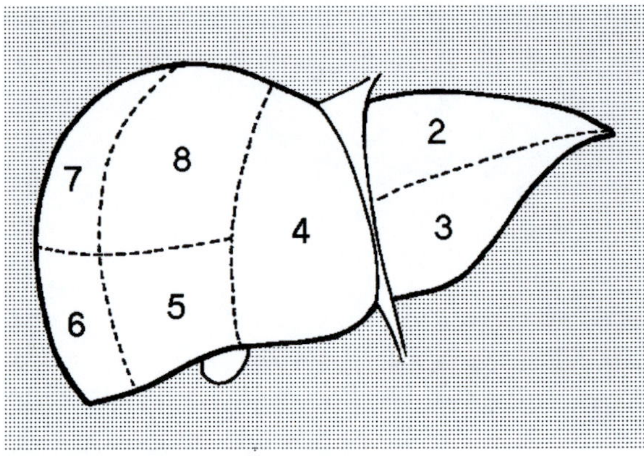

Fig. 10.2 Scheme of liver segments

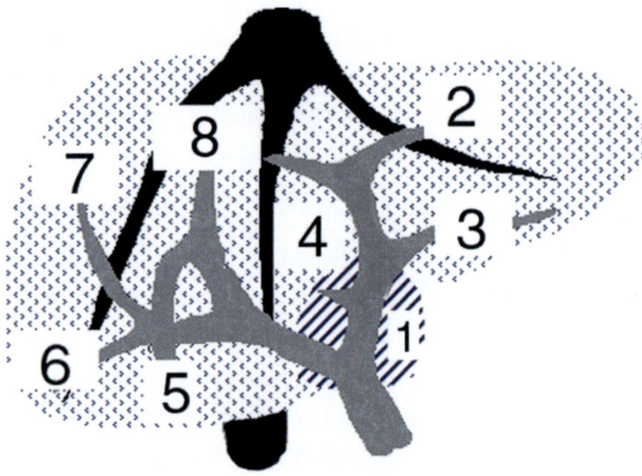

Fig. 10.3 Main vascular structures within the liver

10.3.1 Liver Anatomy and Resectability Assessment

10.3.1.1 Hepatic Anatomy

Good knowledge of hepatic anatomy is essential for any pediatric surgeon planning to perform liver resection. Liver in contrast to most organs has double blood supply: portal and arterial; however, most of malignant liver tumors are fed mainly by arterial vasculature. Classically, according to Couinaud's system, the liver is divided into eight segments including segment 1, which corresponds to the caudate lobe (Fig. 10.2) (Couinaud 1994; Stringer 2007; Roebuck et al. 2006). The left hepatic lobe is formed by segments 2–4 and the right one by segments 5–8. Division between upper and lower segments is marked by the bifurcation of the portal vein horizontally, while the vertical margin between both hepatic lobes is set at the middle hepatic vein or the plane between gallbladder fossa and retrohepatic inferior vena cava (Fig. 10.3). Additionally, the liver can be divided into four sections (previously called sectors): left lateral (seg. 2+3), left medial (seg. 4a and 4b), right anterior (seg. 5+8), and right posterior (6+8) (Fig. 10.4). It is divided according to the course of the right and middle hepatic veins and the umbilical fissure or the umbilical portion of the left portal vein (Figs. 10.3 and 10.4). In many anatomical drawings, the left hepatic vein is mistakenly shown as the borderline between left medial and left lateral sections, while in fact it runs to the left from this boundary (Fig. 10.4) (Roebuck et al. 2006). Caudate lobe is divided anatomically into three regions: the left Spiegel, the process portion, and the paracaval portion (Koga et al. 2009). However, it is only rarely involved in hepatoblastoma.

Unfortunately, liver anatomy can be very variable and segments borders are not quite perfectly correlated with the branching pattern of the portal vein (Roebuck et al. 2006).

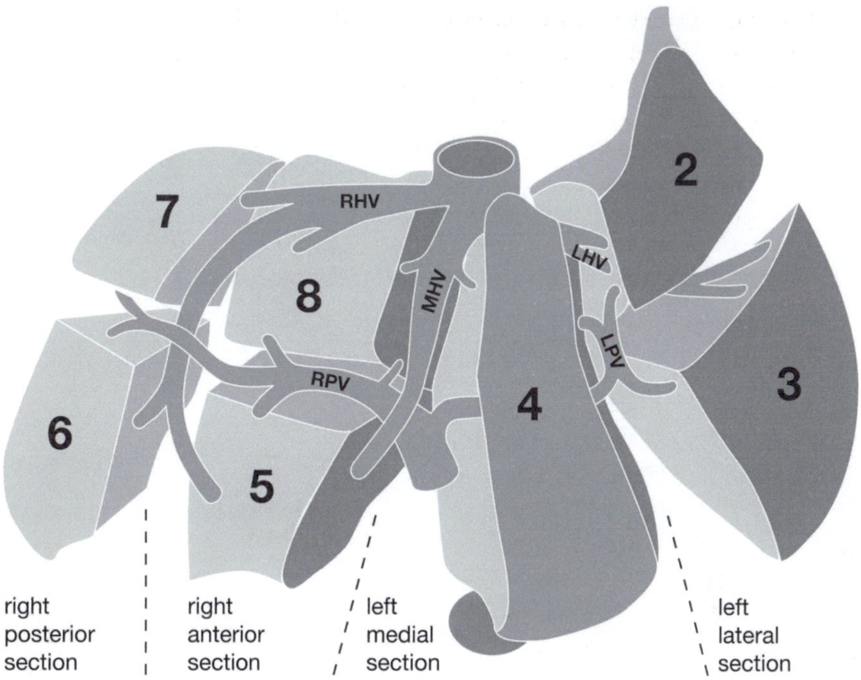

Fig. 10.4 Vascular structures and lines of division of liver parenchyma into segments

10.3.1.2 Resectability

Accurate and adequate assessment of tumor resectability, either at diagnosis or following preoperative chemotherapy depending on overall treatment strategy, is of utmost importance. This requires access to the high-quality cross-sectional *imaging* with contrast-enhanced CT and/or MRI. Ultrasound (with doppler studies) is an especially valuable tool for assessment of hepatic tumor resectability in children, as it allows real-time examination of the mass and its relation to hepatic vessels and may help visualize vascular structures that are not seen on CT because of suboptimal contrast enhancement (Finegold et al. 2008). US can also more easily discriminate actual vascular involvement and presence of neoplastic thrombus from vessel compression only. It is often extremely helpful for the surgeon to be present during the US examination.

Although three *staging systems* exist in pediatric liver tumors, two of them (Clinical Oncology Group staging system and TNM) are postoperative and hence of little use in tumor resectability assessment. Additionally, the *TNM system* is complicated and not very well suited to hepatoblastoma and hence it is rarely used. In 1990, the SIOPEL group introduced the innovative preoperative tumor staging system, which was called *PRETEXT* (PRE-treatment Tumor EXTension) (Pritchard et al. 2000). It was specifically developed to predict tumor resectability and monitor response to preoperative chemotherapy. PRETEXT describes the number of liver sections involved, as well as presence of extrahepatic disease or vascular involvement coded by additional letters: V, P, E, M (Fig. 10.5). The letters V, P, E, and M were added for Venous, Portal, Extrahepatic, and Metastatic involvement. Although extrahepatic and nodal involvement in hepatoblastoma is rare, it was required to confirm this in any case by the biopsy. Vascular involvement was defined as the presence of intravascular thrombus, vessel encasement, or complete occlusion by the tumor. The following table represents definitions of PRETEXT individual categories:

PRETEXT number	Definition
I	One section is involved and three adjoining sections are free
II	One or two sections are involved, but two adjoining sections are free
III	Two or three sections are involved and no two adjoining sections are free
IV	All four sections are involved

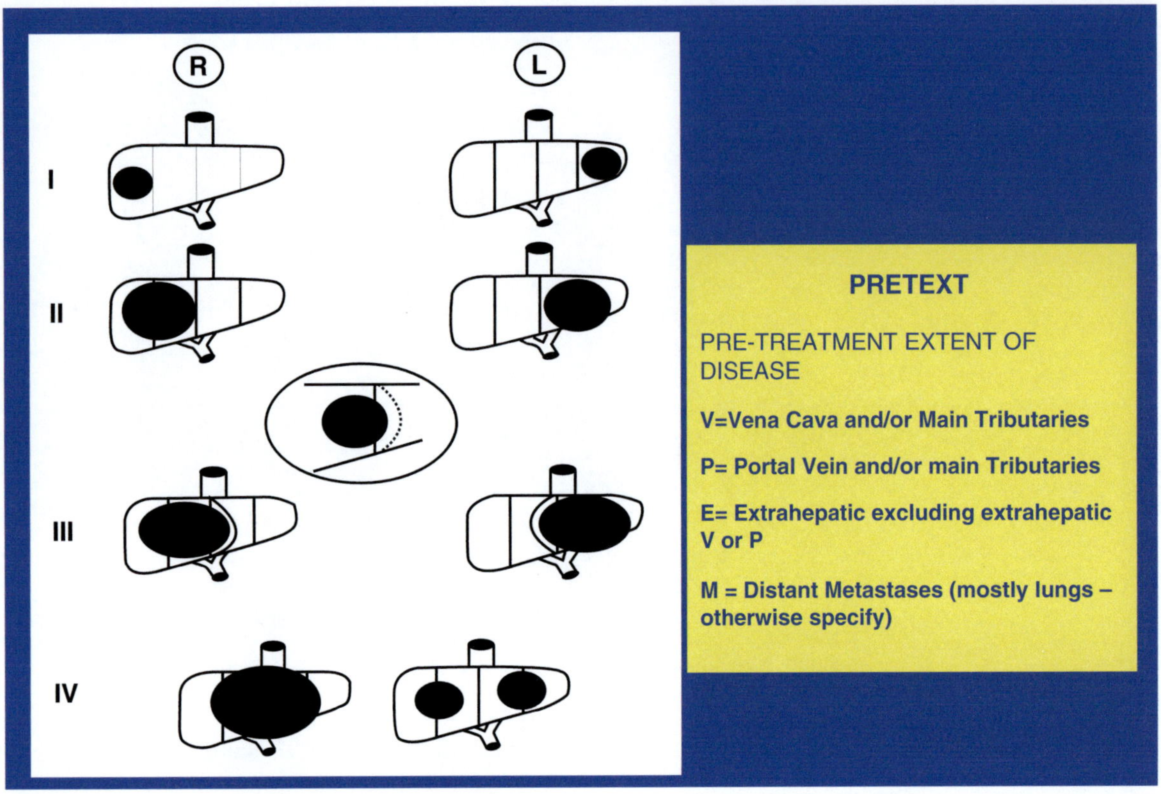

Fig. 10.5 Schematic representation of the PRETEXT staging system

In the year 2005, the PRETEXT system underwent an important modification and was made more detailed with the following changes introduced (Roebuck et al. 2007):

1. Segment 1 involvement was included and coded as "C1" (from caudate lobe). Additionally, by definition, all C1 patients have to be assigned at least to PRETEXT 2 category.
2. For extrahepatic disease, suffix "a" was added, if ascites was present.
3. Tumor focality was added and coded as "F1" (in case of multifocal tumors).
4. Tumor rupture or intraperitoneal hemorrhage at diagnosis was included and coded as "H1." Subcapsular or biopsy-related bleeding is not included and hence coded as "H0."
5. Nodal involvement was coded as "N1," if limited to the abdomen. When extra-abdominal, it was coded as "N2."
6. Finally, involvement of vascular structures was made more specific and coded as "P0," "P1," "P2" (depending on the number of main portal trunks involved) and "V0," "V1," "V2," "V3" (depending on the number of the hepatic veins and/or IVC involved). Additionally, suffix "a" was added in cases of the presence of intravascular tumor.

It was shown that PRETEXT system not only helps to judge tumor resectability at diagnosis and after preoperative chemotherapy but also determines the patient's *prognosis* (Brown et al. 2000). It showed moderate accuracy, good reproducibility, and inter-observer agreement, as well as superior predictive value for survival (in comparison with other staging systems) with a slight tendency to overstage patients (Aronson et al. 2005). Predictive value of PRETEXT system was roughly equivalent to the TNM system but superior to the COG system, when applied retrospectively to the INT-0098 American study (Meyers et al. 2009). Additionally, PRETEXT showed its usefulness in identifying patients amenable to an upfront surgical resection (PRETEXT I and II), as well as those who are potential candidates for liver transplantation (Meyers et al. 2009). Currently it is accepted by all major liver tumors study groups and implied prospectively in their trials (Meyers et al. 2009). However, it needs to be mentioned that some limitations of the PRETEXT system result from the fact that distinction between real invasion beyond the anatomic border of a given hepatic section and its compression and displacement by the tumor can sometimes be very difficult indeed, especially at diagnosis (Otte et al. 2004).

Other factors which influence tumor resectability are *multifocality* and *vascular involvement*: portal and hepatic veins, as well as IVC (D'Antiga et al. 2007).

Due to the impressive regenerative capabilities of the liver, as much as 75–85% of the hepatic parenchyma can be safely resected, provided the remaining liver mass is otherwise healthy (Czauderna et al. 2005; Dicken et al. 2004; Herzog et al. 2000). Within 6 months from major hepatic resection liver mass approaches 80–90% of its original volume (Needham et al. 2008). This regenerative process is limited in patients with liver cirrhosis and decreased functional hepatic reserve. Thus, in cases of preexisting liver disease, especially cirrhosis, preoperative tests measuring hepatic reserve (i.e., Indocyanine Green – ICG – clearance) or remnant liver volume radiographic measurements may be helpful in choosing an operative strategy.

Tumor resectability obviously depends on surgical expertise. For example, some extensive tumors involving both liver lobes can be radically resected by extended hemihepatectomy (trisegmentectomy) provided one lateral hepatic section remains disease-free (Figs. 10.6a, b and 10.7). Even tumor *encasement* or *invasion* of the retrohepatic inferior vena cava does not preclude a radical excision since the IVC can be resected en bloc and replaced by either a prosthetic graft (i.e., Gore-Tex) or a venous autograft (using internal jugular or external iliac vein) (Fig. 10.8) (Fuchs et al. 2002; Hemming et al. 2004). In case of limited involvement, a portion of the IVC wall can be excised and patched using autologous pericardium or Gore-Tex (Fuchs et al. 2002; Hemming et al. 2004). Also, when all three hepatic veins are involved, one of them may be reconstructed with a prosthesis or vascular autograft (i.e., portion of resected portal vein) or even sutured and anastomosed directly to the IVC, if feasible (Fuchs et al. 2002; Hemming et al. 2002). Alternatively, in selected cases of centrally located tumors, *atypical liver resection* with removal of all three hepatic veins leaving the liver remnant dependant on the direct venous drainage to the IVC by accessory retrohepatic veins, as described by Superina, can be used (Fig. 10.9) (Superina et al. 2000). In case of predicted insufficient liver remnant volume, it is possible to apply preoperative portal vein branch embolization, which will lead to hypertrophy of the remaining segments by approximately 25% (Hemming et al. 2004).

However, these "difficult" liver resections, especially those involving vascular reconstructive procedures, have become controversial. Relatively recent worldwide survey has shown excellent results of primary orthotopic liver transplantation (OLT) for hepatoblastoma on the contrary to secondary rescue OLT attempts (Otte et al. 2004). Thus, it has been concluded that very difficult liver resections, which carry a high risk of leaving residual tumor, should be avoided in favor of primary OLT. Liver transplantation in hepatoblastoma is associated with very good long-term survival in the range of 80% (Otte et al. 2004). It is clearly indicated in tumors unresectable by conventional means, predominantly PRETEXT IV tumors. This is supported by

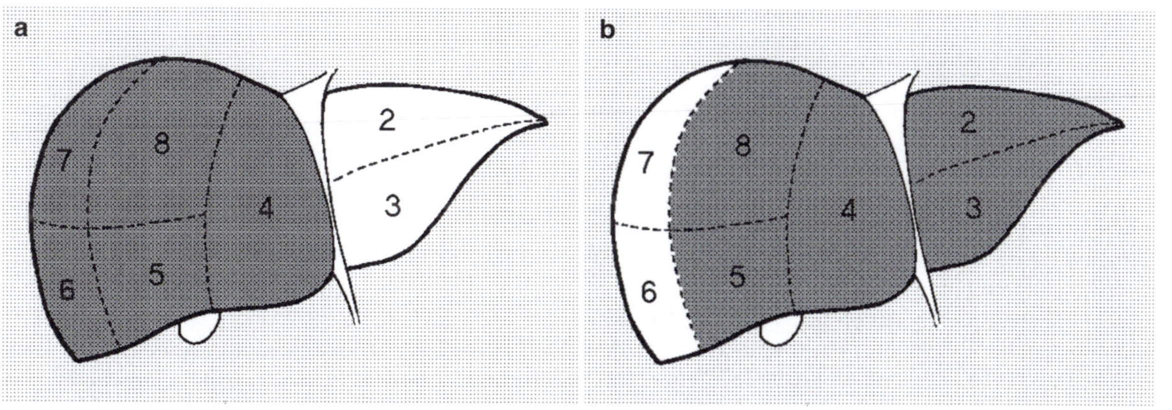

Fig. 10.6 Schematic drawing of the extended right and left hemihepatectomy

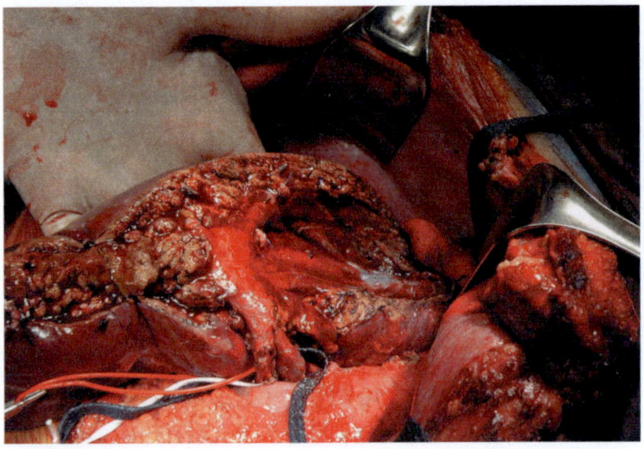

Fig. 10.7 Extended left hemihepatectomy with segments 6 and 7 left. The only remaining right hepatic vein has been peeled off the tumor and is visible at the resection margin. In this case liver transplantation was contraindicated due to HCC histology and presence of pulmonary metastases (Courtesy of Piotr Czauderna)

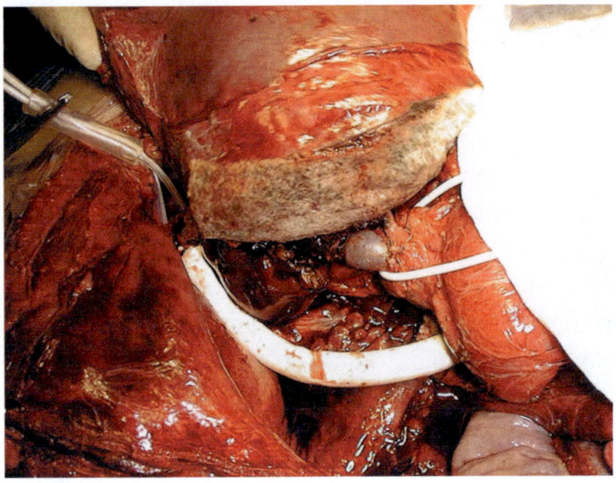

Fig. 10.8 Liver resection with inferior vena cava removal and its replacement with Gore-Tex prosthesis (Courtesy of Piotr Czauderna)

anecdotal reports on local relapse after liver resection in multiple PRETEXT IV tumors in which satellite tumor nodules seemed to be cleared with preoperative chemotherapy (Dall'Igna et al. 2003).

Liver transplantation has also been advised in PRETEXT III tumors located centrally in close proximity to major vascular structures. This issue is somewhat more debatable considering the good outcome for patients with microscopic residuum and difficulties associated with transplant surgery, that is, lack of donors (partly alleviated by living-related OLTs) and the need for life-long immunosuppression. Further studies are warranted taking into account concerns associated with potentially higher risk of tumor recurrence after OLT, especially in cases with initial pulmonary metastases. These doubts will possibly will be alleviated after completion of the *PLUTO* project (Pediatric Liver Unresectable Tumors Observatory) (Kalicinski & Otte 2009).

Difficult liver resections associated with a high chance for tumor residuum should clearly be avoided in localized pediatric HCC. It has been well known for many years that transplantation in adult patients with HCC fulfilling the so-called Conventional Milan Criteria - CMC (less than three tumors, less than 5 cm diameter of the single tumor, less than 3 cm of the largest diameter in case of multiple tumors) is associated with good prognosis with 70% chance for long-term survival (Mazzafero et al. 2008). However, it seems that these criteria are not necessarily ideally suited to children and that they can be safely ignored, at least in some pediatric patients. In the SIOPEL 5 study, designed specifically for pediatric HCC, in transplantation guidelines, there was no upper limit for the lesion size and the number of multiple tumors allowed was increased to 5. In the recent paper of Ismail et al., it was

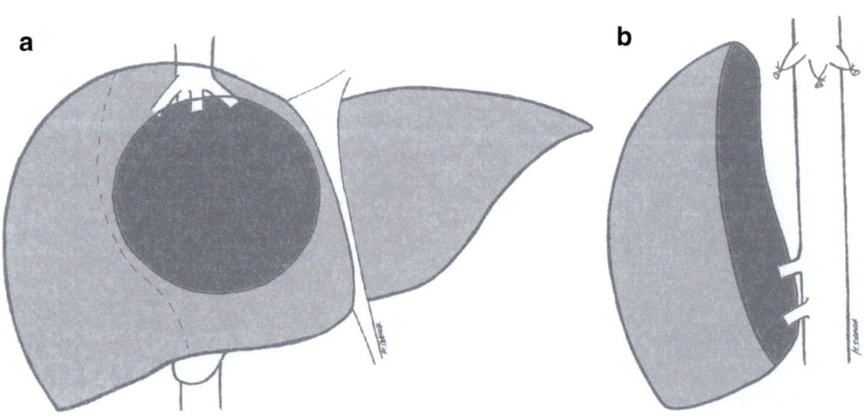

Fig. 10.9 Central atypical hepatectomy based on the direct retrohepatic venous drainage as described by Superina (**a**) Tumor involving all 3 hepatic veins schematically represented; (**b**) Postoperative drawing showing liver remnant based on retrohepatic veins

shown that HCC patients with transplantation (even though 8/11 did not fulfill CMC) had better outcome than resected ones with: 72% versus 30% long-term disease-free survival (Ismail et al. 2009). Moreover, in view of the above findings, it was postulated that in pediatric HCC cases, in which extended lobar resection is required, OLT might be a better option and that resection should be limited to patients in whom wide tumor-free margin can be achieved by standard hemihepatectomy. Of course presence of *metastases* and *extrahepatic disease* are absolute contraindications to OLT. Since numbers in this study are relatively small and originate from a single center only, it is difficult to consider the above suggestions as definite guidelines; however, they merit attention and require future confirmation in major multicenter studies.

In the past, only about 30–40% of liver tumors were resectable but with the above described progress, including introduction of preoperative chemotherapy and liver transplantation, current *resection rates* for standard risk hepatoblastoma are well above 90% (i.e., 97% in SIOPEL 2 study), while for high risk tumors they are in the range of 60–70% (i.e., 67% in SIOPEL 2 study) (Finegold 2002; Czauderna et al. 2006a; Finegold et al. 2008; Brown et al. 2000; Perilongo et al. 2000; Czauderna et al. 2001; Horton et al. 2009). Moreover, SIOPEL studies have shown that 25% of initially inoperable tumors can be converted into being resectable by conventional means (Czauderna et al. 2005). In selected cases, when liver transplantation is not available, intrahepatic *chemoembolization* may render the tumor resectable, when systemic chemotherapy fails to do so (Fig. 10.10) (Czauderna et al. 2006b; Arcement et al. 2000).

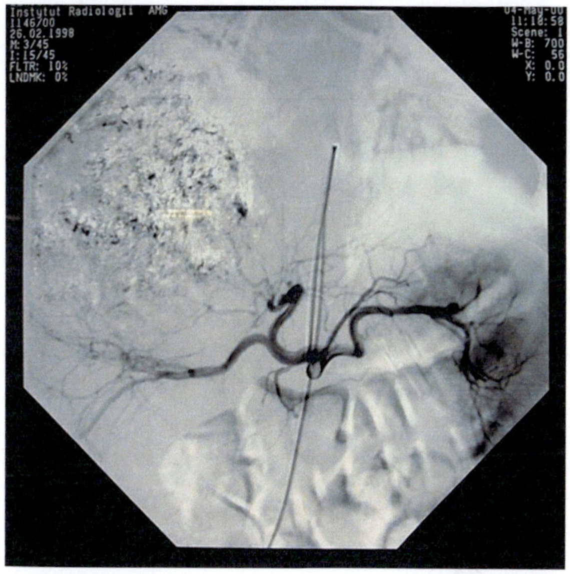

Fig. 10.10 Radiographic picture of hepatic tumor transarterial chemoembolization (TACE). Calcifications from previous TACE procedures are visible within the tumor

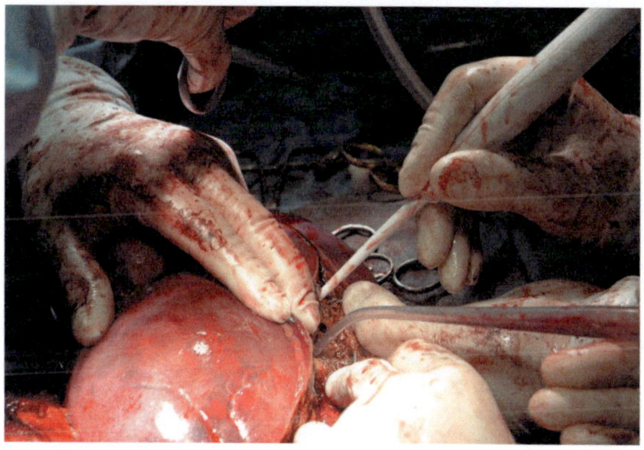

Fig. 10.11 Use of water-knife for parenchymal cleavage (Courtesy of Piotr Czauderna)

10.3.2 Technical Aspects

As already mentioned, because of the rarity of pediatric liver tumors, surgery should be performed in specialist centers that are appropriately experienced and equipped, e.g. ultrasonic CUSA-type dissector, Ligasure (Covidien) or water-knife {Hydro-jet, ERBE}, infrared beamer or argon coagulator, intraoperative ultrasonography. Water-knife seems to have a potential advantage of being quicker than other devices, as well as being associated with much smaller blood loss (half of that in case of CUSA use) and shorter time of Pringle maneuver application (Fig. 10.11) (Rau et al. 2008). Availability of appropriate postoperative care facilities and experienced anesthesiologists is also essential. Even when all these conditions are met, extensive personal experience of hepatic surgery remains important. Patient's cardiac function should be assessed preoperatively by echocardiography to avoid any unexpected cardiac complications during and after surgery.

As there are several techniques applied in hepatic resections, it is very difficult to give detailed surgical guidelines in this field.

Intraoperative ultrasonography may be of significant help in performing liver resection, especially in extensive tumors, that is, multifocal hepatoblastomas or tumors located in close proximity to essential vascular structures (Thomas et al. 1989). It is also very helpful and sometimes even essential, when segmental liver resection is planned.

The first phase of operation is mobilization of the liver from its ligaments and other attachments, which is crucial. Meticulous dissection and control of all vascular structures above and below the liver, including the porta hepatis, as well as liver cleavage using anatomical planes are crucial to assure successful tumor resection and to minimize the chance for complications by providing adequate blood supply and bile drainage for the liver remnant (Fig. 10.12). Usually *porta hepatis* structures are dissected and divided first, which is followed by the dissection, division, and closure of one or two hepatic veins depending on to the extent of resection (Fig. 10.13). This can be done also during parenchymal phase of dissection according to local preference and tumor anatomy. Finally, the liver is divided along the line of ischemia which by that time should be clearly seen (Fig. 10.14).

Whatever technique of liver resection is applied, an important goal is to minimize blood loss and amount of intra-/postoperative transfusions since it is a known factor associated with HCC recurrence, at least in adults (Katz et al. 2009; Huang et al. 2009). Blood loss during the phase of parenchymal resection can be also minimized by the maintenance of a low central venous pressure (in general below 5 cm of water) and by the use of the *Pringle maneuver*

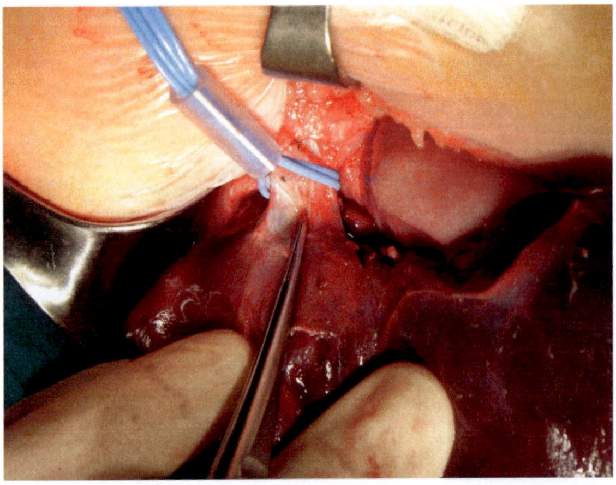

Fig. 10.12 Suprahepatic vena cava encircled by the blue vessel loop, tip of forceps indicates the fissure between left and right hepatic veins (Courtesy of Piotr Czauderna)

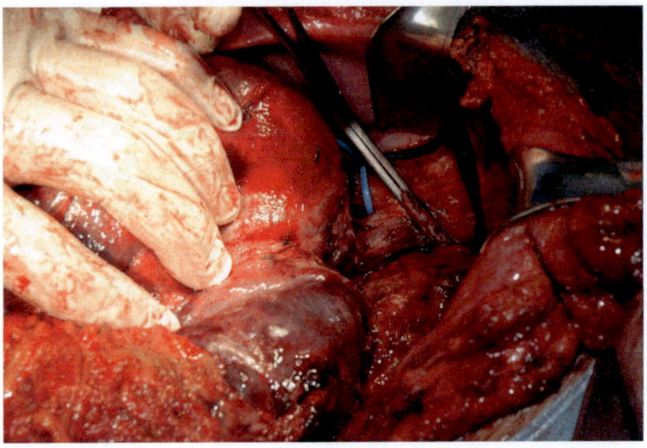

Fig. 10.13 Left and middle hepatic veins being clamped immediately before their suture closure. IVC is seen below (above the blue vessel loop). No clamp placed on hepatic veins distally due to tumor proximity – Pringle maneuver was used to prevent bleeding (Courtesy of Piotr Czauderna)

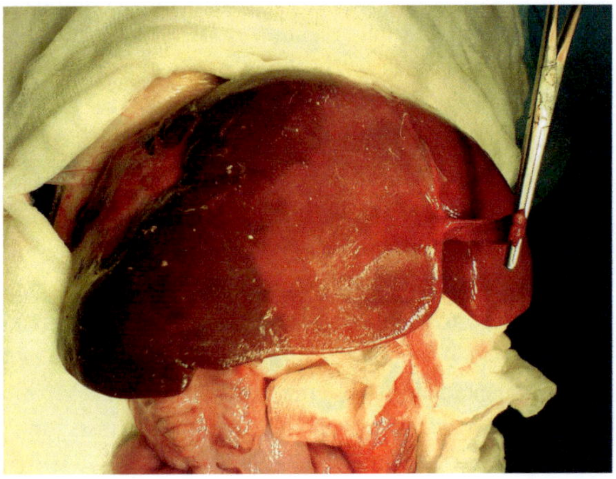

Fig. 10.14 Right hemihepatectomy – line of parenchymal ischemia is clearly seen (Courtesy of Piotr Czauderna)

(compression of the hepato-duodenal ligament) (Hemming et al. 2002; Rau et al. 2008). The latter can be applied safely up to 30–45 min except in small infants in whom severe bowel congestion may be hazardous (Hemming et al. 2004; Liu et al. 2003). However, in many cases, it is possible to perform the resection without occluding the blood flow, which helps preserve an optimal postoperative liver function (von Schweinitz 2006). For the parenchymal phase of resection several methods can be used, that is, ultrasonic aspirator, water knife, finger- or mosquito clamp-fracture technique.

Various techniques of *local hemostasis* can be implied, which include the Ligasure, harmonic scalpel,

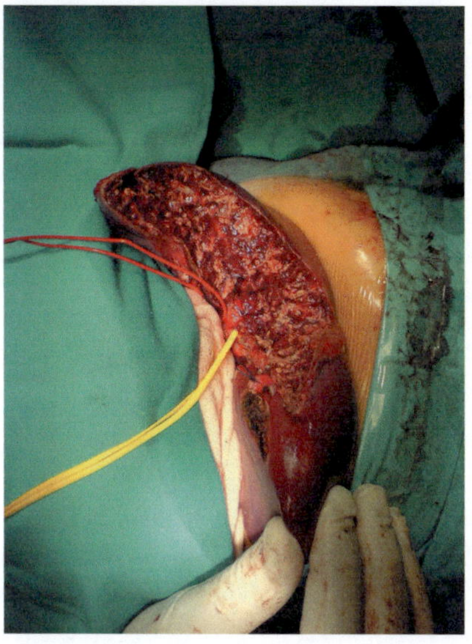

Fig. 10.15 Relatively bloodless liver resection margin (Courtesy of Piotr Czauderna)

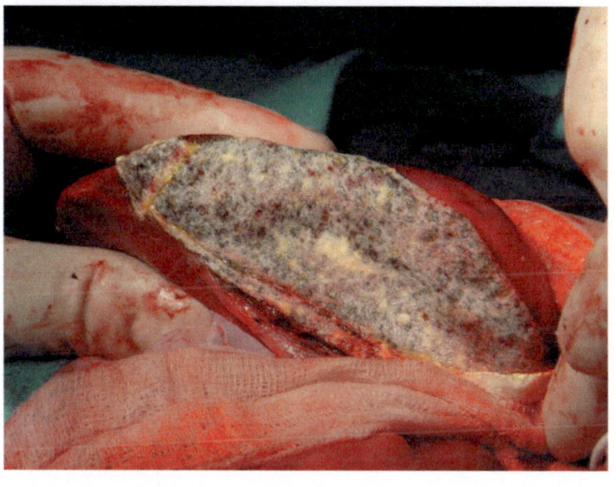

Fig. 10.16 Application of Tachosil to the resection margin (Courtesy of Piotr Czauderna)

vascular clips, bipolar coagulation, argon beamer, infrared coagulation, and local application of thrombostatic materials, that is, Tachosil (Nycomed) or biological sealants, that is, Tissucol or Bioglue (Figs. 10.15 and 10.16). Reduction of central venous pressure during the operation may also decrease blood loss (Tannuri et al. 2009).

Sampling of *lymph nodes* from the hepatoduodenal ligament should be performed in every case as their involvement has a significant impact on prognosis. Extensive lymphadenectomy of the hepatic pedicle is recommended in HCC cases. All extrahepatic intra-abdominal lesions should be biopsied or excised completely, when applicable and feasible.

10.3.2.1 Typical Liver Resections

In most cases of standard risk hepatoblastoma, a typical *hemihepatectomy* is sufficient (Fig. 10.17a and b). Left lateral segmentectomy (excising segments 2 and 3) is rarely used; for example, it was performed only in 5 out of 115 SIOPEL 1 patients (Fig. 10.18) (Schnater et al. 2002). Larger and/or multifocal tumors limited to three hepatic sections may require an extended hepatectomy (trisegmentectomy or *trisectionectomy*) (Figs. 10.6a, b, 10.7, 10.19 and 10.20). Indeed, the percentage of extended resections may reach 40% of resected cases in major multicenter series (Fuchs et al. 2002; Schnater et al. 2002). Some small tumors can be resected by a *segmentectomy* or a bi-segmentectomy.

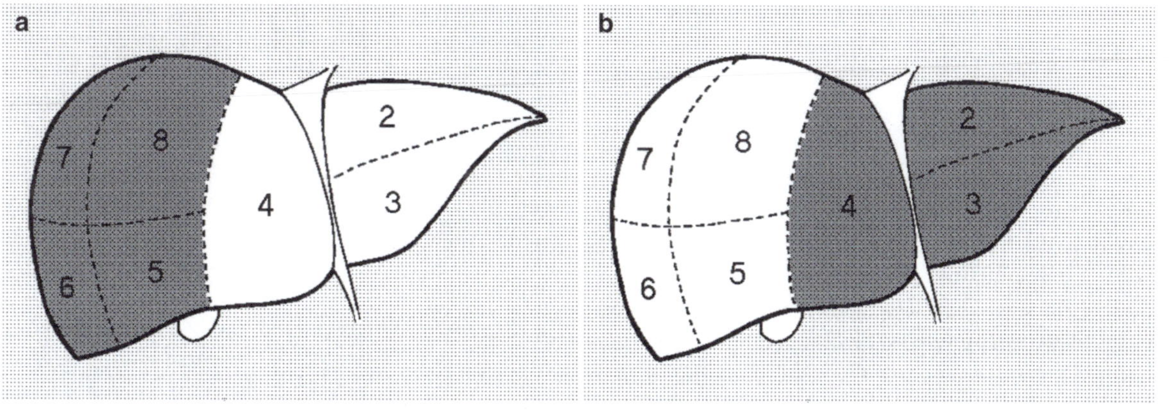

Fig. 10.17 Schematic drawing of the standard right (**a**) and left (**b**) hemihepatectomy

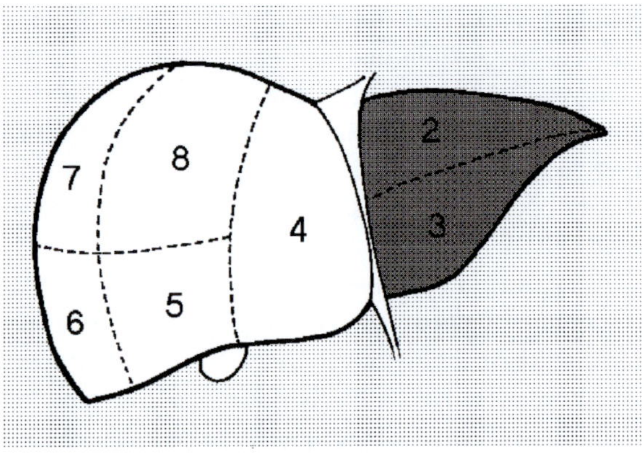

Fig. 10.18 Schematic representation of the left lateral lobectomy (sectionectomy)

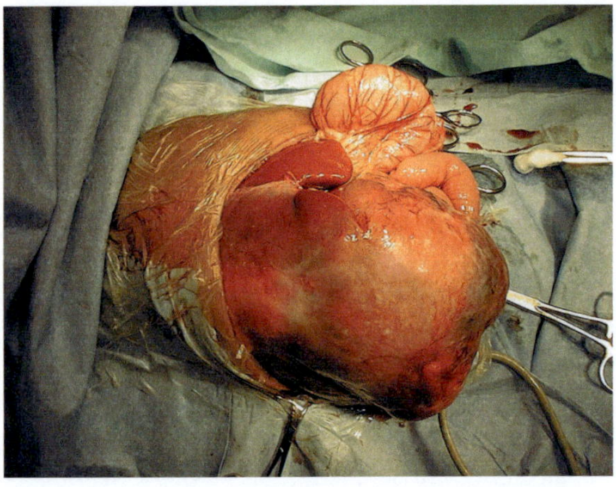

Fig. 10.19 Large tumor of the right lobe and segment 4 requiring extended right hemihepatectomy (Courtesy of Piotr Czauderna)

10.3.2.2 Atypical Liver Resections

In cases of HCC, in common with hepatoblastoma, atypical liver resection techniques should be avoided since they are associated with higher rate of incomplete tumor removal and increased rate of postoperative complications. In two consecutive German Cooperative Liver Tumor studies HB89 and HB94, out of the total 129 liver resections, 36 were atypical and they resulted in 38% of tumor residuum cases in comparison with only 18% in typical liver resections. This difference was statistically significant (Fuchs et al. 2002). It may be partly explained by the dissemination of tumor cells in the liver due to the blood supply pattern after atypical resections and presence of microscopic vascular invasion. Another possibility is that hepatocyte growth factor can stimulate *liver regeneration* and tumor cell proliferation. Standard partial hepatectomy is thus the best surgical practice. Atypical liver resections are justified in very selected cases only, mainly of multifocal tumors, when liver transplantation is not an option.

10.3.2.3 Special Surgical Techniques

When liver transplantation is not available for any reason, special techniques of hepatic resection can be employed in difficult cases, especially when there is a significant vascular involvement and/or infiltration of the central *bile duct*. These include: tumor resection under hypothermia and extracorporeal circulation, total vascular exclusion of the liver (TVE), as well as the central resection (central hepatectomy as described by LaQuaglia) preserving more liver parenchyma but having the potential disadvantage of leaving two raw hepatic surfaces (Fig. 10.21) (Fuchs et al. 2002; Liu et al. 2003; La Quaglia et al. 2002). Another surgical technique is the caudate lobe resection (this tumor location is usually associated with significant intraoperative difficulties) (Koga et al. 2009). Although tumors involve the caudate lobe in children very rarely, its surgical removal tends to be risky because of its anatomy and direct blood outflow to the IVC through very short veins. In general,

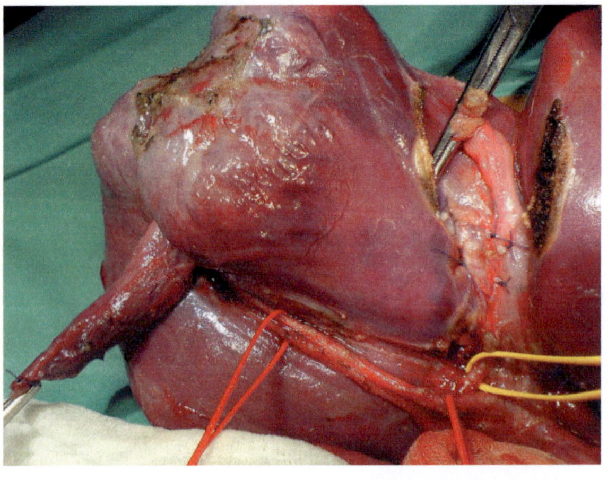

Fig. 10.20 Porta hepatis dissection (to the right of umbilical fissure) during the right extended hemihepatectomy: gallbladder, tumor, and umbilical fissure are clearly seen (Courtesy of Piotr Czauderna)

caudate lobectomy alone may be performed in tumors localized in the left caudate lobe and/or the caudate process (Koga et al. 2009). Tumors involving the entire caudate lobe or located in its paracaval portion require left or right lobectomy. The site of lobectomy is determined by the cranial tumor extent and the origin of its feeding vessels (Koga et al. 2009). Total hepatic vascular exclusion with simultaneous clamping of supra- and infrahepatic IVC, as well as hepato-duodenal ligament, may be particularly useful in cases of IVC wall involvement and the subsequent need for its reconstruction. It has been proven that warm ischemic time can safely be kept as long as 45 min (Liu et al. 2003; Zografos et al. 1999; Delva et al. 1989). Some of the above techniques require significant surgical expertise.

In cases of *portal vein thrombus*, which is particularly common in HCC, portal thrombectomy under conditions of portal clamping may be performed (Aldrighetti et al. 2009). These techniques allow dissection of the tumor from the vessel or with a portion of the vascular wall and its subsequent reconstruction using an autologous venous graft, a strip of peritoneum, or prosthetic patch in a relatively bloodless field. Pediatric experience with these techniques is somewhat limited.

Another possibility available in transplant centers is to resect the tumor with transplantation back-up, in which case the liver can be fully mobilized and dissected beyond a "point of no return" or *ex-vivo* tumor resection with subsequent liver autotransplantation, albeit the latter technique is rarely used nowadays (Hemming et al. 2002; Okajima et al. 2009; Millar et al. 2001).

Recently, laparoscopic techniques have been applied to liver tumors, mainly in adult HCC, as well as in benign pediatric tumors (Dagher et al. 2008; Dutta et al. 2007; Yoon et al. 2006; Han et al. 2009). For a long time, gas embolism risk and difficulty in controlling bleeding were the main obstacles for laparoscopic liver surgery (Han et al. 2009). In most situations, the indications for laparoscopy are limited to anteriorly located, easily accessible tumors occupying mainly segments II, III, V, VI, and partly IV (Han et al. 2009). Also the feasible tumor upper size is considered to be limited to 5 cm in most cases, while pediatric tumors frequently tend to be bigger. The easiest laparoscopic approach is left lateral sectionectomy (Fig. 10.18), which was actually the first pediatric laparoscopic liver resection ever made (Yoon et al. 2006). Laparoscopic techniques require, however, not only access to specialized and costly equipment, for example, laparoscopic ultrasonography, laparoscopic Hydro-Jet and argon beam applicators, harmonic scalpel, or Ligasure, but also vast expertise in minimally invasive surgery.

10.3.3 Tumor Residuum

Incomplete liver tumor resection is usually associated with worse outcome; thus whenever there is any doubt and particularly, when macroscopic residual tumor is found, the surgeon should definitely explore the possibility of immediate re-resection of the margin – taking an "extra slice" of liver (Fig. 10.22a–c).

Even though complete tumor resection should be aimed for at every surgical attempt in case of liver tumor, postoperative microscopic tumor residuum does not seem to confer a worse prognosis for patients with hepatoblastoma after effective chemotherapy. In the SIOPEL 1 trial only 2 of 16 patients (13%), who died, had microscopic residuum after surgery, while in the SIOPEL 2 study microscopic residual disease was found in 13 SR patients and all of them became long-term survivors (Schnater et al. 2002; Perilongo et al. 2004). Interestingly, eight of them did not receive any additional treatment other than standard two postoperative cisplatin (CDDP) courses, as prescribed by the protocol, and one was only observed.

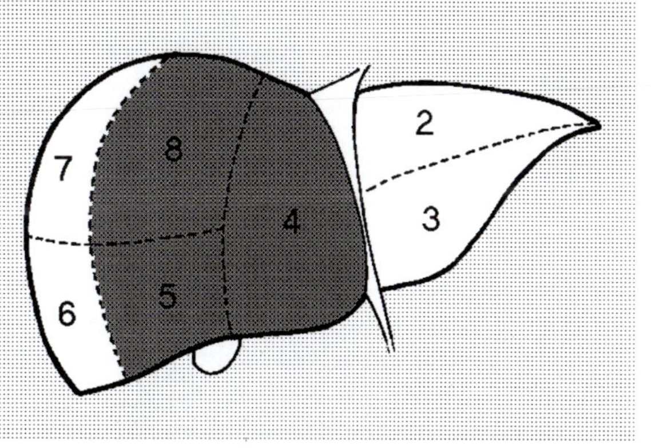

Fig. 10.21 Schematic drawing of the central hepatic resection

In the SIOPEL 3 standard risk arm only 2 out of 28 patients with *microscopical residual* experienced an event and actually 1 of them had initial intraperitoneal tumor spillage (Perilongo et al. 2009). This unexpected finding may be a result of the fact that the resection margin is vacuumed and thus practically ablated in many patients due to the frequent use of CUSA in hepatic resections and/or the residuum cells may not be viable due to the use of preoperative chemotherapy.

Nevertheless, radical tumor excision should always be recommended, especially for HCC and other malignant tumors with poor susceptibility to chemotherapy or radiation.

10.3.4 Complications and Their Management

Postoperative *complications* are relatively frequent in hepatic surgery reaching as many as 15–30% of cases (Pham et al. 2007; Pritchard et al. 2000; Tannuri et al. 2009; Towu et al. 2004). Most frequent intra- and postoperative complications in hepatic surgery include: infection, intraoperative bleeding, intraoperative tumor rupture, cardiac arrest, air embolism, postoperative bile leak or delayed bleeding, transitory hypoglycemia, and finally, bowel obstruction due to adhesions formation (Towu et al. 2004).

10.3.4.1 Bleeding

In SIOPEL 1 study, there were 3 cases of postoperative bleeding among 115 resected cases (Pritchard et al. 2000; Figs. 10.22 and 10.23). Unrecognized anomalous origin of the accessory left or right hepatic artery may contribute to the occurrence of bleeding. In selected cases of severe bleeding, which is the most common intraoperative complication, intravenous recombinant factor VII (Novoseven, NovoNordisk) may be of significant benefit despite its high cost. Use of Pringle maneuver in the parenchymal phase of the dissection may also decrease amount of bleeding. Other techniques like extracorporeal blood circulation, maintaining low central venous pressure and hypothermia can be used in selected cases, too (Fuchs et al. 2002; Ein et al. 1981).

10.3.4.2 Bile Leak and Stricture

Persistent bile leak is one of the most frequent complications in liver surgery occurring in 2–12% of cases and its frequency has not decreased over the years (Vigano et al. 2008; Reed et al. 2002). If it does not resolve in over a week or so, it may require diagnostic hepatic scintigraphy and/or endoscopic retrograde cholangiopancreatography (ERCP) or Cholangio-MRI (MRCP) in order to identify the leak source, which is usually at the resected liver surface (Fig. 10.23). Sometimes it can result from unrecognized biliary anatomy anomalies or excessive skeletonizing of main bile ducts during porta hepatis dissection. In order to prevent this, some advocate biliary duct ligation at the level hilar plate during the parenchymal phase of resection, thus avoiding any dissection of the extrahepatic biliary tree (Tannuri et al. 2009). In most cases, biliary leak can be managed conservatively with the prolonged external drainage and sometimes with additional endoscopic sphincterotomy and internal biliary stenting (Reed et al. 2002). However, leaks draining above 100 cc/day on the tenth day of bile leakage diagnosis are associated with higher chance for conservative management failure (Vigano et al. 2008). If the leak persists, the Roux-en-Y intestinal loop internal drainage may be the procedure of choice (Fig. 10.24). Intraoperative use of normal saline or methylene blue cholangiography may contribute to the decrease in frequency of biliary leaks, although this is not routinely used in children.

Bile leak resulting from the damage to main biliary ducts may lead to the formation of stricture in the process of healing. Otherwise biliary stricture may result from excessive dissection of bile ducts and their subsequent devascularization. This complication seems to be somewhat more common after liver transplantation (reaching 20–30% of patients) than after standard hepatic resection; probably due to biliary anastomosis required during OLT (Mita et al. 2008). Although in adults retrograde endoscopic or antegrade percutaneous transhepatic stricture dilatation may be used, there is little experience with this technique in children (Mita et al. 2008). Thus, choledocho-jejunostomy or hepatico-jejunostomy seems to remain a standard surgical approach.

10.3.4.3 Others

Other complications encountered in liver surgery are: adhesion formation with subsequent ileus,

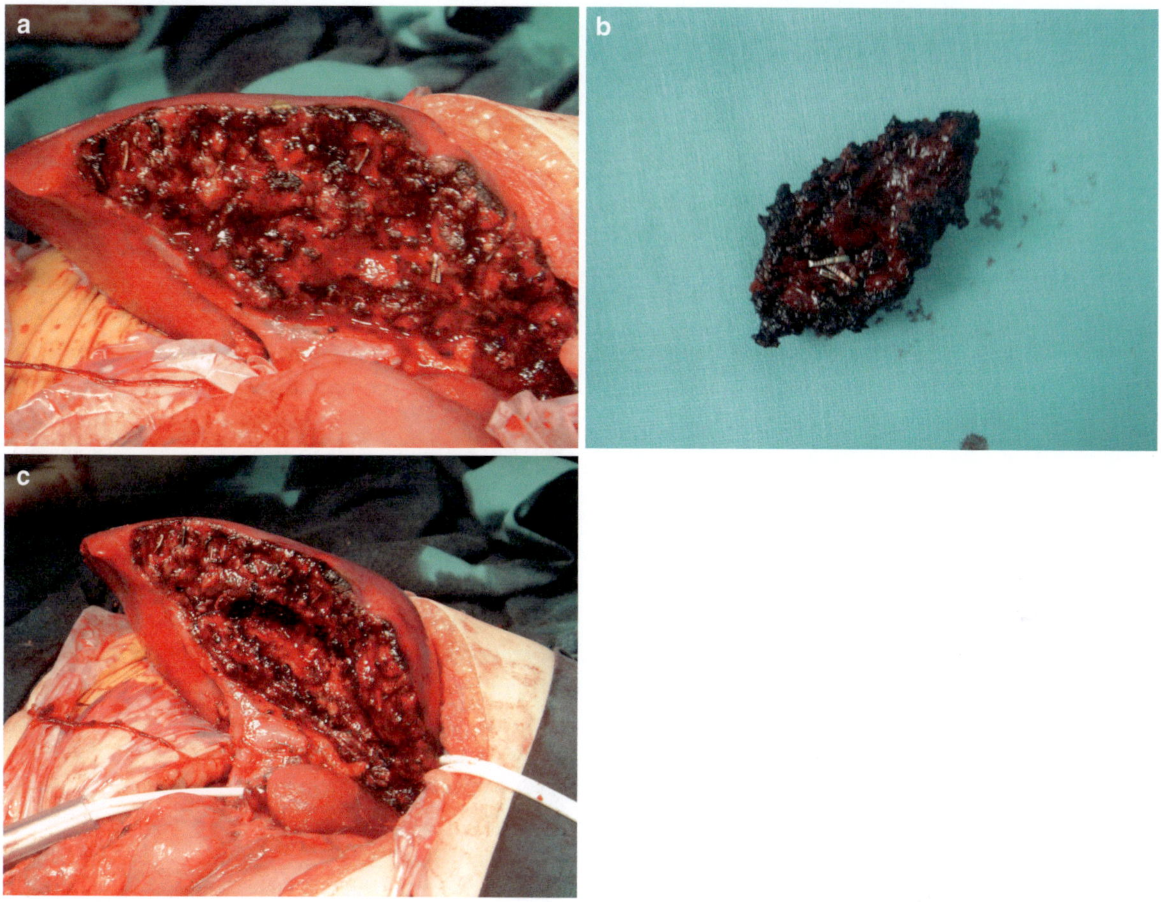

Fig. 10.22 (**a**) Hepatic resection with doubtful margin. (**b**) Re-resection specimen. (**c**) Hepatic margin after re-resection (Courtesy of Piotr Czauderna)

postoperative intussusception, wound infection, intra-abdominal abscess formation. Cardiac arrest may result not only from excessive bleeding but also from tumor material emboli or air emboli. *Air embolism* can be usually prevented by the use of higher PEEP (Positive End-Expiratory Pressure) setting during hepatic veins and IVC dissection.

10.4 Surgery for Metastases

10.4.1 Pulmonary Metastases

Aggressive surgery seems to have an important role in the resection of pulmonary hepatoblastoma metastases, either persisting or relapsed ones (Black et al. 1991; Feusner et al. 1993; Passmore et al. 1995). In the SIOPEL 1 study of 22 children, all 4 who had pulmonary metastases at diagnosis and underwent delayed metastasectomy, survived even though 2 of them had multiple thoracotomies (Schnater et al. 2002). In the Japanese JPLT-1 study, distant metastases were observed in 20 out of 134 cases: 2 them persisted after preoperative chemotherapy and required surgical resection (Matsunaga et al. 2003). In the American Clinical Oncology Group (COG) INT-0098 study, thoracotomy was performed for initial pulmonary metastases in 9 out of 38 children and 8 of them became long-term survivors (Meyers et al. 2007).

Optimal timing of pulmonary metastasectomy is still debatable – among nine patients reported above two were operated before liver resection, fives imultaneously and two afterwards. According to some opinions, however, thoracotomy is preferred before OLT or liver resection in order to avoid the effects of metastases growth stimulation and tumor cell proliferation triggered by hepatic

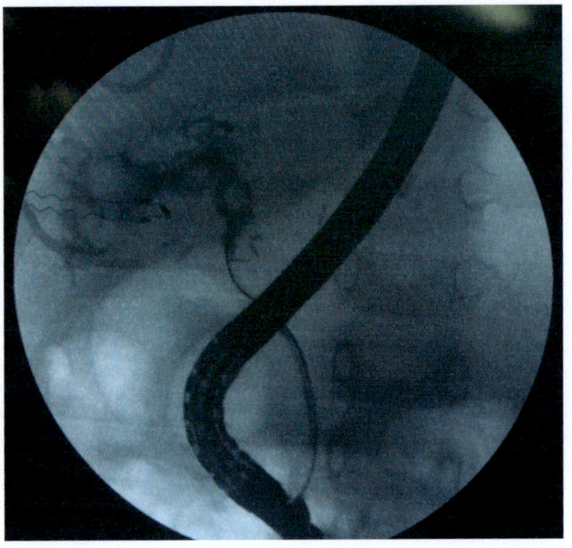

Fig. 10.23 ERCP visualization of the bile leak in the region of the bifurcation of the common hepatic duct probably resulting from necrosis of its wall due to ischemia (Courtesy of Piotr Czauderna)

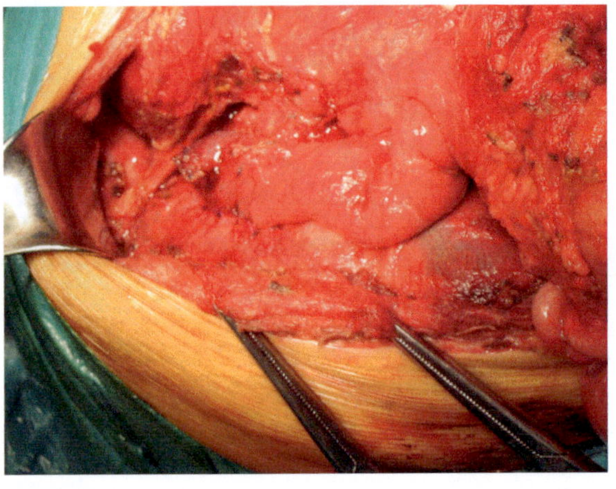

Fig. 10.24 Roux-en-Y ileal limb being sutured to the bile leak source. Post-resection hepatic surface is visible in the left upper corner (Courtesy of Piotr Czauderna)

growth factors secreted after major liver surgery (Fuchs et al. 2002; von Schweinitz et al. 2000).

Regarding optimal approach to pulmonary metastases this is debatable, too. In any case preoperative pulmonary high resolution CT is crucial for adequate operation planning, even though, not infrequently, the number of intraoperatively identified lesions is higher than radiological findings. In the work of Fuchs et al., preoperative imaging detected about 76% of the total number of metastases when compared to intraoperative findings (Fuchs et al. 2008). This was specifically true for lesions smaller than 2 mm of diameter. Metastasectomy, when bilateral lung involvement is present, can be performed either via *sternotomy* or simultaneous *lateral thoracotomies* or in staged fashion via posterolateral thoractomies. All methods have their own advantages and disadvantages. Sternotomy allows for safe and repeated bilateral resection, and it can be even combined with the primary tumor resection; however, access to the posterior part of both pulmonary lower lobes may be compromised with this technique (Fuchs et al. 2008). Necessary luxation of the left lower lobe may result in hemodynamic and ventilation problems (Fuchs et al. 2008). As many as 65 metastases have been removed during single bilateral attempts (Fuchs et al. 2008). When the number of lung metastatic lesions is small, thoracoscopic metastasectomy or video-assisted approach (VATS) may be considered. Usually wedge resection is preferred with the use of staplers or manual suturing. However, in many cases, metastases, especially when deeply seated, can be either enucleated by electrocautery or laser with a safe tissue margin. A lobectomy is rarely indicated.

10.5 Surgery for Recurrent Disease

Surgery may be applied to treat relapsed patients with pulmonary metastases, if numerable and resectable, and/or to liver relapse. Actually, the latter one may be more difficult or even impossible, especially in the setting of previous extended hepatic resections. In the SIOPEL 1 study, two out of five patients who developed recurrent pulmonary disease underwent multiple thoracotomies without any complications (two and three respectively) (Schnater et al. 2002). In the same study five locally relapsed patients underwent liver surgery, all of them were resected completely at the second attempt and two became long-term survivors (Schnater et al. 2002). In the COG experience, three out of ten patients, who developed pulmonary metastases and became long-term survivors, underwent lung surgery with multiple thoracotomies in two of them (Feusner et al. 1993). In the German Cooperative Pediatric Liver Tumor Study HB 94 8 of 14 children (57%) with recurrent tumors survived (Katzenstein et al. 2002a).

All survivors underwent complete resection of their pulmonary metastases or local recurrence. In the Japanese JPLT-1 study surgical resection to preserve liver function was performed in four recurrent liver tumors and all of them were alive with no evidence of disease for at least 17 months (Matsunaga et al. 2003). Similarly, recent Malogolowkin's review of doxorubicin treated INT-0098 patients proved that all relapsed or progressed and subsequently salvaged patients had their tumors surgically resected (Malogolowkin et al. 2008). On the other hand, a relatively recent COG INT-0098 study survey showed that thoracotomy done for tumor relapse is associated with a significant recurrence rate: out of 13 relapsed patients, who underwent thoracotomy with pulmonary metastasectomy (8) or biopsy only (5), only 4 became long-term survivors (Meyers et al. 2007). Thus, it can be concluded that in the setting of recurrent disease the role of surgery is more controversial, particularly regarding pulmonary metastases, although even then it may be the only modality offering the chance for cure. In unresectable liver involvement percutaneous radiofrequency ablation can be considered, although pediatric experience with this technique is very limited (Ye et al. 2008).

References

Aldrighetti L, Pulitano C, Catena M et al (2009) Liver resection with portal vein thrombectomy for hepatocellular carcinoma with vascular invasion. Ann Surg Oncol 16:1254

Arcement CM, Towbin RB, Meza MP et al (2000) Intrahepatic chemoembolization in unresectable pediatric liver malignancies. Pediatr Radiol 30:779–785

Aronson DC, Schnater JM, Staalman CR et al (2005) Predictive value of the pretreatment extent of disease system in hepatoblastoma: results from the International Society of Pediatric Oncology Liver Tumor Study Group SIOPEL-1 Study. J Clin Oncol 23:1245–1252

Black CT, Luck SR, Musemeche CA et al (1991) Aggressive excision of pulmonary metastases is warranted in the management of childhood hepatic tumors. J Pediatr Surg 26:1082–1086

Brown J, Perilongo G, Shafford E et al (2000) Pretreatment prognostic factors for children with hepatoblastoma – results from the International Society of Paediatric Oncology (SIOP) study SIOPEL 1. Eur J Cancer 36:1418–1425

Couinaud C (1994) The paracaval segments of the Liver. J Hepatobiliary Pancreat Surg 2:145–151

Czauderna P, Popadiuk S, Korzon M et al (2001) Multicenter restrospective analysis of various primary pediatric malignant hepatic tumors – management in a series of 47 Polish patients (1985–1995). Eur J Pediatr Surg 11:82–85

Czauderna P, Mackinlay G, Perilongo G et al (2002) Hepatocellular carcinoma in children: results of the first prospective study of the International Society of Pediatric Oncology Group. J Clin Oncol 20:2798–2804

Czauderna P, Otte JB, Aronson DC et al (2005) Guidelines for surgical treatment of hepatoblastoma in the modern era – recommendations from the Childhood Liver Tumour Strategy Group of the International Society of Paediatric Oncology (SIOPEL). Eur J Cancer 41:1031–1036

Czauderna P, Otte JB, Roebuck DJ (2006a) Surgical treatment of hepatoblastoma in children. Pediatr Radiol 36:187–191

Czauderna P, Zbrzezniak G, Narozanski W et al (2006b) Preliminary experience with arterial chemoembolization for hepatoblastoma and hepatocellular carcinoma in children. Pediatr Blood Cancer 46:825–828

D'Antiga L, Vallortigara F, Cillo U et al (2007) Features predicting unresectability in hepatoblastoma. Cancer 110:1050–1057

Dagher I, Lainas P, Carloni A et al (2008) Laparoscopic liver resection for hepatocellular carcinoma. Surg Endosc 22:372–378

Dall'Igna P, Perilongo G, Collins MH et al (2003) Multifocal hepatoblastoma: is there a place for partial hepatectomy? Med Pediatr Oncol 40:113–117

Delva E, Camus Y, Nordlinger B et al (1989) Vascular occlusions for liver resections. Operative management and tolerance to hepatic ischemia: 142 cases. Ann Surg 209:211–218

Dicken BJ, Bigan DL, Lees GM (2004) Association between surgical margins and long-term outcome in advanced hepatoblastoma. J Pediatr Surg 39:721–725

Dutta S, Nehra D, Woo R et al (2007) Laparoscopic resection of a benign liver tumor in a child. J Pediatr Surg 42: 1141–1145

Ein SH, Shandling B, Williams WG et al (1981) Major hepatic tumor resection using profound hypothermia and circulation arrest. J Pediatr Surg 16:339–342

Feusner JH, Krailo M, Haas JE et al (1993) Treatment of pulmonary metastases of initial stage I hepatoblastoma in childhood. Cancer 71:859–864

Finegold M (2002) Chemotherapy for suspected hepatoblastoma without efforts at surgical resection is a bad practice. Med Pediatr Oncol 39:484–486

Finegold MJ, Egler RA, Goss JA et al (2008) Liver tumors: pediatric population. Liver Transpl 14:1545–1556

Fuchs J, Rydzynski J, Hecker J et al (2002) The influence of preoperative chemotherapy and surgical technique in the treatment of hepatoblastoma – a report from the German Cooperative Liver Tumor Studies HB89 and HB94. Eur J Pediatr Surg 12:255–261

Fuchs J, Seitz G, Ellerkamp V et al (2008) Analysis of sternotomy as treatment option for the resection of bilateral pulmonary metastases in pediatric solid tumors. Surg Oncol 17:323–330

Han HS, Cho JY, Yoon YS (2009) Techniques for performing laparoscopic liver resection in various hepatic locations. J Hepatobiliary Pancreat Surg 16:427–432

Hemming AW, Reed AI, Langham MR et al (2002) Hepatic vein reconstruction for resection of hepatic tumors. Ann Surg 235:850–858

Hemming AW, Reed AI, Langham MR et al (2004) Combined resection of the liver and inferior vena cava for hepatic malignancy. Ann Surg 239:712–721

Herzog CE, Andrassy RJ, Eftekhari F (2000) Childhood cancers: hepatoblastoma. Oncologist 5:445–453

Hoffer FA (2000) Liver biopsy methods for pediatric oncology patients. Pediatr Radiol 30:481–488

Horton JD, Lee S, Brown SR et al (2009) Survival trends in children with hepatoblastoma. Pediatr Surg Int 25:407–412

Huang J, Li BK, Chen GH et al (2009) Long-term outcomes and prognostic factors of elderly patients with hepatocellular carcinoma undergoing hepatectomy. J Gastrointest Surg 13:1627–1635

Ismail H, Broniszczak D, Kalicinski P et al (2009) Liver transplantation in children with hepatocellular carcinoma. Do Milan criteria apply to pediatric patients? Pediatr Transplant 13:682–692

Kalicinski P, Otte JB (2009) Editorial: liver transplantation for hepatic malignancies in children – we all need more information. Pediatr Transplant 13:657–658

Katz SC, Shia J, Liau KH et al (2009) Operative blood loss independently predicts recurrence and survival after resection of hepatocellular carcinoma. Am Surg 249:617–623

Katzenstein HM, London WB, Douglass EC et al (2002a) Treatment of unresectable and metastatic hepatoblastoma: a pediatric oncology group phase II study. J Clin Oncol 20:3438–3444

Katzenstein HM, Krailo MD, Malogolowkin MH et al (2002b) Hepatocellular carcinoma in children and adolescents: results from the Pediatric Oncology Group and the Children's Cancer Group Intergroup Study. J Clin Oncol 20:2789–2797

Katzenstein HM, Krailo MD, Malogolowkin MH et al (2003) Fibrolamellar hepatocellular carcinoma in children and adolescents. Cancer 97:2006–2012

Koga H, Ishizaki Y, Fujimura J et al (2009) Complete resection of hepatoblastoma originating in the caudate lobe; case report and literature review. Pediatr Surg Int 25: 1017–1020

La Quaglia MP, Shorter NA, Blumgart LH (2002) Central hepatic resection for pediatric tumors. J Pediatr Surg 37:986–989

Liu DC, Vogel AM, Gulec S et al (2003) Hepatectomy in children under total hepatic exclusion. Am Surg 69:539–541

Malogolowkin M, Katzenstein H, Krailo M et al (2008) Redefining the role of doxorubicin for the treatment of children with hepatoblastoma. J Clin Oncol 26:2379–2383

Matsunaga T, Sasaki F, Ohira M et al (2003) Analysis of treatment outcome for children with recurrent or metastatic hepatoblastoma. Pediatr Surg Int 19:142–146

Mazzafero V, Chun YS, Poon RT et al (2008) Liver transplantation for hepatocellular carcinoma. Ann Surg Oncol 15: 1001–1007

Meyers R, Katzenstein HM, Krailo M et al (2007) Surgical resection of pulmonary metastatic lesions in children with hepatoblastoma. J Pediatr Surg 42:2050–2056

Meyers RL, Rowland JR, Krailo M et al (2009) Predictive power of pretreatment prognostic factors in children with hepatoblastoma: a report from the Children's Oncology Group. Pediatr Blood Cancer 53:1016–1022

Millar AJW, Hartley P, Khan D et al (2001) Extended hepatic resection with transplantation back-up for an unresectable' tumour. Pediatr Surg Int 17:378–381

Mita A, Hashikura Y, Masuda Y et al (2008) Nonsurgical policy for treatment of bilioenteric anastomotic stricture after living donor liver transplantation. Transpl Int 21:320–327

Needham P, Dasgupta D, Stringer DJ (2008) Postoperative biochemical liver function after major hepatic resection in children. J Pediatr Surg 43:1610–1618

Okajima H, Ohya Y, Lee KJ et al (2009) Management of undifferentiated sarcoma of the liver including living donor liver transplantation as a backup procedure. J Pediatr Surg 44:e33–e38

Ortega JA, Douglass EC, Feusner JH et al (2000) Randomized comparison of cisplatin/vincristine/fluorouracil and cisplatin/continous infusion doxorubicin for treatment of pediatric hepatoblastoma: a report from the Children's Cancer Group and the Pediatric Oncology Group. J Clin Oncol 18: 2665–2675

Otte JB, Pritchard J, Aronson DC et al (2004) Liver transplantation for hepatoblastoma: results from the International Society of Pediatric Oncology (SIOP) study SIOPEL-1 and review of the world experience. Pediatr Blood Cancer 1: 74–83

Passmore J, Noblett HR, Wisheart JD et al (1995) Prolonged survival following multiple thoracotomies for metastatic hepatoblastoma. Med Pediatr Oncol 24:58–60

Perilongo G, Shafford E, Plaschkes J (2000) SIOPEL trials using preoperative chemotherapy in hepatoblastoma. Lancet Oncol 1:94–100

Perilongo G, Shafford E, Maibach R et al (2004) Risk adapted treatment for childhood hepatoblastoma; final report of the second study of the International Society of Paediatric Oncology – SIOPEL 2. Eur J Cancer 40:411–421

Perilongo G, Maibach R, Shafford E et al (2009) Cisplatin alone versus cisplatin/doxorubicin for standard risk hepatoblastoma; final report of the randomized international trial, SIOPEL 3 SR-HB. N Engl J Med 361:1662–1670

Pham TH, Iqbal CW, Grams JM et al (2007) Outcomes of primary liver cancer in children: an appraisal of experience. J Pediatr Surg 42:834–839

Pritchard J, Brown J, Shafford E et al (2000) Cisplatin, doxorubicin, and delayed surgery for childhood hepatoblastoma: a successful approach – results of the first prospective study of the International Society of Pediatric Oncology. J Clin Oncol 18:3819–3828

Rau HG, Duessel AP, Wurzbacher S (2008) The use of water-jet dissection in open and laparoscopic liver resection. HPB (Oxford) 10:275–280

Reed DN, Vitale GC, Wrightson WR et al (2002) Decreasing mortality of bile leaks after elective hepatic surgery. Am J Surg 185:316–318

Roebuck DJ, Olsen O, Pariente D (2006) Radiological staging in children with hepatoblastoma. Pediatr Radiol 36:176–182

Roebuck DJ, Aronson DC, Clapuyt P et al (2007) 2005 PRETEXT: a revised staging system for primary liver tumors of childhood. Pediatr Radiol 37:123–132

Schnater JM, Aronson DC, Plaschkes J et al (2002) Surgical view in the treatment of hepatoblastoma – results from the International Society of Pediatric Oncology Liver Tumor Study Group (SIOPEL-1). Cancer 94:1111–1120

Schnater JM, Kohler SE, Lamers WH et al (2003) Where do we stand with hepatoblastoma? A review. Cancer 98:668–678

Stringer MD (2007) The role of liver transplantation in the management of paediatric liver tumours. Ann R Coll Surg Engl 89:12–21

Superina RA, Bambini D, Filler RM et al (2000) A new technique for resecting 'unresectable' liver tumors. J Pediatr Surg 35:1294–1299

Tannuri AC, Tannuri U, Gibelli NE et al (2009) Surgical treatment of hepatic tumors in children: lessons learned from liver transplantation. J Pediatr Surg 44:2083–2087

Thomas BL, Krummel TM, Parker GA (1989) Use of interoperative ultrasound during hepatic resection in pediatric patients. J Pediatr Surg 24:690–693

Towu E, Kiely E, Pierro A et al (2004) Outcome and complications after resection of hepatoblastoma. J Pediatr Surg 39:199–202

Vigano L, Ferrero A, Sgotto E et al (2008) Bile leak after hepatectomy: predictive factors of spontaneous healing. Am J Surg 196:195–200

von Schweinitz D (2006) Management of liver tumors in childhood. Semin Pediatr Surg 15:17–24

von Schweinitz, Faundez A, Teichmann B et al (2000) Hepatocyte growth-factor-scatter factor can stimulate post-operative tumor cell proliferation in childhood hepatoblastoma. Int J Cancer 85:151–159

Ye J, Shu Q, Li M et al (2008) Percutaneous radiofrequency ablation for treatment of hepatoblastoma recurrence. Pediatr Radiol 38:1021–1023

Yoon YS, Han HS, Choi YS et al (2006) Total laparoscopic left lateral sectionectomy performed in a child with benign liver mass. J Pediatr Surg 41:e25–e28

Zografos GN, Kakaviatos ND, Skiathitis S et al (1999) Total vascular exclusion for liver resections: pros and cons. J Surg Oncol 72:55–56

Liver Transplantation for Unresectable Liver Tumors in Children

11

Rebecka L. Meyers and Jean-Bernard Otte

Contents

R.L. Meyers (✉)
Primary Children's Medical Center, University of Utah, 100 N. Mario Cappechi Drive, Suite 2600, Salt Lake City, UT Utah 84113, USA
e-mail: rebecka.meyers@hsc.utah.edu

J.-B. Otte
Department of Paediatric Surgery, Cliniques Universitaires Saint-Luc, Av. Hippocrate 10, 1200, Brussels, Belgium
e-mail: otte@chex.ucl.ac.be

11.1 Introduction

Although the first long-term survivor of liver transplantation described by Starzl in 1968 was a child with biliary atresia and incidental hepatocellular carcinoma (Starzl 1992), it has taken many years for this treatment to evolve. Initial long-term results in many adults with hepatocellular carcinoma (HCC) were disappointing due to the high incidence of tumor recurrence. With this early experience and the high rate of post-transplant tumor recurrence, in the 1980s and early 1990s transplant was relegated to the role of a salvage therapy; something to try after everything else had been tried and failed. In the later 1990s, as effective platinum-based chemotherapy became common, our experience grew, our techniques evolved, and our survival rates improved. During the last decade, liver transplantation has emerged as a valid therapeutic option in many children with unresectable liver tumors. These might be truly malignant neoplasms (hepatoblastoma-HB, hepatocellular carcinoma-HCC, and sarcoma); neoplasms with intermediate malignant potential (infantile epithelioid hemangioendothelioma-IEHE) or benign lesions (diffuse infantile hemangioma with refractory cardiac failure). The experience gained worldwide is the largest and most favorable for HB, which has led the liver tumor study groups of the Children's Oncology Group (COG), the German Pediatric Oncology Hematology Group (GPOH), and the Liver Tumor Strategy Group of the International Society of Pediatric Oncology (SIOPEL) to propose guidelines, which ennumerate current indications and contraindications for transplant in children with HB. Recommendations for transplantation in children with HCC are still evolving as we struggle to modify the adult Milan criteria to better fit the unique biology of pediatric HCC. No set standard of pediatric HCC transplant criteria have yet received

A. Zimmermann et al. (eds.), *Pediatric Liver Tumors*, Pediatric Oncology,
DOI: 10.1007/978-3-642-14504-9_11, © Springer-Verlag Berlin Heidelberg 2011

widespread adoption. For other types of malignant or benign tumors, the experience is anecdotal. Transplant for sarcoma is extremely rare. Transplant for the diffuse form of infantile hemangioma is reserved for those patients with intractable heart failure in whom medical management has failed and lesser surgical interventions are not possible.

Nontransplant options for surgical resection in these patients are occasionally possible with the advances in liver surgery and with techniques such as in-flow occlusion, total vascular exclusion, in situ flush with preservation solution, and complex venous resection and reconstruction of the vena cava. As these surgical techniques have evolved, extensive liver resection with vascular reconstruction is sometimes possible in specialized liver centers with expertise in complex liver surgery. A new term began to appear in the literature describing these heroic liver resections as "extreme liver resection." These "extreme liver resections" are not necessarily safer than transplantation, but as they push the limits of technical feasibility, they make us more clearly reflect on the potential risks and benefits of the different options (Superina and Bilik 1996). Some centers argue that the increase in surgical risk of "extreme resection" might occasionally be justified when balanced against the alternative of transplantation and lifetime immunosuppression. But many questions remain regarding hepatic insufficiency, limits on hepatic regeneration in children receiving chemotherapy, and the potential for increased risk of tumor recurrence, *especially in the case of multifocal tumors*. This chapter will focus on the role of transplantation in the treatment of the most common pediatric liver tumors. We conclude with a plea to all clinicians treating children with potentially unresectable liver tumors to contribute to the international prospective database, PLUTO (Pediatric Liver Unresectable Tumors Observatory). The PLUTO registry will collect comprehensive data that should help guide future recommendations for liver transplant in children with unresectable liver tumors.

11.2 Hepatoblastoma

Cases of "unresectable" hepatoblastoma (HB) due to involvement of the entire liver, extensive multifocality, or major hepatic venous or portal venous involvement still comprise 10–20% of all HB treated in multicenter cooperative group trials (Ortega et al. 2000; Malogolowkin et al. 2006; Fuchs et al. 2002; Von Schweinitz and Haberle 2007; Perilongo et al. 2004; Perilongo and Otte 2009; Sasaki et al. 2002). HB is a rare tumor, which nevertheless accounts for 75% of primary malignant liver tumors in children. The 5-year survival rate of children affected by HB and treated with combination cisplatin-based chemotherapy and complete surgical resection is now in the range of 80–90%, which represents at least a doubling of the survival rate reported in the early 1980s (Ortega et al. 2000; Evans et al. 1982; Plaschkes et al. 1994). Despite these exciting results, epidemiologists estimate the 5-year disease-free survival in the USA to be no higher than 50% suggesting that many children outside of these trials may not be receiving optimal contemporary care (Darbari et al. 2003). Guidelines set forth in the contemporary studies of both COG and SIOPEL are based upon PRETEXT (Pretreatment Extent of disease). For example, those tumors that are recommended for early review by a transplant center in the COG AHEP0731 trial are shown in Fig. 11.1.

11.2.1 PRETEXT and Liver Transplantation for HB in SIOPEL

The PRETEXT system (Pretreatment Extent of disease), originally developed by the Liver Tumor Strategy Group of the International Society of Pediatric Oncology (SIOPEL) (Brown et al. 2000; Aronson et al. 2005), has been used by SIOPEL for many years as a tool for risk stratification. Starting with SIOPEL 2 PRETEXT I, II, and III tumors have been treated as "standard risk" (SR), and PRETEXT IV, +M (metastatic), and those with AFP <100 have been treated as "High Risk" (HR). The recommendations for liver transplant used in the recent study, SIOPEL 3 were as follows: *"The commonest reasons for a tumor being deemed "unresectable" (except via total hepatectomy) are: (a) tumor clearly involving all four sections of the liver as judged by MRI scan +/–angiography; or (b) location so close to the main vessels at the hilum of the liver and/or to the hepatic veins that it is unlikely that a tumor-free excision plane will be achieved. These patients should be identified at diagnosis and their clinical course and imaging followed closely throughout their initial chemotherapy, in conjunction with a liver transplant surgeon."*

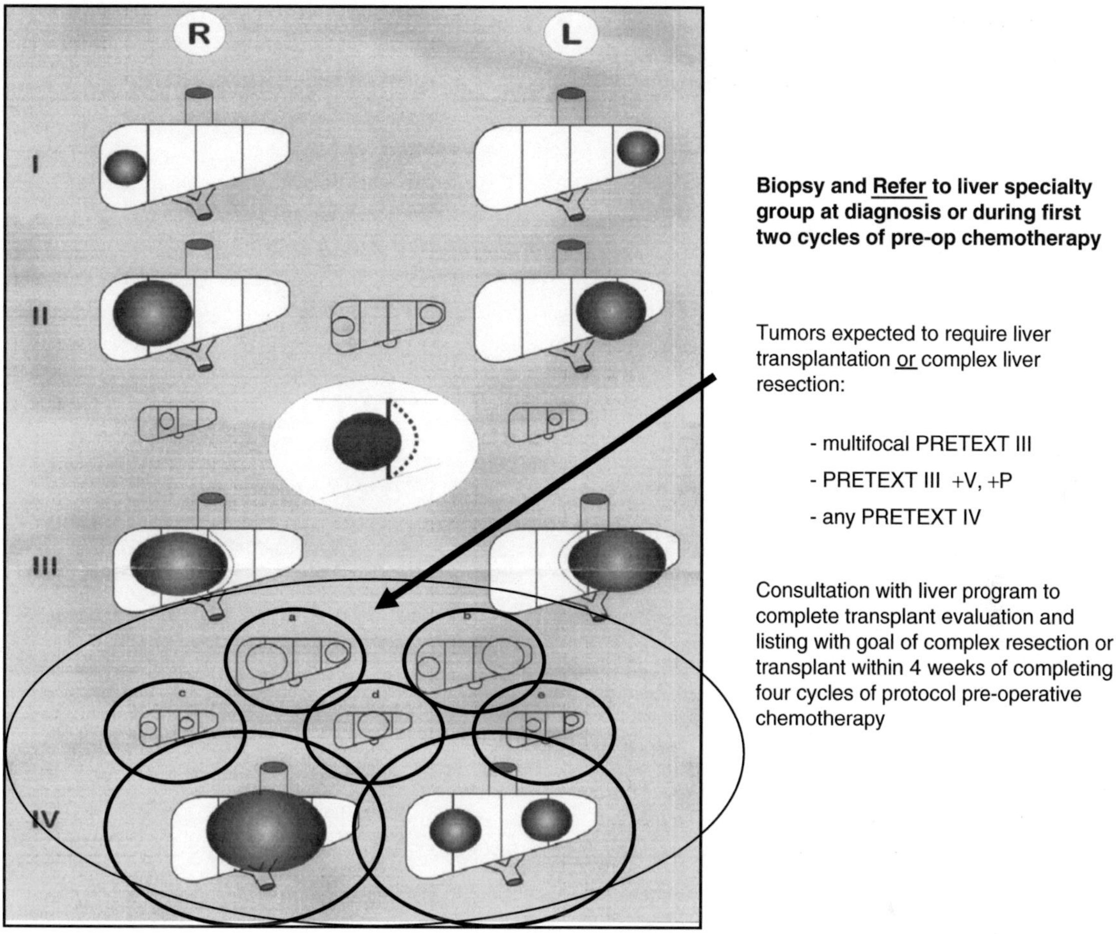

Fig. 11.1 COG AHEP 0731 Surgical resection guidelines (Katzenstein 2009)

In SIOPEL study-1, 12 patients underwent a liver transplantation as the primary surgical option in 7 and as a rescue in 5. The long-term (>10 years) disease-free survival was 85% and 40%, respectively. All eight patients with PRETEXT IV tumors and all six patients with multifocal HB were cured of their disease. Of the seven patients with macroscopic extension into the portal vein and/or the hepatic veins/vena cava, 71% became long-term, disease-free survivors, as well as four of five (80%) children who had lung metastases at presentation with complete clearance of lung lesions after chemotherapy (Otte et al. 2004). In SIOPEL 3 35 high-risk patients underwent a liver transplant; 33 as the primary surgical option and 2 as a "rescue" transplant. Of the 33 patients who underwent primary transplantation, 10 had tumor relapse (31%), 8 died of tumor relapse (24%), and early overall survival was 75%. Of the six patients with metastatic disease at diagnosis who underwent primary transplant, three of six (50%) had a tumor relapse. Although the results of the high risk (HR) arm of SIOPEL 3 have not yet been published as a manuscript, the data from SIOPEL 3 are preliminary data reported at the SIOP meeting in Sao Paulo Brazil 2009 (Casanova et al. 2009). The outcome results for standard and high-risk tumors in SIOPEL 1, 2, and 3 are shown in Table 11.1. The comparative results shown in Table 11.1 (Perilongo et al. 2004; Brown et al. 2000; Casanova et al. 2009; Pritchard et al. 2000; Perilongo et al. 2009) reveal an increase in HR outcome in SIOPEL 3 when compared to SIOPEL 1 and 2 and one reason for this improved outcome is hypothesized to be the more timely and prudent use of primary liver transplant for unresectable tumors over the years.

Table 11.1 Summary results of Liver Tumor Strategy Group of the International Society of Pediatric Oncology (SIOPEL) HB cooperative trials

Study	Chemotherapy	Number of patients	Outcomes
SIOPEL 1 (Perilongo et al. 2004; Brown et al. 2000; Pritchard et al. 2000)	All Patients: PLADO SR: 70% HR: 30%	N=154 at dx (128 surg resection) PRETEXT: I=8; II=57; III=46; IV=6; ?=3 Mets: 31 **Liver Transplant =12 (8% of total)**	**5-year EFS:** I: 100% II: 83% III: 56% IV: 46% Mets: 28%
SIOPEL 2 (Perilongo et al. 2004)	SR: PLADO HR:CDDP/CARBO/DOXO	N=135 (77 SR; 58HR) PRETEXT: I=15; II=63; III=37; IV=21; Mets: 25 **Liver Transplant=7 (5% of total)**	**3-year EFS/OS:** SR: 73%/91% HR: - / 53% HR Mets: 36%/44%
SIOPEL 3 (Zsiros et al. 2010; Perilongo et al. 2009)	SR: CDDP vs PLADO HR: SUPERPLADO	SR=255 PRETEXT I=18;II=133; III=104 HR=151; PRETEXT IV= 74; +VPE=70; mets=70; AFP<100=12 **Liver Transplant=35 (9% of total)**	**3-year EFS/OS:** SR: CDDP 83%/95%; PLADO 85%/93% HR: overall 65%/69% HR mets: 57%/63%

Abbreviations: C5V, cisplatin, fluorouracil and vincristine; CDDP: cisplatin; DOXO: doxorubicin; IFOS: ifosfamide; VP: etoposide; CARBO: carboplatin; IPA: Ifosfamide, cisplatin, adriamycin; SR: standard risk; HR; high risk; PRETEXT: Pretreatment extent of disease staging system; +VPE Mets: metastatic disease; SUPERPLADO: CDDP/CARBO/DOXO; EFS: event-free survival; OS: overall survival.

11.2.2 Outcomes of Transplantation for HB Reported in Literature

Table 11.2 (Penn 1991; Koneru et al. 1991; Tagge et al. 1992; Douglass et al. 1993; Pichlmayr et al. 1994; Stringer et al. 1995; Ehrlich et al. 1997; Achilleos et al. 1996; Al-Qabandi et al. 1999; Reyes et al. 2000; Pimpalwar et al. 2002; Molmenti et al. 2002; Srinivasan et al. 2002; Chardot et al. 2002; Cillo et al. 2003; Tiao et al. 2005; Mejia et al. 2005; Kasahara et al. 2005; Chen et al. 2006; Avila et al. 2007; Austin et al. 2006; Cassas-Medley et al. 2007; Beaunoyer et al. 2007; Faraj et al. 2008; Browne et al. 2008; Kalicinski et al. 2008; Geller et al. 2010) is a compilation of the major published results for liver transplant for HB over the past 20 years. An extensive review of the world experience collected 147 cases of liver transplantation for HB (Otte et al. 2004). Twenty-eight (19% of the total) patients presented with macroscopic venous extension and 12 (8%) with lung metastases. A total of 106 patients (72%) underwent a primary transplant and 41 (28%) received a rescue transplant, either for incomplete resection with partial hepatectomy or for tumor relapse after previous partial hepatectomy. Median follow-up since diagnosis for surviving patients was 38 months (range 1–121 months). Overall disease-free survival at 6 years post-transplant was 82% and 30% for primary transplants and for rescue transplants, respectively. It was 82% and 71% after living-related donor liver transplantation (n=28) and postmortem liver transplantation (n=119), respectively. Multivariate statistical analysis showed no difference in regard to gender, age, and lung metastases at presentation or type of transplant. For primary transplants, the only parameter significantly related to overall survival was macroscopic venous invasion (P=0.045).

The UNOS experience with liver transplantation for HB from 1987 to 2005 was recently reviewed by Rodriguez et al. and is not included in Table 11.1 as it is pending publication [Rodriguez, personal communication]. This review included 180 children; 140 patients (78%) underwent transplantation during the last decade. At a median patient follow-up interval of 24 months, 1-year, 3-year, and 5-year patient and allograft survival rates were 80%, 72%, and 69%, and 71%, 63%, and 61%, respectively. Three-year patient survival rates for deceased donation whole (63.3%), deceased donation segmental (21.8%), and living donor (14.7%) allograft groups were 67.4%, 67.1%, and 84.6%, respectively (p=0.22). Multivariate

Table 11.2 Literature, transplant for HB in children

	# Patients	% Survival	Follow-up(years)
Penn et al. (1991), *Surgery*, multiinsitution	18	50%	
Koneru et al. (1991), *Ann Surg*, multiinstitution	12	50%	2–6
Tagge et al. (1992), *J Pediar Surg*, Pittsburg, PA	6	83%	0.5–2
Douglass et al. (1993), *Clin Oncol*, POG multiinstitution	3	66%	2
Pilchmayer et al. (1994), *Hepatology*,	1	100%	11
Stringer et al. (1995), *Br J Surg*, Leeds UK	1	100%	1.3
Superina et al. (1996), *J Pediatr Surg*, Toronto, ONT	3	66%	1–5
Erlich et al. (1997), *J Pediatr Surg*, Toronto, ONT	2	100%	3.5
Achilleos et al. (1996), *J Pediatr Surg*, Birmingham, UK	2	50%	2–3
Al-Qabandi et al. (1999), *J Pediatr Surg*, Birmingham, UK			
Reyes et al. (2000), *J Pediatr*, Pittsburgh, PA	12	83%	0.1–15.4
Pimpalwar et al. (2002), *J Pediatr Surg*, Birmingham, UK	12	83%	0.1–9.2
Molmlenti et al. (2002), *Am J Transplant*, Dallas, TX	9	55%	0.5–16
Srinivasan et al. (2002), *Transplantation*, London, UK	13	85%	0.1-9
Chardot et al. (2002), *Transplantation*, Paris/Brussels	4	75%	1.1–2
Cillo et al. (2003), *Transplant Proc*, Padua, IT	7	57%	0.2–9
Otte et al. (2004), *Ped Bld Cancer*,			
SIOPEL 1 + "World Experience"			
Primary Transplant	106	82%	
"Rescue" Transplant	41	30%	
Tiao et al. (2005), *J Pediatr*, Cinncinati, OH	9	80%	
Mejia et al. (2005), *Clin Transplant*, San Antonio, TX	10	70%	3.7–18
Kasahara et al. (2005), *Am J Transplantation*, Kyoto, JP	14	71%	3.5+/-?
Chen et al. (2006), *J Ped Gastro Nutr*, St Louis, MO	7	85%	0.6–18
Avila et al. (2006), *Eur J Ped Surg*, Madrid, SP	11	82%	1–14
Austin et al. (2006), *J Pediatr Surg*, UNOS database	135	69%	
Cassas-Medley et al. (2007), *J Pediatr Surg*, Dupont, DE	8	75%	0.6–4.4
Beaunoyer et al. (2007), *Pediatr Transplant*, Stanford CA	15	86%	3.3+/-3.5
Faraj et al. (2008), *Liver Transplant*, London UK	25	78%	0.9–14.9
Browne et al. (2008), *J Pediatr Surg*, Chicago, IL	14	71%	3.8 +/-?
Kalicinski et al. (2008), *Ann Transplantation*, Warsaw ,Poland	6	66%	
Nathan et al, *presented APSA 2009*, Cinncinati, OH	16	100%	

analysis identified ABO match and serum creatinine level (reflecting the global pretransplant medical condition) as the only independent prognostic variables. With regard to allograft type, a trend toward improved survival in the subset of patients receiving a living donor allograft was observed. However, the trend toward improved observed outcomes may, in part, be due to recipient selection for living donation.

Reyes et al. reported 12 children with unresectable HB who underwent transplantation in Pittsburgh between May 1989 and December 1998. Post-transplantation survival rates for 1-year, 3-year, and 5-year were 92%, 92%, and 83%, respectively. Intravenous invasion, positive hilar lymph nodes, and contiguous spread did not have a significant adverse effect on outcome; distant metastasis was responsible for two deaths (Reyes et al. 2000).

Among 52 children (<15 years) treated (1978–2003) at Cliniques Saint-Luc, Brussels, a partial hepatectomy was performed in 39 patients and a transplant in 13 patients. All patients, including transplant ones, were treated with chemotherapy, according to the successive SIOPEL protocols. Overall, disease-free survival was 80% and 89%, respectively (ns). Relapse rate was 23% and 7.6%, respectively (Otte et al. 2005).

In Birmingham, UK, of 34 children with HB treated over a period of 10 years (1991–2000), 12 patients underwent primary liver transplant because the tumor remained unresectable after chemotherapy and 2 patients received a rescue transplant for recurrence after a partial hepatectomy. Disease-free survival rates were 100% after primary transplant and 50% in patients with rescue transplant. The authors concluded that transplantation is a potentially curative option for unresectable HB when chemosensitive (decrease in alpha-fetoprotein and decrease in tumor size) while patients with recurrent or resistant disease are not good candidates (Pimpalwar et al. 2002).

At King's College Hospital, London, UK, orthotopic liver transplantation was performed in 25 children, who were assessed with unresectable HB. Fifteen patients were at level IV in the pretreatment extent of disease staging system (PRETEXT IV) and 10 were level III (PRETEXT III). Preoperative chemotherapy was given according to the risk stratification system for children with HB protocols of the International Liver Tumor Strategy Group of the International Society of Pediatric Oncology (SIOPEL). Eighteen received cadaveric grafts and seven underwent living-related liver transplantation (LRLT). Patient and graft survival after cadaveric transplantation was 91%, 77.6%, and 77.6% at 1, 5, and 10 years, respectively. Patient and graft survival for children undergoing LRLT was 100%, 83.3%, and 83.3%, at 1, 5, and 10 years, respectively. All surviving children but one remain disease-free, with a median follow-up of 6.8 years (range: 0.9–14.9). There were five deaths at a median of 13 months post-transplantation, secondary to tumor recurrence in four patients and respiratory failure in one patient (Faraj et al. 2008).

The Dallas group reported about nine recipients with a diagnosis of unresectable HB who received a transplant. There was one recurrence. Disease-free survival was 66% (median follow-up: 7.7 years). All recipients received preoperative chemotherapy: 67% received postoperative chemotherapy. The only instance in which AFP levels did not decrease to low or undetectable levels post-transplantation was in the patient with recurrent tumor (Molmenti et al. 2002).

Ten cases of unresectable HB who underwent liver transplantation (1985–2003) were reported by the Omaha group (eight deceased donor grafts, two LRLT). Pre-transplant chemotherapy was used in 90% of cases. Post-transplant survival ranges from 3.7 years to 18.6 years. Three patients died of recurrent disease at 4, 14, and 38 months. The two LDLT recipients were able to get pre-transplant chemotherapy with a rapid decision toward transplantation; both are alive and well at 5.5 and 11 years post-transplant (Mejia et al. 2005).

In Kyoto, living donor liver transplantation was performed in 14 patients for unresectable HB (PRETEXT III:7; PRETEXT IV: 7), as a rescue OLT in seven. Actuarial 1- and 5-year patient and graft survival were 78.6% and 65.5%. Four children died from tumor recurrence. The poor prognostic factors were macroscopic venous invasion and extra hepatic involvement with no survivor at 5-year range (Kasahara et al. 2005).

11.2.3 Guiding Principles to Consider for Transplant in HB

A number of guiding principles should be taken into consideration when considering transplantation for HB.

Response to chemotherapy: Patients should be treated with neoadjuvant chemotherapy, whatever the type of resection, before proceeding with surgery, following standardized protocols (Ortega et al. 2000; Fuchs et al. 2002; Pritchard et al. 2000; Pimpalwar et al. 2002; Molmenti et al. 2002; Faraj et al. 2008; Otte and deVille de Goyet 2005). Preoperative chemotherapy renders most tumors smaller, better demarcated from the surrounding liver, and more likely to be completely resected. The majority of the chemotherapy response seems to occur during the first two cycles of chemotherapy with a progressive plateau in response thereafter (Lovorn et al. in press). Lengthy courses of preoperative chemotherapy when tumor is unresectable should be avoided due to diminishing effects on the tumor combined with the substantial risk of inducing chemotherapy resistance with prolonged exposure (Von Schweinitz et al. 1995). Although we still lack evidence, post-transplant chemotherapy should probably be recommended, as long as there is a reasonable chance that any microscopic residual remains chemosensitive.

AFP < 100 poor prognosis. AFP is a reliable marker in most cases presenting with an elevated value and response to chemotherapy is impressive, which is of good predictive value. On the contrary, low AFP (<100) at presentation is a high-risk predictor (Deloris et al. 2008); most likely, transplantation would be best avoided in such an occurrence.

PRETEXT to determine potential need for transplant. PRETEXT has been shown to be a useful way to help identify patients, both at presentation and after chemotherapy, who will need a total hepatectomy and a transplant. Identification at presentation allows timely referral and complete evaluation by a specialty liver center with transplant capability (Aronson et al. 2005; Meyers et al. 2009). Early referral of potentially unresectable HB to a surgical team with liver transplant capability is advised by all three major liver tumor strategy groups: COG, SIOPEL, and GPOH (Fuchs et al. 2002; Czauderna et al. 2005; Meyers et al. 2009). A simplified version of the transplant referral guidelines used in the current COG protocol, AHEP0731, is shown in Fig. 11.2.

Multifocal tumors: Multifocality may be a poor prognostic factor (Meyers et al. 2009; Dall'Igna et al. 2003). Most extensive multifocal tumors may have occult microscopic satellite lesions and are potentially unresectable. Clearance of a lateral section after chemotherapy is most often apparent; it should not mislead the surgeon to perform a partial hepatectomy in truly multifocal PRETEXT IV HB (Dantiga et al. 2007).

Metastatic disease: HB spreads by vascular invasion, typically in the lungs. Most centers feel that patients presenting with lung metastases should not be excluded from OLT if the metastases clear after chemotherapy, completed by surgical resection of remnants if needed (Otte et al. 2005; Otte and deVille de

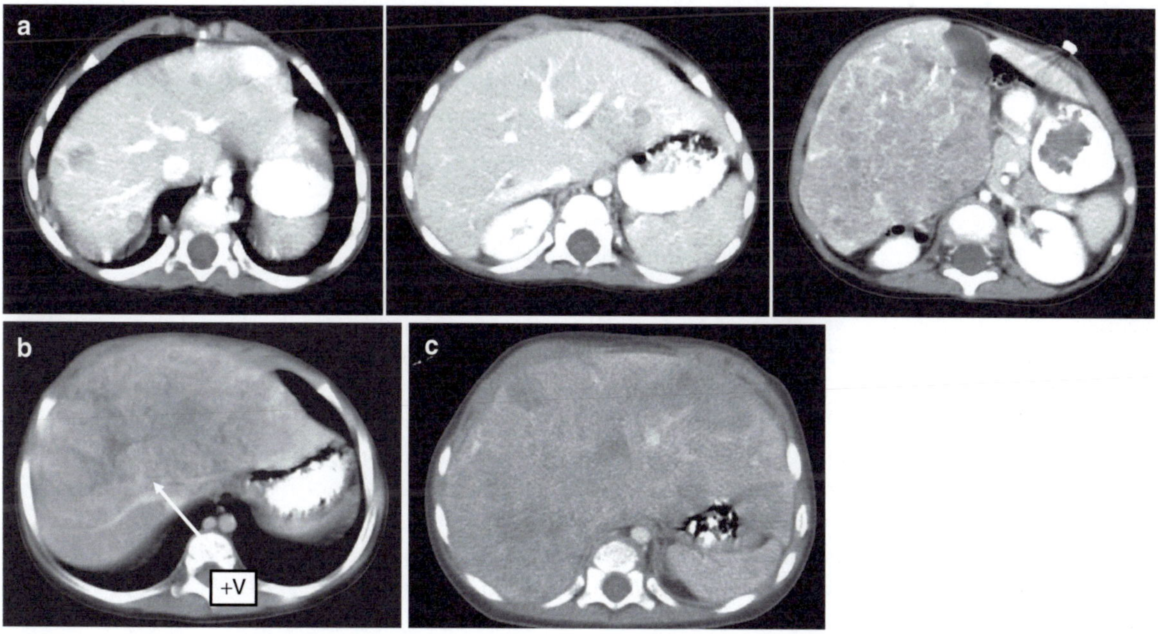

Fig. 11.2 Examples of liver tumors referred for possible liver transplantation (**a**) PRETEXT IV multifocal. (**b**) PRETEXT III, +V: Left lateral section, left medial section, and right anterior section with invasion into all three hepatic veins (+V). (**c**) PRETEXT IV, +V, +P: Tumor involves all four sections and invades vena cava and portal bifurcation

Table 11.3 Literature, transplant for pediatric hepatocellular carcinoma (HCC)

	# Patients	% Survival	Tumor recurrence	[b]Small incidental	[c]Died comp OLT
[a]Olthoff et al. (1990), Arch Surg, UCLA	16	22%	8/16	-	4/16
[a]Penn et al. (1991), Surgery, Transplant Registry	429	-	158/429	31/429	-
Tagge et al. (1992), *J Pediar Surg*, Pittsburgh	9	44%	3/9	-	1/9
Yandza et al. (1993), *Transplat Int*, Paris	2	100%	-	-	-
Broughan et al. (1994), *J Pediatr Surg*, multicenter	4	75%	1/4	0	0
Otte et al. (1996), *Transplant Proc*, Brussels	5	60%	2/5	0	0
Achilleos et al. (1996), *J Pediatr Surg*, Birmingham	2	0	1/2	1/2	1/2
Superina et al. (1996), *J Pediatr Surg*, Toronto	3	100%	0 /3	3/3	0
Reyes et al. (2000), *J Pediatr*, Pittsburgh	19	63%	6/19	7/19	2/12
Tatekawa et al. (2001), *J Pediatr Surg*, Kyoto	2	100%	0	1/2	0
Czauderna et al. (2002), *J Clin Oncol*, SIOPEL 1	2	-	-	1/2	-
Avila et al. (2006), *Eur J Ped Surg*, Madrid	1	100%	-	-	-
Austin et al. (2006), *J Pediatr Surg*, UNOS Database	41	63%	12/41	-	-
Beaunoyer et al. (2007), *Pediatr Transplant*, Stanford	10	83%	1/10	4/10	2/10
Kalicinski et al. (2008), *Ann Transplantation*, Warsaw	8	75%	1/8	-	1/8
Ismail et al. (2009), Ped Transplantation,Warsaw	11	72%	1/11	3/11	2/11

[a]Did not separately analyze pediatric cohort
[b]Most are patients with tyrosinemia, other metabolic liver disease, familial intrahepatic cholestasis, hepatitis, or biliary atresia
[c]Died due to complications of transplant surgery or complications of immunosuppression.

Goyet 2005; Meyers et al. 2007). Table 11.3 shows a meta-analysis of patients with metastatic disease at diagnosis who subsequently had OLT presented by Fecteau, et al, at the Canadian Consensus Conference on the Management of Advanced Pediatric Liver Tumors, 2009 (Superina and Bilik 1996; Perilongo et al. 2004; Casanova et al. 2009; Al-Qabandi et al. 1999; Reyes et al. 2000; Avila et al. 2007; Cassas-Medley et al. 2007; Geller et al. 2010; Schnater et al. 2002; Fectau 2009; Otte 2009). Overall survival appears to be about 60% with no large difference in outcome when lung metastasis cleared completely on chemotherapy versus pulmonary metastasectomy. Interpretation of this data must be done with some caution as this is a highly selected group of patients from centers who have a strong commitment to transplantation. Some techniques that have been suggested to ensure the clearance of lung metastasis prior to transplantation include the use of irinotecan pre-transplant, AFP imaging pre-transplant, PET–CT pre-transplant, median sternotomy with manual palpation of both lungs pre-transplant, lobectomy rather than metastasectomy if lung has more than four nodules in same lobe (Fectau 2009).

Macrovascular invasion: Major venous invasion is a common occurrence in extensive HB. Although it might negatively impact the prognosis (Otte et al. 2004; Kasahara et al. 2005), it should not per se contraindicate transplantation (Reyes et al. 2000). Tumors with persistent major venous invasion after the first two cycles of chemotherapy are potentially unresectable. The current protocol of the Children's Oncology Group (COG) recommends early collaboration with a specialty liver team capable of providing complex resection with immediate availability of transplant backup so that all plans for definitive surgery are in place by the end of the fourth cycle of neoadjuvant chemotherapy.

Living Donor Versus Deceased Allograft: There is a trend to a higher disease-free, patient survival of children receiving a LRLT (Otte et al. 2004; Mejia et al. 2005; Faraj et al. 2008). When a living donor is available, pre-transplant chemotherapy can be scheduled optimally, with a rapid decision toward transplantation (Mejia et al. 2005).

11.2.4 Recommendations for Liver Transplantation in Current Multicenter HB Studies

The following guidelines have been developed over the years and are currently recommended by COG, SIOPEL, and GPOH. It is important that consultation with a transplant center with special expertise in pediatric liver surgery be considered early in the treatment in order to prevent delays and unwanted extended courses of chemotherapy while awaiting resection and transplantation.

Multifocal PRETEXT IV: Multifocal PRETEXT IV HB in the absence of any metastatic disease after chemotherapy (POST-TEXT – M) is a clear indication for liver transplantation. Apparent clearance of tumor from one liver section (multifocal PRETEXT IV – multifocal POST-TEXT III) should not distract from this guideline because of the high probability of persistent microscopic viable neoplastic cells in the now radiographically "clear" section. Clinicians should resist the temptation to intensify chemotherapy in a vain effort to avoid transplantation. These patients should be treated with high-risk protocols of chemotherapy, just as patients with localized tumors amenable to partial hepatectomy, with the same number of cycles of chemotherapy before and after transplantation as patients submitted to partial hepatectomy. Many of these patients with extensive multifocal tumors have had chemotherapy downstage to POST-TEXT III and have undergone trisegmentectomy, only to recur and present for "relapse" transplantation. Prior experience has documented the inferior results achieved in most patients with "relapse," instead of primary transplantation. Similarly, resection of the solitary primary tumor with nonanatomic wedge resection of satellite nodules has been shown to carry a high risk of local relapse.

Solitary PRETEXT IV: Primary liver transplantation may be the best option for large, solitary PRETEXT IV HB, involving all four sections of the liver, unless tumor downstaging to unifocal POST-TEXT III is demonstrated after neoadjuvant chemotherapy. If this were the case, a clear retraction of the tumor from the anatomic border of one lateral sector would allow performance of a trisegmentectomy.

PRETEXT III+V, +P: In a subgroup of PRETEXT III HB, major vascular invasion may preclude standard trisegmentectomy. Resection in the face of major venous invasion runs the risk of leaving viable neoplastic tissue behind if the surgeon must peel off viable tumor directly from the involved vein. Some have argued in favor of venous resection and reconstruction, as opposed to transplantation, in these cases. There are no trials comparing the results of partial resection with extensive venous dissection versus complete resection with transplantation. Partial resection carries an increased risk of surgical complication, including bleeding and/or venous inflow or outflow obstruction, and positive tumor resection margin. The importance of a positive margin remains debatable since a microscopic positive margin, after chemotherapy and surgery, may not always impact prognosis (Aronson 2008).

One thing that is universally recommended is that all patients with these types of tumors should be referred early in the course of their treatment to a surgical team with expertise in *both* radical resection *and* liver transplantation. In the hands of such a team if a major venous resection results in hepatic compromise, the team should be prepared to proceed directly to transplantation. The decision about which form of therapy may be best in a given circumstance can only be made by a surgical team with the expertise and capability to do either, or both.

Macroscopic venous invasion (portal vein, hepatic veins, vena cava) is only a relative contraindication if complete resection of the invaded venous structures can be accomplished. When there is evidence or suspicion of invasion of the retrohepatic vena cava, it should be resected "en bloc" and reconstructed (Chardot et al. 2002). Review of the world's experience shows that venous extent is associated with a significantly shorter survival ($P=0.045$) (Otte et al. 2004). In contrast, 71% of these patients were alive and disease-free >10 years after liver transplantation in the SIOPEL 1 study. Of the nine TNM IV A/IV B patients (eight with major intrahepatic venous invasion) reported by Reyes and associates, seven were alive and disease-free 21–146 months after transplantation (Reyes et al. 2000).

Pulmonary Metastasis at Diagnosis: An absolute contraindication to liver transplant is persistent pulmonary metastases nonresponsive to neoadjuvant chemotherapy and not amenable to surgical resection. The tumor should show at least a partial response to chemotherapy (decrease in tumor size, decrease in serum AFP, and decrease in size or disappearance of pulmonary nodules). Stable or progressive disease is a relative contraindication to transplant (Chardot et al. 2002; Otte et al. 2005; Otte and deVille de Goyet 2005; Stringer 2007). Lung metastases that do not clear completely with chemotherapy should be surgically resected and histologic diagnosis confirmed. Some have advocated sternotomy and bilateral lung palpation, rather than unilateral wedge resection of persistent nodules prior to transplantation although this remains controversial. Lung metastases that disappear completely with chemotherapy with or without surgical resection do not pose a contraindication, yet the risk of post-transplant pulmonary relapse is substantial and therefore the use of liver transplantation for children with metastatic disease remains controversial.

"Rescue" Transplant for Relapse or Persistent Tumors: Multiple series have shown superior outcome after primary transplant (about 80% overall survival) when compared to "rescue" transplant (about 30–40% overall survival) (Otte et al. 2004; Pimpalwar et al. 2002; Avila et al. 2007; Cassas-Medley et al. 2007; Browne et al. 2008). The basis for this is undoubtedly multifactorial, but two important reasons are the likelihood of chemotherapy resistance in relapse tumors, and the debilitated state of the patients when transplanted in the face of end-stage disease. Potential candidates for transplant not only require careful evaluation of their tumor but also a thoughtful consideration of their ability to tolerate the physiologic stress of transplant. Doxorubicin is cardiotoxic and cisplatin is nephrotoxic. A detailed echocardiogram and assessment of renal function is essential prior to transplant, especially a "rescue" transplant. After months, sometimes years of failed therapy, the child's nutritional status may be compromised rendering them more susceptible to infectious complications.

11.2.5 Post-Transplant Immunosuppression

There is concern about the long-term sequelae of the combined nephrotoxicity of cisplatin and calcineurin inhibitors. Children treated with chemotherapy are already suppressed to some degree at the time of transplantation; they might need a tailored reduction of calcineurin inhibitors post-transplant. In the series published by the Brussels' group (Otte et al. 2005), 12 children with a primary transplant were compared with a paired cohort of 12 children transplanted for a non-malignant liver disease during the same period of time (1998–2004). Matching criteria included age, gender, type of graft (ten LRLT grafts and two deceased donor grafts in both groups), and immunosuppression regimen (Tacrolimus-steroids: five versus five; Tacrolimus-Basiliximab: four versus four; Tacrolimus monotherapy: three versus three). Overall patient survival rate was 91% in the first group (1 died of tumor recurrence; the other 11 are alive and disease-free) and 100% in the second group. Rejection-free survival rates up to 5 years post-transplant were 91% and 58%, respectively (p:0.079) despite significantly lower Tacrolimus blood trough levels at 90 days (p:0.004), 6 months (p:0.034), and 1 year (p: 0.019) in HB patients. This limited experience suggests that lower Tacrolimus blood trough levels used in patients transplanted for HB (and likely for other tumors treated with chemotherapy), with the intention to protect the kidneys against the cumulative nephrotoxicity of calcineurin inhibitors and cisplatin, does not increase the rejection incidence during the first year post-transplantation.

11.3 Hepatocellular Carcinoma

In hepatocellular carcinoma (HCC), the cornerstone of therapy is complete tumor resection; however, complete resection is only achieved in about 25% of children (Czauderna et al. 2002; Katzenstein et al. 2002; Katzenstein et al. 2003). Unlike HB, HCC is usually not very sensitive to chemotherapy, is often very advanced at diagnosis, and has a dismal cure rate of less than 30% (Czauderna et al. 2002; Katzenstein et al. 2002; Katzenstein et al. 2003; Reynolds 2001). The role of liver transplantation in pediatric HCC is more controversial than in children with HB and in most cases transplant is not an option because the HCC is too advanced at diagnosis. Because of its chemosensitivity, in HB extrahepatic disease that clears with chemotherapy does not preclude transplant. In HCC, this is NOT true; liver transplant is contraindicated in the presence of any extrahepatic tumor, even in the occasional patient where it clears with chemotherapy. Although HCC is more likely to show some response to chemotherapy in children than in adults, most HCC is chemoresistant. The SIOPEL-1 study included showed a response rate of 49% of pediatric HCC to Cisplatin and Doxorubicin (Czauderna et al. 2002). HCC tumor progression while on chemotherapy is a relative contraindication to transplant since occult extrahepatic micrometastatic disease is increasingly possible in this situation.

Poor prognostic factors for HCC include metastatic spread, large tumor size (PRETEXT IV), extensive multifocality, lymph node metastasis, and major venous invasion. The fibrolamellar variant of HCC has traditionally been regarded as having a higher resection rate and a better prognosis. While this seems to be true in adult HCC, an analysis of ten children with fibrolamellar HCC from the USA showed no difference in outcome compared to typical pediatric HCC. Another distinction between pediatric HCC and adult HCC is the prevalence of cirrhosis, which is much more common in adults. Depending on the series, between 50% and 70% of pediatric HCC presents de novo in the absence of any antecedent liver disease. This is less true in some parts of the world, e.g., Southeast Asia, where hepatitis C is endemic.

11.3.1 Outcomes of Transplantation for HCC Reported in Literature

Table 11.4 (Superina and Bilik 1996; Penn 1991; Tagge et al. 1992; Achilleos et al. 1996; Reyes et al. 2000; Avila et al. 2007; Austin et al. 2006; Beaunoyer et al. 2007; Kalicinski et al. 2008; Olthoff et al. 1990; Ismail et al. 2009) is a compilation of the major published results for liver transplant for HCC over the past 20 years. In his landmark series of 2000, Reyes reported on 19 children with HCC who underwent transplantation (Reyes et al. 2000). In his report a majority of the children transplanted for HCC, 14 of 19 patients, had underlying chronic liver disease, which is just the opposite of what is typically seen in pediatric HCC. The reason for this is twofold. First, many of these patients had "incidental" tumors, meaning that the transplant was performed for the primary indication of the underlying liver disease (e.g., metabolic liver disease) and the HCC was a small focal incidental finding. Second, because metabolic liver disease such as tyrosinemia and glycogen storage disease is known to predispose to the development of HCC, these children are often diagnosed under regular surveillance allowing detection of their HCC at an early stage. Children with cirrhosis from various causes are also included in most other reports of liver transplantation for HCC in children; however, if we are to understand the optimal role of transplantation the results need to be stratified and analyzed separately as (a) de novo tumors in otherwise healthy children; (b) HCC detection during surveillance of chronic liver disease; and (c) truly incidental tumors discovered in the explant of a transplant performed for the underlying liver disease. We tried to separate out these numbers in Table 11.4 and found that in fact it is very difficult, if not impossible, to assign these categories to most cases reported in the literature.

The series from Austin, et al. is particularly problematic in respect to risk stratification of the results (Austin et al. 2006). Data from the United Network for Organ Sharing (UNOS) on standard transplant and research files were analyzed and included pediatric (<18 years) transplant recipients with HCC from 1987 to 2004. A total number of 43 transplants were performed in 41

Table 11.4 Liver transplant in children with HB and pulmonary metastasis at diagnosis, review of literature [56]

Pulmonary metastasis at diagnosis	N =	Post-transplant pulmonary relapse	Alive without evidence of tumor	Died of other causes
Lung lesions disappeared with chemotherapy	24	9 (38%)	14 (58%)	1 (4%)
Pretransplant Pulmonary Metastasectomy	8	3 (38%)	5 (62%)	
TOTAL[a]	32	12 (37%)	19 (60%)	1 (3%)

[a] Patients listed in table have been separately reported in the following series over the past 10 years: Superina et al. (1996), Al-Qabandi et al. (1999), Reyes et al. (2000), Schnater (2002), Perilongo (2004), Avila et al. (2006), Cassas-Medley (2007), Nathan (2009), Casanova (2009), Otte (2009).

children for a diagnosis of HCC. In the discussion, the authors compare their results for HCC, 63% survival, with those of children with HCC in SIOPEL-1, 28% survival, and conclude that the 5-year survival in the UNOS database was significantly better. But this is grossly misleading. SIOPEL 1 is largely a series of children with de novo tumors in otherwise healthy children, whereas the UNOS database includes few, if any, clinical correlative data to help us understand which of these transplants were performed primarily for a new diagnosis of liver tumor, and which were the result of surveillance screening or "incidental" findings in children with baseline liver disease. Indeed the UNOS review data files "contain no center specific information such as tumor staging, chemotherapy regimens, or details about previous surgical resections" and underlying liver disease (Austin et al. 2006).

The contemporary series by Beanoyer (Beaunoyer et al. 2007) and Ismail (Ismail et al. 2009) are more enlightening. Beanoyer et al. report on ten cases of pediatric HCC treated at Stanford between 1988 and 2006. They acknowledge that most cases with HCC in children present with advanced disease and the prognosis is poor (Moore et al. 1997). Median age at transplantation was 10 years (4.4–16.3); seven of ten children had underlying liver disease (4 hepatitis, 1 tyrosinemia, 1 Alagille's, 1 PFIC); three transplants were for denovo tumors in otherwise healthy children, four transplants were for tumors detected in a surveillance program, and three tumors were incidentally diagnosed at the time of transplant. Median size of the tumor was 5.8 cm (2–10.5 cm) with 60% having a lesion of more than 5 cm. Seven patients had more than three lesions; mean AFP at presentation 446,927 ng/mL, five had chemotherapy, and two had chemoembolization. Mean graft survival (14 transplants in 10 patients) was 100% at 1 year and 44% at 5 years, with an actuarial survival of 100% and 83% at 1 and 5 years and a follow-up of 7.9 ± 6.9 years. Two of ten patients died: one from tumor recurrence, and one from multiple recurrent hepatitis B after the third transplant.

Ismail (Ismail et al. 2009) and Kalicinski (Kalicinski et al. 2008) published separate reports from what appears to be the same series of patients in Warsaw Poland. Between 1990 and 2007, 11 children were transplanted for HCC. Median age at transplantation was 10.5 years (3.5–18 years); 5 of 11 children had underlying liver disease (2 hepatitis, 3 tyrosinemia). Six transplants were for de novo tumors in otherwise healthy children; of the five children with underlying liver disease it is unclear in the manuscript, which transplants were for tumors detected in a surveillance program and which tumors may have been incidentally diagnosed at the time of transplant. In 8 or 11 children, the tumor diameter exceeded 5 cm, 5 children had more than three foci of HCC, and three had evidence of vascular invasion. Survival was 72% (8 of 11 children) with follow-up of 4.7 years (32–85 months). Three of 11 patients died: 1 from tumor recurrence, 1 from allograft primary non-function, and 1 from chronic rejection.

11.3.2 Guiding Principles to Consider for Liver Transplant in HCC

A number of guiding principles should be taken into consideration when considering transplantation for HCC.

Response to chemotherapy: Although HCC is more likely to show some response to chemotherapy in children than adults, most HCC is chemoresistant. HCC tumor progression while on chemotherapy is a relative contraindication to transplant since occult extrahepatic micrometastatic disease is increasingly possible in this situation.

PRETEXT to determine potential need for transplant: PRETEXT is primarily useful in predicting tumors that are unresectable by conventional surgical techniques in HB. PRETEXT classification is very useful in stratifying results in pediatric HCC, but the big "unresectable" tumors in HCC are often too advanced at diagnosis to consider transplantation. Nevertheless, any pediatric de novo tumor that is extensive PRETEXT III or IV in the absence of major venous invasion and extrahepatic disease (-V, -P, -E, -M) might be a candidate for transplantation. De novo PRETEXT I and II can probably undergo primary resection although the risk of local relapse is high. In the presence of underlying metabolic disease (e.g., tyrosinemia, glycogen storage disease) or cirrhosis, any PRETEXT -V, -P, -E, -M is a potential transplant candidate.

Multifocal Tumors, Macrovascular Invasion, and Milan Criteria: Outcome for transplant in adult HCC has improved over the years due to our recognition that strict selection criteria can identify candidates with a lower risk of post-transplant tumor relapse. The Milan criteria introduced by Mazzaferro in 1996 restrict transplant in adults with HCC as follows: (a) single tumor diameter < 5 cm; (b) not more than three foci of tumor, each one not exceeding 3 cm; (c) no angioinvasion; (d) no extrahepatic involvement. Since the introduction of these criteria, long-term recurrence free survival after liver transplant in adults with HCC improved from 30% to 75% (Matsunaga et al. 2003; Bismuth et al. 1993; Yao et al. 2001; Leung et al. 2004). There is no distinction between adult and pediatric patients with HCC in terms of the UNOS criteria for assigning the Model/Pediatric for End-Stage liver disease scale (MELD/PELD) scores, which have been based on Milan criteria.

The problem with Milan criteria in children is that 50–70% of children present with large de novo tumors and a large tumor burden in otherwise healthy livers. In contrast, the Milan Criteria were developed in adults with small tumors and underlying cirrhotic liver disease. Furthermore, de novo pediatric HCC often shows features on a continuum with pediatric HB and these transitional tumors may have a more favorable biology (Chen et al. 1998). Kim et al. found the mutation of c-met gene in children with HCC, but not in adults with HCC. Furthermore, they also showed the levels of cyclin D1 expression was significantly lower in childhood HCC than in adults, while loss of heterozygosity on 13q chromosome was higher in childhood HCC than in adults (Kim et al. 2000).

Two recent series of pediatric liver transplantation questioned the relevance of Milan criteria to pediatric HCC. Beaunoyer reported a series of ten cases of transplant for pediatric HCC from Stanford University where the only child who died from tumor recurrence had unrecognized tumor invasion of perihepatic fat, but no vascular invasion (Beaunoyer et al. 2007). Two other children who did have major vascular invasion of the portal vein survived transplantation and have not experienced recurrence with a long-term follow-up. In their series the number of tumors, neither the size of tumors, nor the presence of gross vascular invasion were associated with post-transplant tumor recurrence.

Of the four Milan criteria, Ismail et al. reported a series from Poland where three patients did not fulfill four Milan criteria; three patients did not fulfill two Milan criteria, and two patients did not fulfill one criteria (Ismail et al. 2009). The only child in their series who fulfilled all four Milan criteria was a child with tyrosinemia and a small tumor found on surveillance screening. In view of the lack of improvement in results of conventional treatment of pediatric HCC over the past 2 decades, most clinicians treating pediatric HCC do NOT recommend adherence to Milan criteria in children who present with large de novo tumors and no evidence of extrahepatic disease (Otte 2008).

Metastatic disease: Metastatic disease is considered an *absolute* contraindication to liver transplant in HCC.

Living Donor Versus Deceased Allograft: There is a trend to a higher disease-free, patient survival of children receiving a LRLT for HB (Otte et al. 2004; Mejia et al. 2005; Faraj et al. 2008) it is unclear if this trend would hold true for HCC as well. When a living donor is available, pre-transplant chemotherapy can be scheduled optimally, with a rapid decision toward transplantation (Mejia et al. 2005).

11.3.3 Contemporary Recommendations for Liver Transplantation in HCC in Children

The following guidelines have been formulated by centers with particular expertise in pediatric liver transplantation. They are in a greater state of controversy and evolution than are the guidelines for HB. In most centers, the criteria for transplantation of mutifocal and unifocal HCC are the same as for HB and do *not* follow adult limitations on size and number of nodules. Unlike HB, however, any history of pulmonary metastatic disease, extrahepatic disease, and/or major vascular invasion is considered an absolute contraindication. It is important that consultation with a transplant center with special expertise in pediatric liver surgery be considered early in the treatment in order to prevent delays and unwanted extended courses of chemotherapy while awaiting resection and transplantation.

Multifocal HCC and Milan Criteria: Multifocal HCC in the absence of any metastatic disease both before and after chemotherapy (PRETEXT –M and POST-TEXT –M) is a clear indication for liver transplantation. Apparent clearance of tumor from one liver section (multifocal PRETEXT IV – multifocal POST-TEXT III) should not distract from this guideline because of the high probability of persistent microscopic viable neoplastic cells in the now radiographically "clear" section. Clinicians should resist the temptation to intensify chemotherapy in a vain effort to avoid transplantation. Resection of the dominant primary tumor with nonanatomic wedge resection of satellite nodules carries a high risk of local relapse. In children the number of nodules, as stipulated by Milan criteria, is usually not considered a contraindication to transplantation.

Solitary PRETEXT IV: Primary liver transplantation may be the best option for large, solitary PRETEXT IV HB. Even large solitary PRETEXT III tumors may be best treated by transplantation if a complete tumor-free resection margin is more likely with complete hepatectomy.

PRETEXT III+V, +P: Macroscopic venous invasion (portal vein, hepatic veins, vena cava) is only a relative contraindication if complete resection of the invaded venous structures can be accomplished. When there is evidence or suspicion of invasion of the retrohepatic vena cava, it should be resected "en bloc" and reconstructed. This is an area of great controversy and no established guidelines exist. As long as the tumor is clearly –M and –E many pediatric specialty liver centers would consider these patients for transplantation, many would not.

Pulmonary Metastasis at Diagnosis: An absolute contraindication to liver transplant is pulmonary metastases or extrahepatic disease, whether it responds to chemotherapy or not.

Post-transplant Immunosuppression: Guidelines for post-transplant immunosuppression in HCC are the same as with transplant for HB with one possible difference. Many centers would consider post-transplant adjuvant antiangiogenic therapy with sorafanib in HCC. Sorafanib has clearly been shown to be beneficial in adults in prolonging progression-free survival after conventional resection (Llovet et al. 2008). Experience in the transplant population of patients is limited but in any patient considered to be at high risk for tumor relapse, options for possible antiangiogenic therapy should be discussed. Similarly, many centers have begun to experiment with Rapamycin (Sirolimus) as a post-transplant immunosuppressant because of its antineoplastic and antiangiogenic properties (Chen et al. 2008; Toso et al. 2007). Caution is warranted because of reports suggesting possible increase in post-transplant thrombosis and potential problems with wound healing (www.thedrugmonitor.com), although these have *not* been shown to seriously affect outcome in more recent adult studies (Zimmermann et al. 2008). Experience with Rapamycin (Sirolimus) in *children* transplanted for malignancy is limited.

11.4 Transplant for Other Pediatric Liver Tumors

11.4.1 Infantile Hepatic Hemangioma, Infantile Hemangioendothelioma of the Liver (IHHE), and Angiosarcoma

There is some confusion in the definition and nomenclature of hepatic angiomatous lesions in the pediatric age group. This is in part caused by the noncritical use of the terms hemangioma versus hemangioendothelioma. Infantile hepatic hemangioma is perhaps best classified as focal, multifocal, and diffuse in a clinically oriented approach proposed by Chistison-Lagey et al. (Christison-Lagay et al. 2007). The diffuse subtype of "classical" infantile hepatic hemangioma is sometimes referred to in the literature as hepatic hemangioendothelioma, which can be misleading. Infantile hemangioendothelioma of the liver (IHHE) should be distinguished from "classical" hemangioma whether or not one employs the Boston Vascular Anomalies System, which requires a kaposiform histology and is sometimes referred to as kaposiform hemangioendothelioma. Symptoms seen with these large diffuse lesions may include abdominal distention, hepatomegaly, congestive heart failure, vomiting, anemia, thrombocytopenia, jaundice secondary to biliary obstruction, and associated cutaneous or visceral hemangiomas (Stringer 2000). Unfavorable radiographic features include central varix with arteriovenous shunt, central necrosis or thrombosis, and diffuse hemangiomatous involvement of the liver with abdominal vascular compression (Kassarjian et al. 2994).

In infants who fail medical management, symptomatic solitary tumors may be treated by excision, hepatic arterial ligation, or selective angiographic embolization. Although potentially hazardous, hepatic arterial embolization can be especially helpful in tumors causing high output cardiac failure due to arteriovenous shunts within the tumor (Draper et al. 2008). About 65% of tumors are solitary or unifocal with a survival of 86% and death is usually not caused by the tumor but by a comorbidities (Isaacs 2007). Thirty-five percent of tumors are multifocal or diffuse with a survival somewhere between 60% and 100% with death usually secondary to cardiorespiratory compromise caused by tumors refractory to medical and interventional management (Draper et al. 2008; Isaacs 2007; Dickie et al. 2009). Orthotopic liver transplantation may be life saving for cases with diffuse angiomatous change in which the lesion is progressive with intractable high-output cardiac failure, abdominal compartment syndrome, and failure of lesser treatment options. There are several reports of successful liver transplant in these cases that fail medical management (Kasahara et al. 2005; Egawa et al. 1994; Daller et al. 1999; Walsh et al. 2004). Although the tumor is "benign," not all transplant cases survive due to increased operative complications of bleeding, possible malignant transformation to angiosarcoma (Achilleos et al. 1996), or transplant-related complications (Daller et al. 1999).

IHHE has two subtypes: Type 1 and 2. Type 2 may be an aggressive lesion and has, therefore, been termed low-grade angiosarcoma of the infantile liver [Zimmerman, personal communication]. Apart from this entity, classical adult-type angiosarocma of the liver also exists in childhood, with a histology clearly different from IHHE type 2, but this is a very rare lesion in contrast to IHHE. Case reports document the potential for malignant transformation of infantile hemangioma to angiosarcoma (Awan et al. 1996; Nazir and Pervez 2006; Kirchner et al. 1981). Histologic verification of malignancy may be difficult and this rare entity must be suspected if the biologic behavior of an infantile hemangioma shows unusual progression or recurrence after a period of relative quiescence. Relatively chemoresistant, with angiosarcoma the prognosis is generally poor (Bien et al. 2009). Occasional success after chemotherapy and partial hepatectomy has been reported (Gunawardena et al. 1997). Although there are isolated case reports of transplant for angiosarcoma in children (Awan et al. 1996; Kirchner et al. 1981), adult experience with liver transplant for angiosarcoma has not been good, with very high risk of post-transplant tumor relapse (Penn 1991)

11.4.2 Malignant Epithelioid Hemangioendothelioma

Malignant epithelioid (kaposiform) hemangioendothelioma is a malignant vascular tumor distinct from infantile hemangioma and angiosarcoma (Stringer 2007). It may be slow growing in young women, and very aggressive in children (Awan et al. 1996; Sharif et al. 2004). These tumors are very vascular, large, and diffusely infiltrating and therefore unresectable by conventional technique. No consistently effective chemotherapy is known, but success with an aggressive tumor was recently reported with a four-drug regimen including vincristine, cyclophosphamide, actinomycin D, and methotrexate (Hauer et al. 2007). In a review of five children from three European centers, both patients treated by liver transplantation died within a year, one from viral infection, and the other from recurrent disease (Sharif et al. 2004). In another report, an older child with a slow-growing tumor was successfully treated by liver transplantation (Taege et al. 1999). The operative specimen should be scrutinized for foci of angiosarcoma because recurrence as angiosarcoma has been observed after OLT (Otte et al. 1996). The role of liver transplantation for unresectable malignant epithelioid hemangioendothelioma is therefore uncertain (Stringer 2007).

11.4.3 Mesenchymal Hamartoma

Mesenchymal hamartoma, a fairly common benign tumor is almost always resectable with conventional technique. *Very rarely* a mesenchymal hamartoma is unresectable and liver transplantation may be necessary. There are two reports in the literature. The Pittsburgh group describes two children, both of whom had undergone previous partial hepatectomy with postoperative complications; one died of perioperative bleeding and the other survived (Tepetes et al. 1995). The other case report in the literature had concomitant infantile hemangioma and also had previous unsuccessful conventional resection; transplant was successful (Bejarano et al. 2003).

11.4.4 Inflammatory Myofibroblastic Tumor

These benign tumors may occur anywhere in the body. A handful of cases in the literature document a centrally located and unresectable tumor causing biliary obstruction and portal compression. Inflammatory myofibroblastic tumors are hard and solid, composed of myofibroblasts with an admixture of plasma cells, lymphocytes, and histiocytes in a collagen stroma. Because of their diffuse invasive growth pattern, radiographic imaging often suggests malignancy. Asymptomatic patients may be managed nonoperatively either with simple expectant management or with nonsteroidal inflammatory and antiangiogenic agents. (Applebaum et al. 2005). Some central hilar tumors have been successfully resected and some have required liver transplantation (Stringer 2007; Tepetes et al. 1995; Dasgupta et al. 2004; Kim et al. 1996).

11.4.5 Undifferentiated (Embryonal) Sarcoma

Undifferentiated (embryonal) sarcoma of the liver is a rare childhood hepatic tumor, and has historically been considered an aggressive neoplasm with an unfavorable prognosis. These tumors may arise in a solitary liver cyst (Chowdhary et al. 2004). Survival has improved in recent multimodal approaches, designed for patients with soft tissue sarcomas at other sites, including conservative surgery at diagnosis, multiagent chemotherapy, and second-look operation in cases of residual disease. Using these techniques, several small series have reported survival in up to 70% of children (Bisogno et al. 2002; Kim et al. 2002; Baron et al. 2007). There is a single report of a child with non-metastatic hepatic undifferentiated sarcoma, which was successfully treated by chemotherapy and liver transplant; the key factor in this patient appears to have been the chemosensitivity of the tumor (Dower et al. 2000).

11.5 Pediatric Liver Unresectable Tumor Observatory (Pluto)

Several fundamental questions and controversial issues remain regarding the best use of liver transplantation in children with unresectable liver tumors. (1) What is the optimal treatment of multifocal tumors? (2) What is the role of "extreme resection" versus liver transplant in patients with major venous involvement? (3) What is the role of transplant in patients who present with lung metastasis? (4) Should patients with tumor relapse be offered a "rescue" transplant? (5) What is the role of pre- and post-transplant chemotherapy? (6) How should post-transplant immunosuppression be tailored in children treated with chemotherapy, pre- and post-transplant?

In the hope of answering some of these questions, the SIOPEL study group together with support from COG, GPOH, and the Study of Pediatric Liver Transplantation (SPLIT) has established a worldwide electronic registry for liver transplant in childhood liver tumors: the Pediatric Liver Unresectable **T**umor **O**bservatory called PLUTO (Otte and Meyers 2006). All patients enrolled in the American COG AHEP 0731 study who undergo transplantation will be enrolled into the international PLUTO registry as an integral part of the COG study. All patients on current SIOPEL studies will be enrolled. Enrolment is encouraged from any, and all, pediatric liver transplant centers worldwide. A remote data entry system has been created which is accessible online, worldwide, and free of charge for contributing centers. Information and registration instructions are available on the Web site www.pluto.cineca.org, The aim is to establish a multicenter, international database with prospective registration of pediatric (<18 years) patients presenting with unresectable tumor (HB, HCC, epithelioid hemangioendothelioma, or other rare tumors) undergoing a primary or a rescue transplantation.

All patients treated by liver transplantation will be asked to sign consent within 1 month post transplant giving permission for registration on the PLUTO multicenter international cooperative database for children who receive a liver transplant for tumor. The database collects information about the type of liver tumor, tumor size, number and location of tumors in and outside of the liver, involvement of blood vessels, chemotherapy medications used, lymphocyte blood count, immunosuppression medications used after transplant, side effects of the medications, at what point in the treatment was the transplant performed, complications from the transplant surgery, and outcome of the transplant and the disease-free survival.

11.6 Conclusion

Total hepatectomy and liver transplantation should be considered an integral part of the contemporary treatment of high-risk children with HB. Reliance on chemotherapy to reduce the size or extent of tumors in these high-risk children place them at risk for excess morbidity from chemotherapy, a higher tumor recurrence rate, or death before or during resection. While alternative therapy with "extreme" surgery has been reported with good results in some hands, it remains dependent upon specialized surgical skills and surgical teams with extensive experience. It is these very specialized surgical teams who are best positioned to make a decision regarding transplantation versus "extreme" resection with a transplant safety net. Patients who present with metastatic disease may still benefit from treatment including transplantation but significant questions remain about their optimal treatment. The role of transplant for malignant liver tumors other than HB, i.e., HCC and sarcoma, remains unclear. We strongly urge all physicians and surgeons involved in the care of these high-risk patients to enroll them on available group studies and to register them with the PLUTO registry.

References

Achilleos OA, Buist LJ, Kelly DA et al (1996) Unresectable hepatic tumor in childhood and the role of liver transplantation. J Pediatr Surg 31:1563–1567

Al-Qabandi W, Jenkinson HC, Buckels JA et al (1999) Orthotopic liver transplantation for unresectable hepatoblastoma: a single center's experience. J Pediatr Surg 34: 1261–1264

Applebaum H, Kiernan MV, Coffin CM et al (2005) The rationale for nonsteroidal antiinflammatory drug therapy for inflammatory myofibroblastic tumors: a Children's Oncology Group Study. J Pediatr Surg 40:999–1003

Aronson DC (2008) Liver tumours and the SIOPEL story. In: SIOP education book 2008. International Society of Pediatric Oncology, Berlin, pp 68–75

Aronson DC, Schnater JM, Staalman CR et al (2005) Predictive value of the pretreatment extent of disease system in hepatoblastoma: results from the international society of pediatric oncology liver tumor study group SIOPEL-1 study. J Clin Oncol 23:1245–1252

Austin MT, Leys CM, Feusner ID et al (2006) Liver transplant for childhood hepatic malignancy: a review of the United Network of Organ Sharing (UNOS) database. J Pediatr Surg 41:182–186

Avila LF, Encinas JL, Leal N et al (2007) Liver transplantation for malignant tumors in children. Cir Pediátr 20:189–193

Awan S, Davenport M, Portmann B et al (1996) Angiosarcoma of the liver in children. J Pediatr Surg 31:1729–1732

Baron PW, Majiessipour F, Bedros AA et al (2007) Undifferentiated embryonal sarcoma of the liver successfully treated with chemotherapy and liver resection. J Gastrointest Surg 11:73–75

Beaunoyer M, Vanetta JM, Ogihara M et al (2007) Outcomes of transplantation in children with primary hepatic malignancy. Pediatr Transplant 12:1–3

Bejarano PA, Serrano MR, Casillas J et al (2003) Concurrent infantile hemangioendothelioma and mesenchymal hamartoma in a developmentally arrested liver of an infant requiring hepatic transplantation. Pediatr Dev Pathol 6: 552–557

Bien E, Stachowicz-Stencel T, Balcerska A et al (2009) Angiosarcoma in children: still uncontrollable oncologic problem. Report of Polish Pediatric Rare tumor Study. Eur J Cancer Care 18:411–420

Bismuth H, Chiche L, Adam R et al (1993) Liver resection versus transplantation for hepatocellular carcinoma in cirrhotic patients. Ann Surg 218:145–151

Bisogno G, Pilz T, Perilongo G et al (2002) Undifferentiated sarcoma of the liver in childhood: a curable disease. Cancer 94:252–257

Broughan TA, Esquivel CO, Vogt DP et al (1994) Pretransplant chemotherapy in pediatric hepatocellular carcinoma. J Pediatr Surg 29:1319–1322

Brown J, Perilongo G, Shafford E et al (2000) Pretreatment prognostic factors for children with Hepatoblastoma – results from the International Society of Pediatric Oncology (SIOP) Study SIOPEL 1. Eur J Cancer 36:1418–1425

Browne M, Sher D, Abramson IL et al (2008) Survival after liver transplantation for hepatoblastoma: a two center experience. J Pediatr Surg 43:1973–1981

Cassas-Medley AT, Malatack J, Consoliai D et al (2007) Successful liver transplant for unresectable hepatoblastoma. J Pediatr Surg 42:184–187

Chardot C, Sant Martin C, Gilles A et al (2002) Living related liver transplantation and vena cava reconstruction after total hepatectomy including the vena cava for hepatoblastoma. Transplantation 73:90–92

Chen JC, Chen CC, Chen WJ et al (1998) Hepatocellular carcinoma in children: clinical review and comparison with adult cases. J Pediatr Surg 33:1350–1354

Chen LE, Shepherd RW, Nadler ML et al (2006) Liver transplantation and chemotherapy in children with unresectable primary hepatic malignancy: development of a management algorithm. J Pediatr Gastroent Nutr 43:487–493

Chen JB, Sun YA, Gong JP et al (2008) Effects of rapamycin in liver transplantation. Hepatobiliary Pancreat Dis Int 7:25–28

Chowdhary SK, Trehan A, Das A et al (2004) Undifferentiated embryonal sarcoma in children: beware of the solitary liver cyst. J Pediatr Surg 39:9–12

Christison-Lagay ER, Burrows PE, Alomari A et al (2007) Hepatic hemangiomas: subtype classification and development of a clinical practice algorithm and registry. J Pediatr Surg 42:62–68

Cillo U, Ciarleglio FA, Bassanello M et al (2003) Liver transplant for the management of hepatoblastoma. Transplant Proc 35:2983–2985

Czauderna P, MacKinley G, Perilongo G et al (2002) Hepatocellular carcinoma in children: results of the first prospective study of the international society of pediatric oncology group. J Clin Oncol 20:2798–2804

Czauderna P, Otte JB, Aronson DC et al (2005) Guidelines for surgical treatment of hepatoblastoma in the modern era: recommendations from the childhood Liver Tumour Strategy Group of the International Society of Paediatric Oncology (SIOPEL). Eur J Cancer 41:1031–1036

Dall'Igna P, Cecchetto G, Toffolutti T et al (2003) Multifocal hepatoblastoma: is there a place for partial hepatectomy? Med Pediatr Oncol 40:113–117

Daller J, Bueno J, Guitierrez J et al (1999) Hepatic hemangioendothelioma: clinical experience and management strategy. J Pediatr Surg 34:98–106

Dantiga L, Vallortigara F, Cillou et al (2007) Features predicting unresectability in hepatoblastoma. Cancer 110:1050–1058

Darbari A, Sabin KM, Shapiro CN, Schwarz KB (2003) Epidemiology of primary hepatic malignancies in US children. Hepatology 38:560–566

Dasgupta D, Guthrie A, McClean P et al (2004) Liver transplantation for a hilar inflammatory myofibroblastic tumor. Pediatr Transplant 8:517–521

DeIoris M, Brugieres L, Zimmermann A et al (2008) Hepatoblastoma with a low serum alpha-fetoprotein level at diagnosis; the SIOPEL group experience. Eur J Cancer 44:545–550

Dickie B, Dasgupta R, Rair R et al (2009) Spectrum of hepatic hemangiomas: management and outcome. J Pediatr Surg 44:125–133

Douglass EC, Reynolds M, Finegold M et al (1993) Cisplatin, vincristine and uorouracil therapy for hepatoblastoma: a Pediatric Oncology Group Study. Clin Oncol 11:96–99

Dower NA, Smith LJ, Lees G et al (2000) Experience with aggressive therapy in three children with unresectable malignant liver tumors. Med Pediatr Oncol 34:132–135

Draper H, Diamond IR, Temple M et al (2008) Multimodal management of endangering hepatic hemangioma. J Pediatr Surg 43:120–125

Egawa H, Berquist W, Garcia-Kennedy R et al (1994) Respiratory distress from benign liver tumors: a report of two unusual cases treated with hepatic transplantation. J Pediatr Gastroenterol Nutr 19:114–117

Ehrlich PF, Greenberg MI, Filler RM (1997) Improved survival with preoperative chemotherapy for hepatoblastoma. J Pediatr Surg 32:999–1002

Evans AE, Land VJ, Newton WA et al (1982) Combination chemotherapy (vincristine, adriamycin, cyclophosphamide, and 5-fluorouracil) in the treatment of children with malignant hepatoma. Cancer 50:821–826

Faraj W, Dar F, Marangoni G et al (2008) Liver transplantation for hepatoblastoma. Liver Transplant 14:1614–1619

Fectau A (2009) Liver transplant in children with hepatoblastoma presenting with metastatic disease. In: Transplant symposium: controversies in liver transplantation for hepatoblastoma. Toronto, Ontario

Fuchs J, Rydzynski J, von Schweinitz D et al (2002) Pretreatment prognostic factors and treatment results in children with hepatoblastoma: a report from the German Cooperative Pediatric Liver Tumor Study HB94. Cancer 95:172–182

Geller J, Nathan J, Wagner L, et al (2010) Chemotherapy and liver transplanation for unresectable hepatoblastoma: The Cinninati childrens Hospital Medical Center (CCHMC) Experience. Ped Bld Cancer 55: 905–906

Gunawardena SW, Trautwein LM, Finegold MJ et al (1997) Hepatic angiosarcoma in a child: successful treatment with surgery and adjuvant chemotherapy. Med Pediatr Oncol 28: 139–143

Hauer J, Graubner U, Konstantopoulos N et al (2007) Effective treatment of kaposiform hemeangioendothelioma associated with Kasabach–Merritt phenomenon using four drug regimen. Pediatr Blood Cancer 49:852–854

Isaacs H Jr (2007) Fetal and neonatal hepatic tumors. J Pediatr Surg 42:1797–1803

Ismail H, Broniszcak D, Kalicinski P et al (2009) Liver transplant in children with HCC: Do Milan criteria apply to pediatric patients? Pediatr Transplant 13:682–692

Kalicinski P, Ismail H, Broniszczak D et al (2008) Non-resectable hepatic tumors in children-role of liver transplantation. Ann Transplant 13:37–41

Kasahara M, Ueda M, Haga H et al (2005) Living-donor liver transplantation for hepatoblastoma. Am J Transplant 5: 2229–2235

Kassarjian A, Zurakowski D, Dubois J et al (2994) Infantile hepatic hemangioma: clinical and imaging findings and their correlation with therapy. Am J Roentgenol 18:785–789

Katzenstein HM (2009) Biology and treatment of children with all stages of hepatoblastoma: COG protocol AHEP-0731. Approved by CTEP and NCI 2008, open for enrollment. www.childrensoncologygroup.org

Katzenstein HM, Krailo MD, Malogolowkin MH et al (2002) Hepatocellular carcinoma in children and adolescents: results from the Pediatric Oncology Group and the Children's Cancer Group Study. J Clin Oncol 29:2789–2797

Katzenstein HM, Krailo MD, Malogolowkin MH et al (2003) Fibrolamellar hapatocellular carcinoma in children and adolescents. Cancer 97:2006–2012

Kim HB, Maller E, Redd D et al (1996) Orthotopic liver transplantation for inflammatory myofibroblastic tumor of the liver hilum. J Pediatr Surg 31:840–842

Kim H, Lee MJ, Kim MR et al (2000) Expression of cyclin D1, cyclin E, cdk4 and loss of heterozygosity of 8p, 13q, 17p in heptocellular carcinoma: comparison study of childhood and adult hepatocellular carcinoma. Liver 20:173–178

Kim DY, Kim KH, Jung SE et al (2002) Undifferentiated (embryonal)sarcoma of the liver: combination treatment by surgery and chemotherapy. J Pediatr Surg 37:1419–1423

Kirchner SB, Heller Rm, Kasselberg AG et al (1981) Infantile hepatic hemangioendotheolioma with subsequent malignant degeneration. Pediatr Radiol 11:42–45

Koneru B, Flye MW, Bussuttil R et al (1991) Liver transplantation for hepatoblastoma: the American experience. Ann Surg 213:118–121

Leung JY, Zhu AX, Gordon FD et al (2004) Liver transplantation outcomes for early-stage hepatocellular carcinoma: results of a multicenter study. Liver Transplant 10:1343–1354

Llovet JM, Ricci S, Mazzaferro V et al (2008) Sorafenib in advanced hepatocellular carcinoma. NEJM 359:378–390

Lovorn HN, Ayers D, Zhaoz et al (2010) Defining hepatoblastoma responsiveness to induction therapy as measured by tumor volume and serum L-fetoprotein kinetics. J Pediatr Surg 45:121–128

Malogolowkin MH, Katzenstein HM, Krailo M et al (2006) Intensified platinum therapy is an ineffective strategy for improving outcome in pediatric patients with advanced hepatoblastoma. J Clin Oncol 24:2879–2884

Matsunaga T, Sasaki F, Ohira M et al (2003) Analysis of treatment outcome for children with recurrent or metasatic hepatoblastoma. Pediatr Surg Int 19:142–146

Mejia A, Langnas AN, Shaw BW et al (2005) Living and deceased liver transplant for unresectable hepatoblastoma at a single center. Clin Transplant 19:721–725

Meyers RL, Katzenstein HM, Krailo M et al (2007) Surgical resection of pulmonary metastatic lesions in hepatoblastoma. J Pediatr Surg 42:2050–2056

Meyers RL, Rowland JH, Krailo M et al (2009) Pretreatment prognostic factors in hepatoblastoma: a report of the Children's Oncology Group. Pediatr Blood Cancer 53:1016–1022

Molmenti EP, Wilkinson R, Molmenti H et al (2002) Treatment of unresectable hepatoblastoma with liver transplantation in the pediatric population. Am J Transplant 2:535–538

Moore L, Bourne AJ, Preston H, Byard RW (1997) Hepatocellular carcinoma following neonatal hepatitis. Pediatr Pathol Lab Med 17:601–610

Nazir Z, Pervez S (2006) Malignant vascular tumors of liver in neonates. J Pediatr Surg 41:e49–e51

Olthoff KM, Millis JM, Rosove JH et al (1990) Is liver transplant justified for the treatment of hepatic malignancy? Arch Surg 125:1261–1268

Ortega JA, Douglass EC, Feusner JH et al (2000) Randomized comparison of cisplatin/vincristin/5-fluorouracil and cisplatin/doxorubicin for the treatment of pediatric hepatoblastoma (HB): a report from the Children's Cancer Group and the Pediatric Oncology Group. J Clin Oncol 18:2665–2675

Otte JB (2008) Should the selection of children with hepatocellular carcinoma be based on Milan criteria? Pediatr Transplant 12:1–3

Otte JB (2009) Pluto. In: IPTA 5th congress workshop. Istanbul, 3 April 2009

Otte JB, deVille de Goyet J (2005) The contribution of transplantation to the treatment of liver tumors in children. Sem Ped Surg 14:233–238

Otte JB, Meyers RL (2006) Liver transplantation. J Pediatr Surg 41:607–608

Otte JB, Aronson D, Vraux H et al (1996) Preoperative chemotherapy, major liver resection, and transplantation for primary malignancy in chldren. Transplant Proc 28:2393–2394

Otte JB, Pritchard J, Aronson DC et al (2004) Liver transplantation for hepatoblastoma: results from the international society of pediatric oncology (SIOP) study SIOPEL-1 and review of the world experience. Pediatr Blood Cancer 42:74–83

Otte JB, deVille de Goyet J, Reding R (2005) Liver transplantation for hepatoblastoma: indications and contraindications in the modern era. Pediatr Transplant 9:557–656

Penn I (1991) Hepatic transplantation for primary and metastatic cancers of the liver. Surgery 110:726–738

Perilongo G, Otte JB (2009) Autologous peripheral blood stem cell transplantation with a double conditioning regimen for recurrent hepatoblastoma after liver transplant: a valid therapeutic option or just too much? Pediatr Transplant 13:148–149

Perilongo G, Shafford E, Maibach R et al (2004) Risk adapted treatment for childhood hepatoblastoma: final report of the second study of the internal society of pediatric oncology, SIOPEL 2. Eur J Cancer 40:411–421

Perilongo G, Maibach R, Shafford E et al (2009) Cisplatin versus cisplatin plus doxorubicin for standard risk hepatoblastoma. NEJM 361:1662–1670

Pichlmayr R, Weiman A, Ringe B (1994) Indications for liver transplant in hepatobiliary malignancy. Hepatology 20: 33–40

Pimpalwar AP, Sharif K, Ramani P et al (2002) Strategy for hepatoblastoma management: transplant versus nontransplant surgery. J Pediatr Surg 37:240–245

Plaschkes J, Perilongo G, Shafford EA et al (1994) SIOP trial report – overall preliminary results of SIOPEL-I for the treatment of hepatoblastoma (HB) with preoperative chemotherapy - continuous infusion cisplatin and doxorubicin (PLADO). Med Pediatr Oncol 23:170

Pritchard J, Brown J, Shafford E et al (2000) Cisplatin, doxorubicin, and delayed surgery for childhood hepatoblastoma: a successful approach – results of the first prospective study of the international society of pediatric oncology. J Clin Oncol 18:3819–3828

Reyes JD, Carr B, Dvorchik I et al (2000) Liver transplant and chemotherapy for hepatoblastoma and heptocellular carcinoma in childhood and adolescence. J Pediatr 136: 795–804

Reynolds M (2001) Pediatric liver tumors. Semin Pediatr Surg 10:140–145

Sasaki F, Matsunaga T, Iwafuchi M et al (2002) Outcome of hepatoblastoma treatment with JPLT-1 Protocol-1: a report from the Japanese study group for pediatric liver tumor. J Pediatr Surg 37:851–856

Schnater JM, Aronson DC, Plaschkes J et al (2002) Surgical view of the treatment of patients with hepatoblastoma. Cancer 94:1111–1120

Sharif K, English M, Ramani P et al (2004) Management of hepatic epithelioid haemangioendothelioma in children: what option? Br J Cancer 90:1498–1501

Srinivasan P, McCall J, Pritchard J et al (2002) Orthotopic liver transplantation for unresectable hepatoblastoma. Transplantation 74:652–655

Starzl TE (1992) The puzzle people: memoirs of a transplant surgeon. University of Pittsburgh Press, Pittsburgh, p 168

Stringer MD (2000) Liver tumors. Semin Pediatr Surg 9:196–208

Stringer MD (2007) The role of liver transplantation in the management of paediatric liver tumours. Ann R Coll Surg Engl 89:12–21

Stringer MD, Hennayake S, Howard ER et al (1995) Improved outcome for children with hepatoblastoma. Br J Surg 82:386–391

Superina R, Bilik R (1996) Results of liver transplant in children with unresectable liver tumors. J Pediatr Surg 31:835–839

Taege C, Haltzhausen H, Gunter G et al (1999) Malignant epitheloid hemangioendothelioma of the liver: a very rare tumor in children [German]. Pathologe 20:345–350

Tagge E, Tagge DU, Reyes J et al (1992) Resection, including transplantation for hepatoblastoma and hepatocellular carcinoma: impact on survival. J Pediatr Surg 27:292–296

Tatekawa Y, Asanuma K, Uemotos et al (2001) Liver transplant for biliary atresia associated wtih malignant hepatic tumors. Pediatr Surg 36:436–439

Tepetes K, Selby R, Webb M et al (1995) Orthotopic liver transplantation for benign hepatic neoplasms. Arch Surg 130: 153–156

Tiao GM, Bobey N, Allen S et al (2005) The current management of hepatoblastoma: a combination of chemotherapy, conventional resection, and liver transplant. J Pediatr 146: 204–211

Toso C, Meeberg GA, Bigan DL et al (2007) De novo sirolimus based immunosuppression after liver transplant for hepatocellular carcinoma: long term outcome and side effects. Transplantation 83:1162–1168

Von Schweinitz D, Haberle B (2007) German liver tumor study: HB 99. In: First international symposium childhood hepatoblastoma. Gdansk, Poland

Von Schweinitz D, Hecker H, Harms D et al (1995) Complete resection before development of drug resistance is essential for survival from advanced hepatoblastoma – a report from the German cooperative pediatric liver tumor study HB-89. J Pediatr Surg 30:845–852

Walsh R, Harrington J, Beneck D et al (2004) Congenital infantile hepatic hemangioendothelioma type II treated with orthotopic liver transplantation. J Pediatr Hematol Oncol 26:121–123

Yandza T, Alvarez F, Laureat J et al (1996) Pediatric liver transplant for primary hepatocelllar carcinoma associated with hepatitis. Transplant Int 6:95–98

Yao FY, Ferrell, Bass NM et al (2001) Liver transplantation for hepatocellular carcinoma: expansion of the tumor size limits does not adversely impact survival. Hepatology 33: 1394–1403

Zimmermann MA, Trotter JF, Wachs M et al (2008) Sirolimus based immunosuppression following liver transplantation for hepatocellular carcinoma. Liver Transplant 14:633–635

Zsiros J, Maibach R, Shafford E, et al (2010) Successful treatment of childhood high risk hepatoblastoma with dose intensive multi agent chemotherapy and surgery: Final results of the SIOPEL 3HR study. J Clin Oncol 28:2584–2590

Chemotherapy for Childhood Hepatoblastoma and Hepatocellular Carcinoma

12

Giorgio Perilongo, Bruce Morland, and Marcio Malogolowkin

Contents

G. Perilongo (✉)
Pediatric Department, University of Padua, Padua, Italy and Department of Pediatrics "Salus Pueri", University-Hospital of Padua, Italy, Via Giustiniani 3, 35128 Padua, Italy
e-mail: giorgio.perilongo@unipd.it

B. Morland
Birmingham Children's Hospital, Steelhouse Lane, Birmingham B4 6NH, United Kingdom

M. Malogolowkin
Division of Hematology-Oncology, Children's Hospital Los Angeles, 4650 Sunset Blvd., MS #54, Los Angeles, CA 90027, USA

12.1 Hepatoblastoma

Currently, systemic chemotherapy plays a fundamental role in the cure of children affected by hepatoblastoma. Unquestionably, surgery remains the cornerstone of any therapeutic strategy directed to the cure of these children, and indeed, it is universally accepted that complete tumor resection is the single most important prognostic factor. However, the best chances of cure can be achieved only with a multidisciplinary treatment strategy based on surgery and systemic chemotherapy.

12.1.1 Why Chemotherapy?

The first evidence of the curative role of chemotherapy for children diagnosed with hepatoblastoma can be traced to the early 1970s. At that time, members of the Children's Cancer Study Group (CCSG) and of the Pediatric Division of the Southwest Oncology Group (SWOG) launched the very first cooperative group studies for the treatment of children with malignant liver tumors (Evans et al. 1982). In this first study, patients with disease limited to one lobe and completely resected tumors (Stage I) received no further chemotherapy, while those with residual disease received sequential chemotherapy with actinomycin-D, vincristine, and cyclophosphamide for 18 months with or without radiation therapy. Seven of the 11 patients (64%) in Stage I developed metastatic disease, and only 7 of the 40 patients entered in this study survived. All survivors had either complete surgical resection of the tumor or minor residual disease treated with concomitant radiation. No tumor response was observed in patients treated with chemotherapy alone.

A. Zimmermann et al. (eds.), *Pediatric Liver Tumors*, Pediatric Oncology,
DOI: 10.1007/978-3-642-14504-9_12, © Springer-Verlag Berlin Heidelberg 2011

Due to the lack of chemotherapy response with this regimen, the second trial used a new and more aggressive regimen consisting of vincristine, cyclophosphamide, doxorubicin, and 5-fluorouracil in six weekly cycles given for one year (Evans et al. 1982). All patients including those with completely resected tumors received chemotherapy. Twenty-four patients had no measurable disease following initial surgical treatment and 27 patients had measurable disease at the time of study entry. The response rate to chemotherapy was 44% (12/27 patients), and 20 of the 24 with no measurable disease following initial surgical resection continued relapse-free for more than 20 months. In this study, only 1 of 16 patients (6%) in Stage I developed metastatic disease. This was significantly lower than the 64% metastatic rate observed for similar patients on the first study who did not receive adjuvant chemotherapy.

These historical trials served to produce the first evidence that systemic chemotherapy is effective in reducing tumor volume and thus making originally unresectable tumors amenable to surgical resection (Fig. 12.1), and perhaps most importantly, reducing the subsequent risk of metastatic disease after radical surgery. Since then, chemotherapy has, in the majority of cases, continued to be included in the treatment of hepatoblastoma.

12.1.2 When Chemotherapy?

Since its inception, the North American Cooperative Study Groups on Hepatoblastoma have adopted as its treatment strategy the use of chemotherapy after an

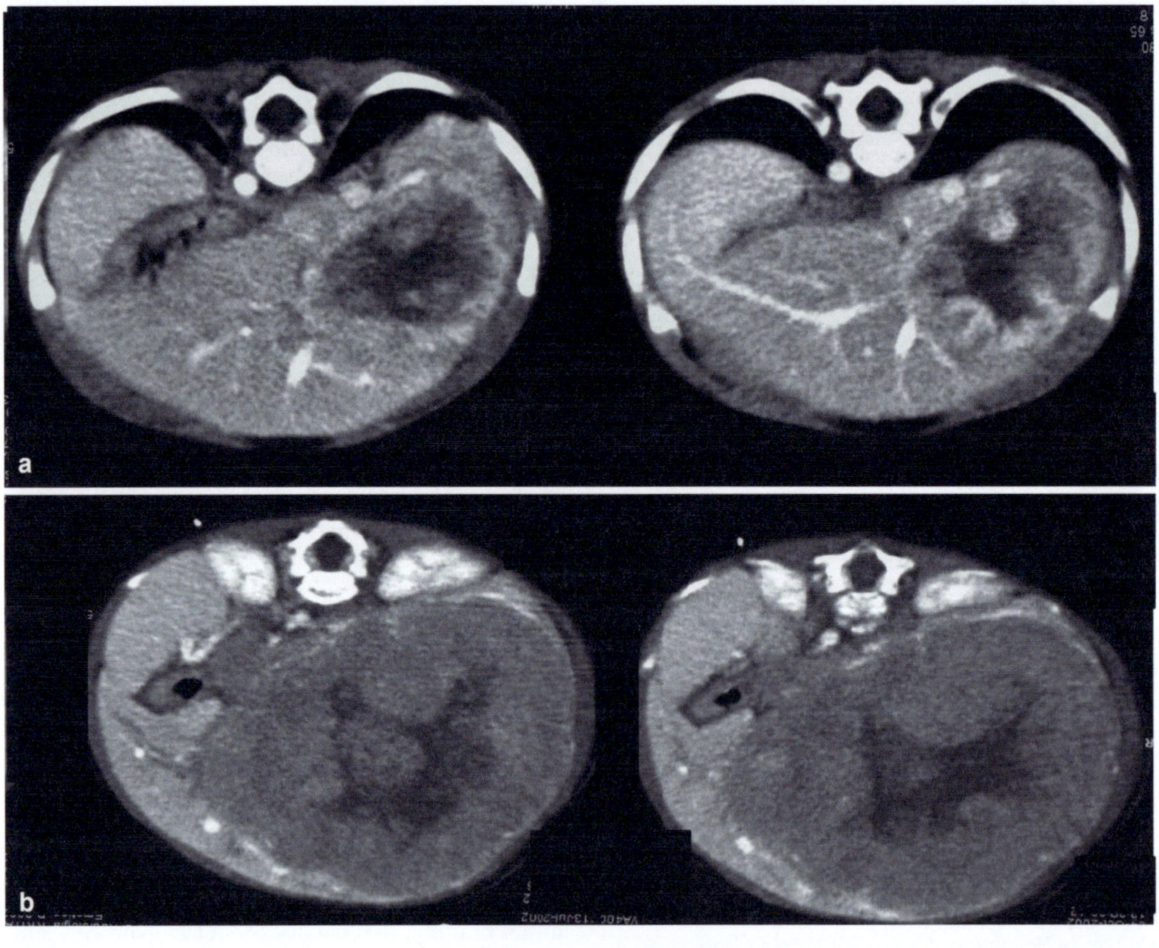

Fig. 12.1 (**a**) Computed tomography scan of a huge hepatoblastoma (PRETEXT III) at diagnosis occuring in a 2-year-old boy; (**b**) the same tumor after four cycles of preoperative chemotherapy with cisplatin alone

initial upfront attempt at surgical resection (adjuvant chemotherapy) for all cases of hepatoblastoma regardless of the tumor extension within and/or outside the liver. In contrast, the European Study Group – which in the early nineties initiated its history of running clinical trials under the umbrella of the International Society of Pediatric Oncology (SIOP) assuming the name of SIOPEL Group – has adopted a treatment strategy based on the use of preoperative chemotherapy before definitive surgical resection (neo-adjuvant chemotherapy) for all patients presenting with hepatoblastoma. The results of these two strategies have been comparable with a 3 to 5 year overall and event-free survival of over 70% (Tables 12.1 and 12.2).

12.1.3 Which Chemotherapy?

The prognosis for children affected by hepatoblastoma changed dramatically since the introduction of cisplatin to the therapeutic armamentarium of these tumors. The response rates of hepatoblastoma to cisplatin-based chemotherapy range from 80% to 100% and the resection rate from 67% to 80%, with a corresponding 3-year overall survival over 70% (Douglass et al. 1991; Katzenstein et al. 2002a, 2002c, 2009; Ortega et al. 1991, 1998, 2000; Perilongo et al. 2004, 2009; Pritchard et al. 2000; von Schweinitz et al. 1997).

Cisplatin-based chemotherapy has become the gold-standard for the treatment of hepatoblastoma. Consecutive international clinical trials conducted

Table 12.1 Results of the North American trials for childhood hepatoblastoma

Trial [reference]	Type of trial/ inclusion criteria	Regimen	Number of patients	Outcome
CCG 862 (Evans et al. 1982)	Single arm/all patients	Vincristine+ cyclophosphamide/ doxorubicin alternating with vincristine, cyclophosphamide, 5-fluorouracil	61	Three-years OS Stage I = 94 Stage II = 57% Stage III = 20% Stage IV = 14%
CCG 823F (Ortega et al. 1991)	Single arm	Cisplatin/doxorubicin	33	Two-years OS Stage II = 86% Stage III = 58% Stage IV = 32%
POG 8697 (Douglass et al. 1991)	Single arm	Cisplatin/vincristine/ 5-fluorouracil	60	Four-years OS Stage I/PFH = 100%* Stage I/II = 90% Stage III = 67% Stage IV = 12 %
INT 0089 (Ortega et al. 2000)	Prospective randomized trial	Cisplatin/vincristine/ 5-fluorouracil versus cisplatin/doxorubicn	Stage I/II 50 Stage III 83 Stage IV 40	Four-years OS Stage I/II 100% versus 96% Stage III 66% versus 71% Stage IV 33% versus 42%
POG 9345 (Ortega et al. 1998)	Single arm Stage III/IV	Carboplatin followed by carboplatin/vincristine/ 5-fluorouracil	Stage III 22 Stage IV 11	Four-years OS Stage III =73% Stage IV = 27%
COG P9645 (Malogolowkin et al. 2006)	Prospective randomized Stage III/IV	Cisplatin/vincristine/ 5-fluorouracil versus cisplatin/carboplatin	Stage III 38 Stage IV 50	Three-years OS All patients = 75% versus 56%

Stage I = microscopic complete resection; Stage II = microscopical residuals; Stage III macroscopical residual; Stage IV = presence of metastases; OS = Overall survival

Table 12.2 Results of the International Childhood Liver Tumor Strategy Group – SIOPEL- trials for childhood hepatoblastoma

Trial [reference]	Type of trial inclusion criteria	Regimen	Number of patients	Outcomes
SIOPEL 1 (Pritchard et al. 2000)	Single arm/all patients	Cisplatin/ doxorubicin	130	Five-years OS 66% Three-years EFS 75%
SIOPEL 2 SR (Perilongo et al. 2004)	Single arm SR-HB	Cisplatin alone	77	Three-years OS 91% (±7%) Three-years PFS 89% (±7%)
SIOPEL 2 HR (Perilongo et al. 2004)	Single arm HR-HB	Cisplatin and carboplatin/ doxorubicin	58	Three-years OS 53% (±13%) Three-years PFS 48% (±13%)
SIOPEL 3 SR (Perilongo et al. 2009)	Prospective randomized trial SR-HB	Cisplatin/ doxorubicin versus cisplatin alone	255	Cisplatin/doxorubicin Three-years OS 93% (±5%) Three-years EFS 85% (±7%) Cisplatin alone Three-years OS 95% (±4%) Three-years EFS 83% (±7%)
SIOPEL 3 HR (Zsíros et al. in press)	Single arm HR-HB	Cisplatin and carboplatin/ doxorubicin	151	Three-years OS 69% (±7%) Three-years EFS 65% (±8%)

SR-HB = Standard-risk hepatoblastoma: tumor confined to the liver, involving at most three hepatic sectors associated with alpha-fetoprotein >100 ng/mL; HR-HB = high-risk hepatoblastoma: tumor involving the entire liver, and/or presenting with metastases; and/or with vascular invasion and/or with extrahepatic abdominal disease and/or with alpha-fetoprotein <100 ng/mL; OS = overall survival; EFS = event-free survival

since early 1970s have helped the identification of prognostic factors associated with the risk of treatment failure leading to the development of different risk groups and therapeutic strategies.

12.2 The North American Experience (Table 12.1)

The Intergroup North American study group (INT-0098), using a treatment strategy based on upfront surgery was able to document that children with completely resected (Stage I) pure fetal hepatoblastoma with low mitotic index (<2 mitoses/ten high power microscopic fields) could be cured with four cycles of doxorubicin alone (Ortega et al. 2000). In the recently completed Children's Oncology Group (COG) study (P9645), these patients were treated with surgery followed only by observation. Preliminary analysis documents that all nine patients with Stage I pure fetal histology hepatoblastoma were alive and free of disease at the time of last contact (Finegold 2002)

On the INT-0098 study, children with all other histological subtypes of hepatoblastoma completely resected with or without microscopic residual disease (Stage I and II unfavorable histology) were randomized to receive either a regimen consisting of the combination of cisplatin (90 mg/m^2 infusion over 6 h) followed by doxorubicin (80 mg/m^2 continuous infusion over 96 h) or a regimen with the combination of cisplatin (90 mg/m^2 infusion over 6 h on day 1), vincristine (1.5 mg/m^2 on day 2), and 5-fluorouracil (600 mg/m^2 on day 2). This study demonstrated that the overall survival for patients treated according to either regimen was almost 100% (Ortega et al. 2000).

The 5-year event-free survival for all patients (except Stage I with pure fetal histology) was 57% for patients enrolled on the INT-0098 study and treated with cisplatin/vincristine/5-fluorouracil and 69% for those treated with cisplatin/doxorubicin (Ortega et al. 2000). Although the difference in outcome between the two regimens was not statistically significant, the types of events associated with each regimen were notably different. While tumor progression accounted for 86% of all reported events for patients treated with cisplatin/vincristine/5-fluorouracil, it represented only 56% of all events observed in those patients treated with cisplatin/doxorubicin. However, this latter combination was associated with an increased number of treatment complications and toxic deaths. Based on these results, the COG investigators adopted the cisplatin/vincristine/5-fluorouracil as the standard for the treatment of children with hepatoblastoma. These results also suggested that cisplatin was the most effective chemotherapeutic agent for the treatment of hepatoblastoma.

Despite the overall improvement in the outcome of children with hepatoblastoma, this trial also highlighted the fact that those patients with macroscopic residual disease at diagnosis (Stage III) and/or with metastases (Stage IV) continued to have a poor prognosis with an overall survival of approximately 50% and 30%, respectively (Ortega et al. 2000). In an attempt to further improve the prognosis of these patients, the subsequent COG P9645 study investigated whether a more intensified use of platinum-derived drugs, mainly based on the introduction of carboplatin, could improve the survival of these patients (Malogolowkin et al. 2006). This research hypothesis was based on the experience acquired with the intensification of cisplatin in germ cell tumors (Cushing et al. 2004) and a limited pilot experience for hepatoblastoma patients (Ortega et al. 1998). This hypothesis was tested in a prospective randomized trial – COG trial P9645 – opened in March 1999, designed to compare the standard "cisplatin/vincristine/5-fluorouracil" combination to a regimen consisting of cisplatin alternating with carboplatin administered every 2 weeks (Malogolowkin et al. 2006). On this trial, patients received four cycles of the assigned chemotherapy followed by response evaluation. Patients with unresectable disease at that time were considered treatment failures. Patients who had their tumors resected went on to receive two more cycles of their assigned therapy. The 1-year event-free survival was 37% for patients receiving the cisplatin/carboplatin regimen and 57% for those receiving cisplatin/vincristine/5-fluorouracil ($p = 0.017$). Patients randomized to cisplatin/carboplatin required more blood product support. There were no differences between the regimens when the other toxicities were compared. The randomization was discontinued after 3 years of enrollment, because the projected improvement in long-term outcome associated with cisplatin/carboplatin was statistically excluded as a possible outcome of this trial (Malogolowkin et al. 2006).

On the P9645 study, stage I and II patients received four cycles of cisplatin/vincristine/5-fluorouracil after their upfront surgery. In addition, all patients enrolled in this study were randomized to receive or not amifostine at a dose of 740 mg/m^2 intravenously over 15 min before each administration of a platinum agent with the goal of reducing the toxicities associated with cisplatin therapy (Katzenstein et al. 2009). In October 2003, the randomization to receive amifostine was terminated as a result of an interim toxicity analysis that determined that amifostine in the dose and schedule used did not provide significant benefit with respect to the amelioration of hematological toxicity or ototoxicity associated with platinum agents. This analysis included 82 patients randomized to receive platinum-containing therapy with or without amifostine. The disease outcome for patients who received amifostine was similar to the outcome for patients who did not receive amifostine ($p = 0.22$). The incidence of significant hearing loss (>40 dB) according to the modified Brock criteria (Brock et al. 1995; Blouin et al. 2004) was similar for patients who received (38% – 14/37 patients) or did not receive amifostine (38% – 17/45 patients; $p = 0.68$). There were no differences in the incidence of renal or bone marrow toxicities evaluated; however, patients who received amifostine had a higher incidence of hypocalcemia (5% versus 0.5%; $p = 0.00006$).

In order to further determine the role of doxorubicin, the COG investigators reviewed the outcomes of the patients with hepatoblastoma entered in the INT-0098 study with emphasis on the postevent survival time for both regimens (cisplatin/vincristine/5-fluorouracil and cisplatin/doxorubicin) (Malogolowkin et al. 2008). Fifty-five of the 173 randomized patients experienced tumor progression or recurrence after initial treatment. Eleven (31%) of the 36 patients treated with cisplatin/vincristine/5-fluorouracil were successfully retrieved with a doxorubicin-containing regimen and surgery and remained alive at last contact, whereas only one (6%) of the 18 patients treated with cisplatin/doxorubicin was alive after retrieval therapy. In summary, they concluded that doxorubicin is effective in rescuing patients with recurrent disease after cisplatin/vincristine/5-fluorouracil treatment and should be incorporated as a means of intensifying therapy for advanced-stage, nonmetastatic hepatoblastoma.

The current COG study for children with newly diagnosed hepatoblastoma (AHEP0731) builds on the results of previous North American clinical trials. The main hypothesis of this study is that a risk-based treatment approach will maintain or improve event-free survival (EFS), decrease acute and long-term chemotherapy toxicity, and identify new agents in the treatment of children with hepatoblastoma. On this study, patients with Stage I Pure Fetal Histology hepatoblastoma will be treated with surgery only. Patients with Stage I non- Pure Fetal Histology hepatoblastoma, non-Small Cell Undifferentiated hepatoblastoma, or with Stage II non- Small Cell Undifferentiated hepatoblastoma will be treated with two adjuvant cycles of cisplatin, 5-flouorouracil, and vincristine, while patients with Stage I, II Small Cell Undifferentiated SCU, or any Stage III hepatoblastoma will be treated with an intensified regimen consisting of the addition of doxorubicin to the cisplatin, 5-flouorouracil, and vincristine combination. All patients with any Stage IV hepatoblastoma as well as patients with any stage of hepatoblastoma and initial AFP <100 ng/mL will be treated with two cycles of "upfront" vincristine/irinotecan window therapy. Patients who respond to vincristine/irinotecan will continue to receive these agents, and will receive a total of six cycles of cisplatin, 5-flouorouracil, and vincristine and doxorubicin with two more cycles of vincristine and irinotecan (total of four).

12.3 The SIOPEL Experience (Table 12.2)

The cornerstone of the treatment strategies of the SIOPEL group has always been based on a preoperative chemotherapy approach and with the combination cisplatin/doxorubicin.

The first trial the group ran – SIOPEL 1 – was a single-arm prospective study which did not include any patient stratification by clinical and/or histological characteristics (Pritchard et al. 2000). The study design included, after the initial diagnosis, four cycles of cisplatin/doxorubicin (cisplatin 80 mg/m² in 24 h continuous infusion and doxorubicin 60 mg/m² in 48 h continuous infusion on day 2 and 3) followed by definitive surgery and then by two further cycles of the same therapy. One hundred and fifty-four patients were registered in the study, and 138 received preoperative chemotherapy. One hundred and thirteen (82%) showed a partial response with tumor shrinkage and serial decrease of serum alpha-fetoprotein levels. One hundred and fifteen patients had delayed surgery, and 106 had complete resection of primary tumor; the 5-year event-free survival was 66%, and overall survival was 75%. These excellent results confirmed the feasibility of the therapeutic approach based on preoperative chemotherapy and this strategy has continued to be advocated by the SIOPEL group for all patients with hepatoblastoma.

This population of children, homogenously staged and treated, allowed investigation of clinical prognostic factors (Brown et al. 2000). The presence of lung metastases and the extent of tumor at diagnosis as defined by the PRETETX system (Aronson et al. 2005) were found to be statistically significant factors associated with 2-year overall survival (p = 0.004 respectively) and event-free survival (p = 0.001 respectively). The 2-year overall and event-free survival for children without and with (lung) metastases were 83% versus 66% and 77% versus 32%, respectively. Among the four PRETEXT categories, the PRETEXT IV group (i.e., tumor involving all four hepatic sections at diagnosis) had the worst 2-year overall and event-free survival (68% and 44%, respectively) (Brown et al. 2000; Perilongo et al. 2000). At that time, no other clinical or tumor characteristic was consistently identified as a potential prognostic factor for overall and event-free survival. Subsequently, the poor outcome for children with a low alpha-fetoprotein at diagnosis was demonstrated to be a further risk factor from this study (De Ioris et al. 2008).

The subsequent studies run by the SIOPEL group were based on these data and have stratified patients according to two risk groups: *standard-risk hepatoblastoma*, represented by those tumors exclusively limited to the liver involving at most three hepatic sectors (PRETEXT I to III) and with an elevated alpha-fetoprotein (>100 ng/mL); while all the other patients were placed in the *high-risk hepatoblastoma.*

For children with standard-risk hepatoblastoma, the SIOPEL group addressed the issue if Cisplatin (80 mg/m² in24 h continuous infusion) alone could maintain the same outcome for this population of children when compared to the combination cisplatin (as per above)/doxorubicin (60 mg/m² in 48 h continuous infusion on day 2&3) as determined by the rate of complete resection, overall and event-free survival. For this purpose and based on the results of pilot studies (– SIOPEL2 – which showed the feasibility of this approach) (Perilongo et al. 2004), the SIOPEL group conducted a randomized prospective trial between 1998 and 2006 to address this issue, comparing the standard combination cisplatin/doxorubicin to a regimen based on Cisplatin alone (Perilongo et al. 2009). The same study design as the SIOPEL 1 trial was adopted, which included a preoperative phase with four cycles of the randomized regimen followed by definitive surgery and then by two postoperative cycles of the same therapy. Two-hundred and fifty-five patients from 92 institutions worldwide were randomized. The complete resection rates were 95% and 93%, respectively, in the Cisplatin/doxorubicin and Cisplatin arm, with a 3-year event-free-survival and overall survival of 83% (95% CI 77–90%) and 95% (95% CI 91–99%) in the CDDP arm and 85% (95% CI 79–92%) and 93% (95% CI 88–98%) in the Cisplatin/doxorubicin arm (with a median follow-up of 46 months). Based on these data, the SIOPEL group concluded that compared with cisplatin plus doxorubicin, cisplatin monotherapy achieved similar rates of complete resection and survival for children with standard-risk hepatoblastoma and thus, doxorubicin can be safely omitted (Perilongo et al. 2009). While awaiting further refinement of the prognostic profile of this subgroup of patients, the SIOPEL group is currently looking into the possibility of reducing the cisplatin-related organ toxicity by adding sodium thiosulphate, an oto-protective agent, in a randomized setting.

Similar to the approach taken by COG investigators in advanced stage hepatoblastoma, the SIOPEL group also looked at the impact of an intensive use of platinum-derived drugs in improving the survival of high-risk hepatoblastoma (PRETEXT IV, metastatic disease, low alpha-fetoprotein). The SIOPEL 4 study adopted a regimen consisting of alternating courses of cisplatin and the combination of carboplatin/ doxorubicin (Zsíros et al. in press). Of the 151 eligible patients who were entered into the trial, 79% had an overall partial response and 76% achieved complete resection of the liver tumor either by partial hepatectomy (56%) or by liver transplant (21%); 70% achieved complete resection of both liver and lung metastases. In 45% of the patients with PRETEXT-IV, the tumor could be completely resected with partial hepatectomy, while 35% of the patients underwent liver transplantation. Fifty-two percent of the patients with initial lung metastases achieved complete remission of the lung lesions with chemotherapy alone. Event-free and overall survival estimates at 3 years were 65% (57–73%) and 69% (62–77%) for the whole group, for patients with PRETEXT-IV tumor 75% and 77%, and for those with lung metastasis 57% and 63%, respectively. This is a major improvement when compared to the 5-year event-free and overall survival obtained in the SIOPEL 1 trial, i.e., 46% and 57%, respectively, for patients with PRETEXT IV and 28% and 44%, respectively, for children presenting with lung metastases (Brown et al. 2000; Perilongo et al. 2000; Pritchard et al. 2000). In the most recent generation of clinical trials directed toward children with advanced hepatoblastoma, the SIOPEL group is looking into a further intensification in the use of cisplatin, based on the weekly administration of the drug.

12.4 Other Regimens

Cisplatin, doxorubicin (as well as other members of the anthracycline family, such as epirubicin, and tetrahydropyranyl-Adriamycin [Blouin et al. 2004; Casanova et al. 2005; Hou et al. 2004; Suita et al. 2004]), vincristine, 5-fluorouracil, and carboplatin are the agents most commonly included in the chemotherapeutic armamentarium of childhood hepatoblastoma. Evidence exists for the inclusion of other agents. Ifosfamide has been used in combination with cisplatin and doxorubicin by the Study Committee of the Cooperative Pediatric Liver Tumor Study HB89 of the German Society for Pediatric Oncology and Hematology (von Schweinitz et al. 1997). Despite the small number of patients entered in this study, the treatment results achieved seem similar to those produced by the larger cooperative groups. Etoposide has been used in combination with cisplatin and carboplatin (Casanova et al. 2005; Katzenstein et al. 2002b; von Schweinitz et al. 1997). In the North American Trial – POG 9345 – children with hepatoblastoma who did not respond to an initial course of carboplatin, vincristine, and 5-fluorauracil were candidates to be treated with high-dose cisplatin and etoposide (Katzenstein et al. 2002b). Out of the 12 patients treated with this regimen, 9 (75%) had some response, indicating a potential role of this drug combination in treating hepatoblastoma. In the most recent German cooperative group trial, nine patients with a high-risk hepatoblastoma (three with unresectable tumors and six presenting with metastases) were treated with two courses of carboplatin (800 mg/m^2) and etoposide (400 mg/m^2). Patients who had tumor responses received one or two courses of high-dose chemotherapy with carboplatin (2,000 mg/m^2) and etoposide (2,000 mg/m^2) with peripheral stem cells rescue, followed by resection of the primary tumor and metastases, whenever possible. Six of these nine patients were good responders to carboplatin/VP16 and five of these have been reported to be alive with no evidence of disease. Only one of three children with no tumor response received a liver transplant. In four of the six patients presenting with lung metastases, the primary could be removed completely or, in one case, they had vanished in the computer tomography scan under chemotherapy (Häberle et al. 2003). Irinotecan has been shown to induce tumor response by SIOPEL and other investigators (Zsiros 2010, personal communication; Bomgaars et al. 2007). No other conventional agents, used alone or in combination, at standard or high dose have been proven to be effective in this neoplasm (Cacciavillano et al. 2004).

12.5 Hepatocellular Carcinoma

Due to the rarity of hepatocellular carcinoma (HCC) in the pediatric age and its intrinsic chemotherapy resistance (Thomas and Zhu 2005; Varela et al. 2003), the history of the clinical research for this tumor is much less rich than the one on hepatoblastoma.

12.5.1 The North American Experience

The North American investigators enrolled 46 patients with HCC in the prospective randomized trial, INT-0098, that compared the treatment with cisplatin/doxorubicin against cisplatin/vincristine/5-fluorouracil regimen (Katzenstein et al. 2002b). Tumor was resected successfully upfront only in eight children (17%). For the entire cohort, the event-free survival at 5 years was 19% (SD = 6%). The event-free survival for children with a completely resected tumor (stage I) was 88% (SD = 12%), for the ones with macroscopic residual disease (Stage III) 8% (SD = 5%), and for those presenting with metastases 0%. The corresponding 5-year overall survival was similar to the event-free-survival: 88%, 23%, and 10%, respectively. There was no statistically significant difference in survival between both chemotherapy regimens. Due to small numbers, no formal prognostic factors analysis was performed, although there was a trend toward better survival in patients with initially low AFP level (<20 ng/mL). In summary, the study confirmed the expected poor prognosis of children diagnosed with HCC and that systemic chemotherapy did not make unresectable tumors amenable to resection These observations confirmed the extreme chemotherapy resistance of these tumors and the failure of such therapeutic strategy.

12.5.2 The SIOPEL Experience

The first cooperative clinical trial run by the SIOPEL group – SIOPEL 1 – was also open to patients less than 16 years of age diagnosed with HCC. The overall survival for the 40 patients entered into that trial was 40% (95% CI 24–55) at 2-years and 28% (95% CI 14–43) at 5-years (Czauderna et al. 2002). Event-free-survival at 2-years was 23% (95% CI 10–37%), while at 5-years, it was 17% (95% CI 6–30). The extent of pretreatment intrahepatic disease, as defined by the PRETEXT grouping and metastases were identified as predictors of overall survival (hazard ratios 0.16 (95% CI 0.04, 0.68) and 1.82 (95% CI 1.01, 3.2)). Presence of metastases and vascular invasion in a univariate analysis were significant predictors for event-free survival, two factors were significant at the 10% level ($p = 0.0001$ and $p = 0.08$, respectively).

The subsequent SIOPEL Group trial for high-risk hepatoblastoma – SIOPEL 2 – including the use of cisplatin alternating with courses of carboplatin/doxorubicin also enrolled patients with HCC (Czauderna et al. 2002). Twenty-one patients diagnosed with HCC were registered. Thirteen of the 16 treated patients received preoperative chemotherapy. Partial response to preoperative chemotherapy was observed in 6 of the 13 cases (46%) treated. Tumor resection was achieved in eight patients (47%) (including one liver transplantation). Three of them underwent primary tumor excision. Six of the eight operated patients received between two and ten courses of postoperative chemotherapy. Nine cases (53%) never became operable. One patient was lost to follow-up just before planned surgery. Four of the resected patients were alive at a median follow-up time of 53 months (35–73). Twelve patients died due to progressive disease, one from surgical complications. In summary, even with this more intensified regimen, the overall treatment results of HCC patients remained extremely poor (22% survival).

12.6 The German Experience

In the cooperative studies of the German Society for Pediatric Oncology and Hematology, childhood HCC were submitted to upfront surgery when feasible and then treated with the same regimen as the one used for patients with hepatoblastoma (von Schweinitz et al. 1997). In the first study, HB89 (1989–1993) neo-adjuvant and adjuvant chemotherapy consisted of conventional dosed ifosfamide, cisplatin, and doxorubicin without substantial effect. Of the 12 patients enrolled in the study only 4 with resectable tumour survived. In the second study, HB94 (1994–1998) patients with nonresectable HCC received conventional dosed carboplatin and etoposide in addition to Ifosfamide, cisplatin, and doxorubicin (von Schweinitz et al. 1997). This regimen showed a short-term partial effect. Of the 25 patients entered in the study, 5 had complete upfront tumor resection (Stage I), 9 had nonresectable tumors (Stage III), and 11 had metastases at diagnosis. A total of eight patients were alive without evidence of disease (8/25 = 32%, 4 Stage I, 3 Stage III, and 1 Stage IV). In the most recent study, HB99, nonresectable HCC is treated neo-adjuvantly with conventional dosed and high-dosed carboplatin and etoposide (Häberle et al. 2003 May-Jun). Since 1999, 33 patients were entered in the study. Seven patients with primary complete resection, one of two patients with primary microscopic residual disease, and all of six with presumed tumor spillage at primary operation are alive and disease free. All five patients with unresectable tumour as well as 8 of 11 with metastases at diagnosis died of disease. Of the remaining three patients, one is still undergoing therapy and two are alive at the time of last follow-up. Carboplatin and etoposide seem to have activity against HCC; however, the outcome for these patients remains dismal.

12.6.1 Other Experiencees

A large study from Taiwan of 55 children with HCC showed even worse results with only two long-term survivors and resectability rate at diagnosis of 10% (Chen et al. 1998). However, this population of patients was different from the one in the SIOPEL or the North American Intergroup studies as virtually all of them had hepatitis B infection and 75% had liver cirrhosis. In this group of children, neither standard systemic chemotherapy nor transhepatic arterial embolization was successful. Thus, most children received supportive treatment only. Average duration of survival in nonresectable cases was 8–18 weeks.

Other pediatric HCC reports deal with very small number of nonuniformly treated cases, and hence are difficult to interpret (Ahn et al. 2001; Chang 1998; Tagge et al. 1992).

In summary, although chemotherapy has demonstrated some activity against childhood HCC, it has not significantly increased tumor resectability and therefore, it has not altered the outcomes for these patients.

Promising data, coming from adult experiences on HCC, on biologically driven therapy are expected to be reproduced in children. Reference is made mainly to sorafenib, a broad-spectrum tyrosine kinase inhibitors, for which there is now robust evidence in favor of its role in patients with advanced HCC with preserved liver function (Verslype et al. 2009).

12.6.2 Overall Conclusive Remarks

Systemic chemotherapy has been proven to be quite effective for the treatment of hepatoblastoma, while for childhood HCC it is of limited benefit. It is difficult to anticipate significant improvement in the prognosis of both these tumors by further refinement of this treatment modality. At this time, investigators of all cooperative groups are working in identifying prognostic factors based on clinical, histological, and biological characteristics that can help risk stratify patients and therefore tailor therapy more effectively in hopes to improve survival and reduce treatment-associated long-term side effects. In order to continue to improve outcomes of children diagnosed with these tumors, the development of novel, effective, and less toxic therapies are needed. International cooperation will be key for further advancements in the outcomes of these rare tumors.

References

Ahn SI et al (2001) Hepatocellular carcinoma with lung metastasis in a 9-year-old boy. J Pediatr Surg 36:1599–1601

Aronson DC, Schnater JM, Staalman CR et al (2005) Predictive value of the pretreatment extent of disease system in hepatoblastoma: results from the International Society of Paediatric Oncology Liver Tumour Study Group SIOPEL-1 study. J Clin Oncol 23:1245–1252

Blouin P, Brugières L, Tabone M et al (2004) Carboplatin–epirubicin regimen for the treatment of hepatoblastoma. Pediatr Blood Cancer 42(2):149–154

Bomgaars LR, Bernstein M, Krailo M et al (2007) Phase II trial of Irinotecan in children with refractory solid tumors; a Children's Oncology Group Study. J Clin Oncol 25(29):4622–4627

Brock PR, Bellman SC, Yeomans EC et al (1995) Cisplatin ototoxicityin children: a practical grading system. Med Pediatr Ocol 19:295–300

Brown J, Perilongo G, Shafford E et al (2000) Pretreatment prognostic factors for children with hepatoblastoma – results from the International Society of Paediatric Oncology (SIOP) study SIOPEL 1. Eur J Cancer 36(11):1418–1425

Cacciavillano WD, Brugières L, Childs M et al (2004) Phase II study of high dose cyclophosphamide in resistant/relapsing hepatoblastoma in children a study from the SIOPEL group. Eur J Cancer 40(15):2274–2279

Casanova M, Massimino M, Ferrari A et al (2005) Etoposide, cisplatin, epirubicin in the treatment of pediatric liver tumours. Pediatr Hematol Oncol 22(3):189–198

Chang MH (1998) Hepatocellular carcinoma in children. Acta Paed Sin 39:366–370

Chen JC, Chen CC, Chen WJ et al (1998) Hepatocellular carcinoma in children: clinical review and comparison with adult cases. J Pediatric Surgery 33:1350–1354

Cushing B, Giller R, Cullen JW et al (2004) Randomized comparison of combination chemotherapy with etoposide, bleomycin, and either high-dose or standard-dose cisplatin in children and adolescents with high-risk malignant germ cell tumors: a Pediatric Intergroup Study – Pediatric Oncology Group 9049 and Children's Cancer Group 8882. J Clin Oncol 22:2691–2700

Czauderna P, Mackinlay G, Perilongo G, Brown J, Shafford E, Aronson D, Pritchard J, Chapchap P, Keeling J, Plaschkes J, Otte JB (2002) Hepatocellular carcinoma in children; results of the first prospective study of the International Society of Pediatric Oncology. J Clin Oncol 20(12): 2798–2804

De Ioris M, Brugieres L, Zimmermann A et al (2008) Hepatoblastoma with a low serum alpha-fetoprotein level at diagnosis: the SIOPEL group experience. Eur J Cancer 44: 545–550

Douglass EC, Reynolds M, Stalen JP (1991) Effectiveness and toxicity of cisplatin, vincristine and fluorouracil therapy for hepatoblastoma. A Pediatric Oncology Group Study. J Clin Oncol 11:96–99

Evans AE, Land VJ, Newton WA Jr (1982) Combination chemotherapy in the treatment of children with malignant hepatoma. Cancer 50:821–826

Finegold MJ (2002) Chemotherapy for suspected hepatoblastoma without efforts at surgical resection is a bad practice. Med Pediatr Oncol 39:484–486

Häberle B, Bode U, von Schweinitz D (2003) Differentiated treatment protocols for high- and standard-risk hepatoblastoma – an interim report of the German Liver Tumor Study HB99. Klin Padiatr 215(3):159–165

Hou JY, Liu HC, Yeh TC et al (2004) Improved survival outcome for hepatoblastoma based on an optimal chemotherapeutic regimen – a report from the study group for pediatric solid malignant tumors in the Kyushu area. J Pediatr Surg 39(2):195–198

Katzenstein HM, London WB, Douglass EC et al (2002a) Treatment of unresectable and metastatic hepatobalstoma: a Pediatric Oncology Group Phase II Study. J Clin Oncol 20:3438–3444

Katzenstein HM et al (2002b) Hepatocellular carcinoma in children and adolescents: results from the Pediatric Oncology Group and the Children's Cancer Group Intergroup Study. J Clin Oncol 20:2789–2797

Katzenstein HM, Rigsby C, Shaw PH et al (2002c) Novel therapeutic approaches in the treatment of children with hepatoblastoma. Pediatr Hematol Oncol 24(9):751–755

Katzenstein HM, Chang K, Krailo M et al (2009) Amifostine does not prevent platinum-induced hearing loss associated with the treatment of children with hepatoblastoma. A report of the Intergroup Hepatoblastoma Study P9645. Cancer 115(24):5828–5835

Malogolowkin MH, Katzenstein H, Krailo MD et al (2006) Intensified platinum therapy is an ineffective strategy for improving outcome in pediatric patients with advanced hepatoblastoma. J Clin Oncol 24(18):2879–2884

Malogolowkin MH, Katzenstein HM, Krailo M et al (2008) Redefining the role of doxorubicin for the treatment of children with hepatoblastoma. J Clin Oncol 26(14):2379–2383

Ortega JA, Krailo MD, Haas JE et al (1991) Effective treatment of unresectable or metastatic hepatoblastoma with cisplatin and continuous infusion doxorubicin chemotherapy: a report from the Children's Cancer Study Group. J Clin Oncol 9: 2167–2176

Ortega JA, Rios P, Malogolowkin MH (1998) Successful treatment of hepatoblastoma (HB) with an intensified platinum regimen. Proc ASCO 17:545a

Ortega JA, Douglass EC, Feusner JH et al (2000) Randomized comparison of cisplatin/vincristine/fluorouracil and cisplatin/continuous infusion doxorubicin for treatment of pediatric hepatoblastoma: a report from the Children's Cancer Group and the Pediatric Oncology Group. Journal of Clinical Oncology 18(14):2665–2675

Perilongo G, Brown J, Shafford E et al (2000) Hepatoblastoma presenting with lung metastases: treatment results of the first cooperative, prospective study of the International Society of Paediatric Oncology on childhood liver tumors. Cancer 89(8):1845–1853

Perilongo G, Shafford E, Maibach R et al (2004) Risk-adapted treatment for childhood hepatoblastoma. Final report of the second study of the International Society of Paediatric Oncology – SIOPEL 2. Eur J Cancer 40:411–421

Perilongo G, Maibach R, Shafford E, Childs M, Widing E, Laithier V, Plaschkes J, Pritchard J, Scopinaro M, MacKinlay G, Czauderna P (2009) Cisplatin versus cisplatin plus doxorubicin for standard risk hepatoblastoma. N Engl J Med 361(17):1662–1670

Pritchard J, Brown J, Shafford E et al (2000) Cisplatin, doxorubicin, and delayed surgery for childhood hepatoblastoma: a successful approach-results of the first prospective study of the international society of pediatric oncology [In Process Citation]. J Clin Oncol 18:3819–3828

Suita S, Tajiri T, Takamatsu H et al (2004) Improved survival outcome for hepatoblastoma based on an optimal chemotherapeutic regimen – a report from the study group for pediatric solid malignant tumors in the Kyushu area. J Pediatr Surg 39:195–198, discussion 195–198

Tagge EP et al (1992) Resection, including transplantation, for hepatoblastoma and hepatocellular carcinoma: impact on survival. J Pediatr Surg 27:292–297

Thomas MB, Zhu AX (2005) Hepatocellular carcinoma: the need for progress. J Clin Oncol 23:2892–2899

Varela M, Sala M, Llovet JM et al (2003) Treatment of hepatocellular carcinoma: is there an optimal strategy? Cancer Treat Rev 29:99–104

Verslype C, Van Cutsem E, Dicato M et al (2009) The management of hepatocellular carcinoma. Current expert opinion and recommendations derived from the 10th World Congress on Gastrointestinal Cancer, Barcelona, 2008. Ann Onc 20(Suppl 7):vii1–vii6

von Schweinitz D, Byrd DJ, Hecker H et al (1997) Efficiency and toxicity of ifosfamide, cisplatin and doxorubicin in the treatment of childhood hepatoblastoma. Study Committee of the Cooperative Paediatric Liver Tumour Study HB89 of the German Society for Paediatric Oncology and Haematology. Eur J Cancer 33:1243–1249

Zsíros J, Maibach R, Shafford E et al (2010) Successful treatment of childhood high risk hepatoblastoma with dose intensive multiagent chemotherapy and surgery – final results of the SIOPEL-3HR study of the childhood Liver tumor strategy group. J Clin Oncol 28(15):2584–2590

Salvage Strategies

13

Jozsef Zsiros and Laurence Brugières

Contents

J. Zsiros
Département de Pédiatrie, Service d'Oncologie Pédiatrique, Institut Gustave Roussy,, 11 Rue Camille Demoulins, 94805 Villejuif, France

L. Brugières (✉)
Service d'Oncologie Pédiatrique, Institut Gustave Roussy, Dept. de Pédiatrie, 11, Rue Camille Desmoulins, F-94805 Villejuif, France
e-mail: brugiere@igr.fr

13.1 Failures in Hepatoblastoma

The introduction of cisplatin-based chemotherapy in the 1980s resulted in a dramatic improvement in the survival of children affected by hepatoblastoma (HB). Large (inter)national studies conducted in the last 3 decades have provided solid evidence for the efficacy of neo-adjuvant and/or adjuvant chemotherapy in improving resectability and survival, and pre- and/or postoperative chemotherapy has become an essential part of the treatment strategy for all patients (Ortega et al. 1991, 2000; Perilongo 1999, 2000; Sasaki et al. 2002; Von Schweinitz et al. 1997). The importance of complete surgical resection of all (residual) tumor lesions (after preoperative chemotherapy), as prerequisite for cure, is highly appreciated (Czauderna et al. 2005, 2006; Otte et al. 2004, 2005; Schnater et al. 2002; Von Schweinitz et al. 1987, 1995). The prognosis of patients with localized, resectable disease at diagnosis is very good with administration of limited amount of chemotherapy and tumor resection with partial hepatectomy (Haberle et al. 2003; Ortega et al. 2000; Perilongo et al. 2004, 2009). The use of intensive neo-adjuvant chemotherapy and aggressive surgery (liver transplantation and [multiple] metastectomy, if necessary), leads to a strongly improved survival of patients with locally advanced or metastatic disease (Katzenstein et al. 2002a; Zsíros et al. 2010). Most recent data from the large cooperative studies confirm that chemotherapy can be successfully stratified according to the presence of initial risk factors giving us the possibility to limit the (long-term) toxicity of chemotherapy in patients with good prognosis (Brown et al. 2000; Fuchs et al. 2002; Malogolowkin et al. 2008; Ortega et al. 2000; Perilongo et al. 2004, 2009).

Despite the improving results, in a significant number of patients, the treatment of HB remains

A. Zimmermann et al. (eds.), *Pediatric Liver Tumors*, Pediatric Oncology,
DOI: 10.1007/978-3-642-14504-9_13, © Springer-Verlag Berlin Heidelberg 2011

challenging and patients may fail to achieve cure with standard treatment alone. The main clinical situations in which salvage therapy can be considered are: (a) progressive disease or (b) unresectable, refractory disease, both on first line treatment and (c) recurrent disease. Most of the patients who experience progression or recurrence initially have a high risk of advanced disease or unfavorable biological features (low APF, small cell undifferentiated HB histology) (De Ioris et al. 2007; Haas et al. 2000; Zsíros et al. 2010).

Although, we have learned from the large cooperative studies that the prognosis for children with progressive disease or with unresectable, viable, refractory residual tumor during first line treatment is dismal (Haberle et al. 2008; Katzenstein et al. 2002a; Zsíros et al. 20100), the prognosis of patients with recurrent disease is much less known. Only very little data are available in the literature on patients with recurrent disease regarding the applied treatment strategy and the outcome.

Feusner et al. reported that 6 of 33 patients with initial stage 1 tumor experienced a tumor relapse confined to the lung, and 3 of the 6 patients were long-term survivors after a pulmonary metastasectomy (Feusner et al. 1993).

Matsunaga reported on 12 of 134 patients who experienced recurrence (four liver, eight lung) after treatment according to the JPLT-1 protocol. All 12 patients were treated with chemotherapy and 11 underwent surgery. Nine patients had NED at last follow-up (13–106 months; four with liver relapse, five with lung metastases). Chemotherapy varied greatly among the patients (cyclophosphamide + THP-adriamycin + cisplatin ± etoposide; ifosfamide + etoposide; carboplatin + etoposide; high-dose melphalan; ifosfamide + carboplatin, THP-adriamycin + etoposide; carboplatin + etoposide + THP-adriamycin). All four patients with liver relapse received chemotherapy and underwent radical tumor resection and were cured. Complete surgical resection was performed in six cases with unilateral pulmonary relapse. Five of them were alive and well more than a year after recurrence. One patient experienced a second relapse and died. Patients without complete resection died. In five of seven cases who were treated with chemotherapy before or without surgery, chemotherapy was not effective in reducing tumor size. The authors conclude that surgical resection of recurrent tumor is necessary to achieve cure but not always sufficient (Matsunaga et al. 2003).

Meyers et al. described 20 patients who experienced pulmonary relapse of their tumor (two initial stage I, nine stage III, nine stage IV). Twelve patients also had tumor relapse at other sites including the liver, mediastinum, or bone. All 20 patients had salvage chemotherapy, and 13 underwent at least one thoracotomy. In only eight of the patients did the thoracotomy achieve complete eradication of all radiographically identifiable relapse disease. Only three of these eight children were long-term survivors. Five of the 13 lung resection patients had persistent tumor present postoperatively in either lung, liver, or bone. Only one of these five children was a long-term survivor (Meyers et al. 2007).

Semerano et al. analyzed the clinical and follow-up data of patients who experienced a first relapse after having been enrolled on one of the previous SIOPEL studies. Fifty-six (7.4%) relapsed, with a median time from initial diagnosis to relapse of 21 months (2–116 m). The site of relapse was: liver in 21 patients, lung metastases in 27, both liver and lung in 3, and other sites in 3. At initial diagnosis 33 patients had high risk HB (including 17 patients with lung metastases). The relapse treatment strategy included surgery and chemotherapy for 25 patients, surgery alone for 7, chemotherapy alone for 17, and only palliative treatment in 5 (2 unknown). Thirty-four patients (61%) achieved a second complete remission (CR). With a median follow-up of 46 months, 26 patients were alive (20 in second CR, 6 after a further relapse including 4 patients alive with disease) and 30 patients died (28 from disease and 2 from complications). Three year event-free survival and overall survival (OS) were respectively 26% and 38%. Only three patients are alive without surgery (Semerano et al. 2009).

As demonstrated by the above reports, currently, no standard treatment is available for these patients and no consensus exists on the best treatment modalities. Due to the rarity of the cases, most patients receive individual therapy regimens with different drugs and schedules based on the decision of the local physician. Children are treated in many different centers and data on clinical features, applied treatment strategy, and response to therapy are not collected systematically. This prevents the accumulation of sufficient knowledge and experience with the management of this difficult problem and makes the launching of a common worldwide study for patients with refractory or recurrent HB an urgent need.

13.2 Salvage Modalities

Based on the literature data, unpublished clinical experience existing within the large cooperative groups, and the principles learned from and applied in the first-line treatment, the following general rules can be drawn for salvage situations. In the salvage treatment both treatment modalities (chemotherapy and surgery) has to be considered. The timing of the modalities depends mainly on two factors: the actual tumor status and the previous treatments given.

Complete eradication of the tumor (primary and metastatic), similar to the first line treatment, is a prerequisite for cure, which makes an aggressive surgical approach necessary and justified. For locally unresectable tumors LTX has to be considered early in the treatment. For the eradication of residual lung metastasis/recurrences, multiple thoracotomies may be necessary. In some cases, small residual lesions represent merely posttreatment changes without vital tumor cells. In case of doubt, (multiple) biopsies can help to prove viable tumor residuals.

In patients with unresectable disease, the administration of chemotherapy is inevitable and the only option to achieve clearance or resectability of the lesions. Second line or salvage chemotherapy, preferably with drugs that were not used in the initial treatment, result in objective response in a significant number of the patients, which can be sufficient to achieve resectability. Additionally, effective chemotherapy also decreases the chance of a new recurrence after radical resection. These arguments make the use of chemotherapy in the salvage setting reasonable even when radical resection can be done.

13.3 Chemotherapeutic Agents in Salvage Treatment

The armamentarium of HB treatment is limited to a few drugs. From these drugs, only a few have been tested for activity in HB as single agent. For cisplatin, doxorubicin, and carboplatin, literature data provide solid evidence for antitumor activity (Black et al. 1991; Champion et al. 1982; Douglass et al. 1985; Katzenstein et al. 2002a; Lockwood et al. 1993, Neglia and Woods 1986). The other drugs have never been tested as single agent in HB since they have been used only in combinations with other drugs, mainly with cisplatin (Douglass et al. 1993; Evans et al. 1982; Von Schweinitz et al. 1997).

Cisplatin is the most active drug in HB and is extensively used in all first-line regimens. Due to the considerable and cumulative toxicity of cisplatin, and the observed or assumed development of drug resistance against cisplatin, the administration of this drug is mostly limited to first-line treatment.

Carboplatin has a clear activity in HB and has a different toxicity profile from cisplatin which makes it a good candidate for use in a multidrug combination (Katzenstein et al. 2002a). It is important to realize, however, that its antitumor activity in HB is lower than that of cisplatin (Blouin et al. 2004; Dall'Igna et al. 2001; Fuchs et al. 1998; Malogolowkin et al. 2006). Due to its proven activity in primary HB, the fact that it is used less extensively in the first-line regimens, and its ability to be administered for patients with decreased glomerular function, carboplatin is a good candidate for second-line treatment. Little is known, however, about its antitumor activity in patients with recurrent or progressive disease who previously received cisplatin-containing chemotherapy.

Doxorubicin is assumed to be the second most effective drug in HB with proven activity as a single drug. In some early studies, it has been extensively used in first line treatment for all patients (Pritchard et al. 2000; Ortega et al. 1991). Recent data show, however, that patients with standard risk or resectable localized disease can be cured with an excellent prognosis without doxorubicin treatment. In the current treatment protocols, the administration of doxorubicin is limited to patients with high risk or advanced HB, reducing the long-term toxicity in patients with standard risk or resectable localized disease (Malogolowkin et al. 2008; Perilongo et al. 2009). This provides the opportunity to use doxorubicin in the second line (salvage treatment) for patients who have not received this drug previously.

In HB, *etoposide* is used almost exclusively in combination with other drugs (mostly with carboplatin) and only in second-line treatment. This is presumably caused by the fact that no sufficient data exist on its activity as single agent in HB.

The activity of the combination *carboplatin* ± *etoposide* (CARBO/VP16) in HB is better characterized. In the German Cooperative Pediatric Liver Tumor HB-99 study, patients with newly diagnosed high-risk

HB were first treated with two courses of carboplatin (800 mg/m^2) and etoposide (400 mg/m^2). The reported response rate was 84% (Haeberle 2008). The activity of the combination carboplatin+ etoposide in patients with advanced or recurrent disease was first described by Fuchs et al. In the HB-89 study, 14 children with recurrent or advanced HB were additionally treated with CARBO/VP16, the reason being observation of drug resistance after four or more courses of ifosfamide, cisplatin, adriamycin (IPA) therapy. Two patients underwent CARBO/VP16 chemotherapy for advanced HB at first operation: all were alive and well. Five patients with local relapse and/or distant metastases responded partially to CARBO/VP16 therapy, and a complete remission was achieved in one patient. In five patients, progressive disease was observed during therapy with CARBO/VP 16. One patient, with stable disease on CARBO/VP16 chemotherapy, had a successful resection. Acute toxicity of chemotherapy was observed in seven patients (50%). Tumor resection was attempted in 13 children but, in only three cases, was a complete tumor resection achieved in one operation. Seven of the patients (50%) were in remission at last follow-up (Fuchs et al. 1999a). In the subsequent HB 94 study, the authors reported on eighteen children with advanced or recurrent HB who underwent VP16/CARBO chemotherapy, with a response achieved in 12 children (Fuchs et al. 2002). Although, in both reports, the limited number of patients and the lack of important clinical data prevent the full understanding of the exact role of this combination in the salvage situation, the data suggest that some patients may benefit from the use of CARBO/VP16 with acceptable toxicity.

In the most recent SIOPEL trial for high-risk HB (SIOPEL-4) two cycles of *Carboplatin* (AUC 10.6 mg/mL.min) + *doxorubicin* (75 mg/m^2) were used as salvage treatment for those patients whose tumor remained unresectable after initial chemotherapy with cisplatin (560 mg/m^2) and doxorubicin (180 mg/m^2). The study was recently completed, and results regarding response and resection rate in this salvage situation are awaited.

Irinotecan (CPT-11), a semisynthetic topoisomerase-I inhibitor, is an important and attractive new chemotherapeutic agent that can be used in the treatment of (relapsed or refractory) HB.

Irinotecan demonstrated high activity against a broad spectrum of malignancies, including different childhood tumors, both in preclinical xenograft models for rhabdomyosarcoma, neuroblastoma, primitive neuroectodermal tumor, medulloblastoma, ependymoma, and malignant glioma (Hare et al. 1997; Thompson et al. 1997a, b; Vassal et al. 1996, 1997; Furman et al. 1999) and in subsequent clinical phase I and II studies for newly diagnosed and recurrent rhabdomyosarcoma, neuroblastoma, and brain tumors (Blaney et al. 2001; Bomgaars et al. 2007; Cosetti et al. 2002; Furman et al. 1999; Mugishima et al. 2002; Raymond et al. 2003; Shitara et al. 2006; Turner et al. 2002; Vassal et al. 1998, 2003, 2007, 2008).

A variety of schedules of irinotecan administration has been used in the preclinical and clinical phase I–II studies. Data suggest that the efficacy of irinotecan is strongly schedule dependent and that smaller doses of irinotecan administered repeatedly may result in greater antitumor activity than large doses administered intermittently (Furman et al. 1999; O'Leary et al. 1998; Pazdur et al. 1998; Vassal et al. 1997, 2007). Accordingly, a protracted schedule of intravenous irinotecan administration ([every day ×5] ×2) has been associated with better disease response. However, the optimal schedule of administration of irinotecan in different childhood tumors remains uncertain.

The phase I–II trials with different dose regimens have extensively evaluated the toxicity and safety of irinotecan both in adults and children (Blaney et al. 2001; Bleiberg et al. 1996; Hecht et al. 1998; Langevin et al. 1998; Saliba et al. 1998; Vassal et al. 2003, 2007, 2008). Depending on the schedule, the primary dose-limiting toxicity is diarrhea and myelosuppression, where diarrhea is associated with the protracted schedule.

In the early pediatric trials, one patient with HB was reported to have a complete response, and another heavily pretreated patient with refractory HB had a one-log reduction in AFP level after three cycles (Blaney et al. 2001; Bomgaars et al. 2007).

In the last years, the SIOPEL group conducted a prospective multicenter phase II study in children with refractory or recurrent HB to assess the clinical activity of irinotecan in HB and test the feasibility of irinotecan single drug treatment as salvage therapy. Irinotecan was administered on a prolonged schedule: 20 mg/m^2/day i.v. infusion (60 min) daily for 5 consecutive days, followed by 2 days off, for 2 weeks out of 3 ([(d5)2]2×). Patients were treated with a total of four courses of irinotecan as single agent chemotherapy unless tumor progression occurred or resectability of the tumor is achieved. Twenty-five patients were included. The preliminary results show that irinotecan has significant antitumor activity with acceptable toxicity in patients with relapsed hepatoblastoma, making irinotecan a very attractive drug for use in salvage chemotherapy (Zsiros et al. 2009). Detailed analysis of the study is under way.

A few case reports further underline these encouraging results.

Katzenstein reports on three patients who were treated with irinotecan. The first paient was treated for a second pulmonary relapse with 20 mg/m^2 × 5 days for 2 weeks. He had a decline in the AFP level, demonstrating efficacy, and then underwent resection of the tumor lesion. Postoperatively, the patient continued to receive irinotecan for a total of 22 cycles. One month after discontinuation of irinotecan, a recurrent tumor has been detected that was unresectable. Despite new chemotherapy, the patient died of tumor progression. The second patient experienced a recurrence after treatment for a stage I HB. For the relapse, for an unresectable tumor with extrahepatic growth, chemotherapy was initiated with cisplatin, carboplatin, etoposide, doxorubicin, and cyclophosphamide. After three cycles, progression was observed and treatment with irinotecan was started (65 mg/m^2 × 5 days, every 3 weeks). The patient's clinical status improved dramatically and the AFP level declined promptly. After 12 courses, the tumor showed shrinkage and there was no evidence of extrahepatic disease. The patient underwent liver transplantation (LTX). Four month after LTX, a new relapse (in the liver and lungs) was detected and the patient died of tumor progression. The third patient had initial stage IV disease and was treated with cisplatin and carboplatin followed by resection of the primary tumor and the remaining lung lesions. The treatment was completed with tandem high-dose chemotherapy (HDT) and peripheral blood stem cell transplantation (PBSCT) rescue. Six months after the second HDT, the patient experienced a relapse in the lungs and mediastinum. The patient was then administered irinotecan (50 mg/m^2 × 5 days) and had a decrease in the AFP level. After 11 cycles of irinotecan, her AFP level was normal and had no evidence of disease (Katzenstein et al. 2002b).

Palmer et al described a child with multiply relapsed HB who previously received multiple, intensive chemotherapy regimens. His AFP level fell dramatically in response to single agent irinotecan treatment (600 mg/m^2/day at 3 weeks interval). After six courses the APF level normalized. He received in total eight courses and remained in remission for more than 7 months off treatment (follow-up time). After the first course, he experienced nausea, vomiting, and abdominal cramp, but the other cycles were exceptionally well tolerated (Palmer and Williams 2003).

Ijichi et al. described a heavily pretreated patient with relapsed HB after LTX who was treated with irinotecan (35 mg/m^2 daily for 3 days/week for 2 consecutive weeks, and repeated every 28 days). After four courses of irinotecan, metastatic lesions were remarkably reduced in size, and the serum level of AFP decreased from 0.7 million to 927 ng/mL. Diarrhea and neutropenia were observed as side effects. After the sixth cycle AFP level began to rise. These results suggest that irinotecan may be safely given to a patient with relapsed HB after LTX without serious side effects (Ijichi et al. 2006).

In the report of Qayed, patient 1 presented with stage IV HB with unresectable primary tumor and was treated with standard chemotherapy and tumor resection. CR was achieved. Seven month off therapy a recurrence in the liver was detected. He received one cycle of ifosfamide, carboplatin, and etoposide with only a transient decline in the AFP and therapy was switched to iritnotecan (20 mg/m^2/day × 5, after two courses 50 mg/m^2) and VCR (1.5 mg/m^2/day) in 3 week cycles. After three cycles, 60% decrease of the tumor size was observed and the AFP declined. The patient underwent LTX and 2 months posttransplant the AFP normalized. Subsequently, the patient received 15 cycles of oral irinotecan + VCR. The patient remained relapse free for the follow-up time (8 month off therapy). Patient 2 had stage IV disease and was treated with standard first-line treatment. AFP was normal following four cycles but the primary tumor remained unresectable and there was persistence of pulmonary lesions. His therapy was augmented to include irinotecan (50 mg/m^2/day × 5) and VCR (1.5 mg/m^2). No decrease in tumor size or decline of the AFP was observed. A right thoracotomy was performed with resection of 16 pulmonary nodules, and no evidence of viable tumor at histology was found. For the primary tumor, a partial hepatectomy has been done with negative margins. Patient no 3 had stage IV disease and was treated with standard first-line chemotherapy. Six months off therapy pulmonary and mediastinal recurrence was detected and irinotecan therapy was started (50 mg/m^2/day × 5). AFP normalized and radiological findings resolved following two cycles. A total of 32 cycles were given over 2 years. She remained in CR for the follow-up of 6 years (Qayed et al. 2010).

Based on these results, irinotecan can be highly recommended for the treatment of recurrent, refractory or progressive HB. In case of good tumor response, repeated administration of irinotecan should be considered. Whether prolonged (maintenance) treatment after tumor clearance is reasonable and contributes to an improved survival remains unknown and requires further study. Although Katzenstein and Qayed reported that prolonged administration of irinotecan was well tolerated in heavily pretreated children, the efficacy of long-term maintenance use of irinotecan is difficult to assess in such a limited series (Katzenstein et al. 2002b; Qayed et al. 2010) and has to be explored further.

The combination of *irinotecan and vincristine* is well tolerated and has shown better activity in rhabdomyosarcoma than irinotecan alone (Pappo et al. 2007). These data and the sporadic observations in HB make the use of this combination attractive and reasonable in a salvage situation, although, due to lack of sufficient data, no evidence-based support can be given for this approach. Ongoing and upcoming studies investigate the role of this combination, and results are awaited.

Topotecan, another topoisomerase I inhibitor, demonstrated in-vitro and clinical activity in various childhood tumors and is increasingly used, either alone or in combination, in both first and second-line setting in the treatment of many pediatric tumors. Based on preclinical observations, it could also be an interesting drug in HB (McCrudden et al. 2002; Nitschke et al. 1998; Warman 2001; Zhang et al. 2008). However, no data have been published yet on clinical use of topotecan in HB.

13.4 High-Dose Chemotherapy

The efficacy of high-dose (HD) chemotherapy followed by autologous stem cell rescue has been increasingly studied and used in the last decades in various childhood malignancies. As a result, HD chemotherapy has been established as part of the standard treatment strategy (first or second line) for some childhood tumors. In HB, the role of HD chemotherapy – either as first line or as salvage treatment – is unknown. Based on the assumption that the development of drug resistance against cisplatin and/or other drugs during neo-adjuvant treatment may play a role in treatment failures, it would seem an attractive strategy to use HD chemotherapy as part of the salvage strategy.

The issue of HD chemotherapy in HB has been addressed only in very few studies and in rather different clinical situations.

The multicentric prospective study HB99 of the German Society for Pediatric Oncology and Hematology (GPOH) attempted to improve the results in high-risk patients by using HD chemotherapy as part of the first-line treatment. Patients with unresectable multifocal tumors or infiltration of large vessels and patients with distant metastases at diagnosis were considered high-risk. First, they were treated with two courses of conventional dose carboplatin (800 mg/m^2) and etoposide (400 mg/m^2). In case of tumor response, one or two courses of high-dose carboplatin (2,000 mg/m^2) and high-dose etoposide (2,000 mg/m^2) were administered with autologous peripheral stem cell rescue. Chemotherapy was followed by delayed surgery or liver transplantation. Nonresponders were treated with salvage chemotherapy containing ifosfamide, cisplatin, and doxorubicin (IPA). Twenty-one of the 37 high-risk patients received HD chemotherapy with a response rate of 75%. In 13 patients the tumor could be completely resected (60%). Twelve of the 21 patients survived tumor free (57%). After HD chemotherapy, thrombocytopenia and neutropenia was seen in 80% and 90% of the courses, respectively. Mucositis and temporary elevation of liver enzymes occurred in 30% and 27%, respectively. The rate of the gross total tumor resection was 70% (26/37) and 54% (20/37) for microscopical complete resection. The tumor-free survival of all high-risk patients was 51% (19/37).

The authors concluded that the overall results were comparable to those of other cooperative studies, and no special benefit of high-dose carboplatin/etoposide chemotherapy was observed in comparison to conventional-dose cisplatin-containing chemotherapy (Haberle et al. 2008).

In the POG 9345 study, patients with stage III or IV HB were initially treated with one cycle of carboplatin alone (700 mg/m^2) and three cycles of carboplatin (700 mg/m^2), vincristin (1.5 mg/m^2, weekly, 3×), and 5-fluorouracil (3,000 mg/m^2). For those patients whose tumor remained unresectable high-dose (HD) cisplatin (200 mg/m^2) and etoposide (300 mg/m^2) were administered for a total of two courses. Of the 33 patients (22 stage III, 11 stage IV) 12 received high-dose cisplatin. Of these 12 patients (six stage III, three stage IV), 9 had partial response and two experienced progressive disease. Five patients underwent complete tumor resection and achieved CR. All five were free of tumor at last follow-up (minimum 5.5 years). Among the 12 patients who received HD cisplatin, 5-year EFS was 42% ± 14%. The 5-year EFS estimates for the whole group (33 patients) was 59% ± 11% for stage III and 27% ± 16% for stage IV disease, respectively. These results are comparable or even inferior to the results of other cooperative studies that use conventional-dose cisplatin, suggesting that the use of HD cisplatin – at least within this treatment strategy – does not provide benefit for these patients (Katzenstein et al. 2002a).

In the first prospective multicenter trial in children with refractory or recurrent HB, the SIOPEL group assessed the efficacy of HD cyclophosphamide in 17 patients who failed on or after treatment with SIOPEL-1 or -2 protocols (9 patients with progressive disease, 2 with refractory unresectable disease, and 6 with recurrent disease, all heavily pretreated with cisplatin-containing chemotherapy). Patients were treated with one to four cycles of HD cyclophosphamide (4 mg/m^2) until progression occurred. Only one patient responded, achieving PR after two cycles and CR after three cycles. One patient had SD after two cycles. All patients died, 17 of disease progression, 1 patient of surgical complication. The low response rate and the severe side effects demonstrated that this approach is not useful and feasible in the treatment of heavily pretreated recurrent or refractory HB (Cacciavillano et al. 2004).

A number of case reports provide some information on sporadic use of HD chemotherapy in individual patients.

Hara et al. reported on four patients with HB (within a group of 28 patients in total with "high risk" solid tumor) who received HD chemotherapy and autologous stem cell rescue. Patients received a double-conditioning regimen, consisting of two cycles of a combination of thiotepa (300–600 mg/m^2) plus melphalan (70–150 mg/m^2) with a 1-week interval, followed by a single grafting. Although the procedure was tolerable, renal toxicity and mucositis (predominant toxicity) was significant and occasionally severe. Treatment-related deaths in the whole group was 7% (fungal pneumonia and renal tubular acidosis). One patient with a third relapse of HB (no other chemotherapy given for this relapse) showed PR but experienced further progression and ultimately died of disease. The other three children who initially had localized HB (stage II and III) were treated previously with conventional chemotherapy and underwent partial hepatectomy, but did not achieve CR, which was the reason for inclusion in the HD program. Unfortunately, no information is given in the report regarding the cause of not being in CR (microscopic or macroscopic residual disease or elevated AFP). After HD therapy, all three patients achieved CR and remained tumor free for the last follow-up (19, 34, and 50 months, respectively). Although, this report underlines the experience that even heavily pretreated patients can demonstrate some response to (new) drugs, it is, due to lack of essential information, impossible to judge the specific value of high-dose treatment in this situation (Hara et al. 1998).

Yoshinari reported on a 9-month-old boy with stage III B hepatoblastoma of caudate lobe origin. Surgical resection was attempted following six courses of chemotherapy, but viable tumor cells remained microscopically at resection margins. Subsequently, the patient received HD chemotherapy consisting of carboplatin, etoposide, tetrahydropyranyl adriamycin, and melphalan followed by peripheral blood stem cell transplantation (PBSCT). The patient showed no local or metastatic relapse without any further chemotherapy. The authors concluded that PBSCT for patients with postoperative residue may improve the outcome of advanced HB (Yoshinari et al. 1998). This conclusion needs, however, some comments. The SIOPEL group has repeatedly shown in large prospective studies that microscopical residual disease after liver resection without any other residual disease does not have an unfavorable effect on (event free) survival (Perilongo et al. 2004, 2009, Warmann et al. 2001, 2010). These patients have an excellent prognosis and do not need any additional treatment for the microscopical residue in the liver. Accordingly, the use of HD chemotherapy in this situation does not seem to be justified and its value in improving survival cannot be judged with these data.

Katzenstein et al. described three children who received HD chemotherapy with autologous stem cell rescue. The first patient had a localized HB, stage II, and was treated with tumor resection and adjuvant chemotherapy. The patient achieved CR, but 1 month after the completion of therapy AFP began to rise, although no recurrent lesion could be detected on imaging studies. Chemotherapy was initiated with etoposide, ifosfamide, and carboplatin which resulted in a decrease of AFP. The patient then underwent tandem HDT with PBSCT rescue. After the administration of the first HDT regimen (etoposide 2,400 mg/m^2, carboplatin 2,000 mg/m^2, and cyclophosphamide 3,600 mg/m^2), the patients developed neurological symptoms, and the presumptive diagnosis of Guillain–Barre syndrome was made. The second regime was given 1 month after the first one and consisted of thiotepa (900 mg/m^2) and cyclophosphamide (6,000 mg/m^2). Two years after the HDT, the patient presented with a solitary lung nodule, and underwent surgical resection (histology: viable HB). After resection, AFP returned to normal without any further treatment and the patient remained tumor free until the last follow-up (5.5 years). The second patient was initially treated for stage IV HB including resection of the liver tumor. Due to residual tumor in the lung the patient underwent tandem HDT with PPBSCT rescue. The first regimen (etoposide 2,400 mg/m^2, carboplatin 2,000 mg/m^2, and cyclophosphamide 3,600 mg/m^2) caused mild neuropathy. The second regimen was given 1 month later (thiotepa 900 mg/m^2 and cyclophosphamide 180 mg/kg). Three month after the second HD treatment the patient was diagnosed with a recurrent lung lesion. The third patient had initial stage IV disease and was treated with cisplatin and carboplatin followed by resection of the primary tumor and the remaining lung lesions. The treatment was completed with tandem HDT and PBSCT rescue. The two regimens consisted of etoposide (2,400 mg/m^2) + carboplatin (2,000 mg/m^2) + cyclophosphamide (3,600 mg/m^2) and melphalan (180 mg/m^2) + cyclophosphamide (6,000 mg/m^2), respectively. Six month after the second HDT, the patient experienced a relapse in the lungs and mediastinum (Katzenstein et al. 2002b).

In the paper of Nishimura, three patients with metastatic HB are described who received HD chemotherapy with autologous bone marrow rescue. In patient 1, who had an initial stage IV disease, treated with primary surgery and six cycles of adjuvant chemotherapy, HD chemotherapy was given at first pulmonary relapse after resection of the pulmonary metastases and extensive conventional-dose chemotherapy with different combinations (one cycle of carboplatin, doxorubicin, and etoposide, two cycles of cisplatin, 5-fluorouracil, cyclophosphamide, and etoposide, and one cycle of etoposide and ifosfamide). The patient developed a new pulmonary relapse 6 months after HD chemotherapy and was than treated by resection of the metastasis. About 30 months later, the child developed a new lung metastasis that was resected surgically. At both relapses after HD chemotherapy vital tumor cells have been found in the resected tumor. After the last thoracotomy, the child has been without tumor for more than 6 years (last follow-up). The second patient presented initially with multiple pulmonary metastases. He was treated with seven cycles of conventional chemotherapy (cisplatin, doxorubicin, carboplatin, and etoposide) and gross resection of the primary tumor and the metastases. His treatment was completed with HD chemotherapy (melphalan, L-PAM/VP-16/5-FU) with A-BMT. At the time of transplant his AFP was 20 ng/mL. However, 1 month later, a new pulmonary lesion was detected with elevated AFP and the child underwent excision of pulmonary metastasis (histology showed vital tumor). Although, his AFP level decreased to normal and no other metastases were detected on the CT scan, a second round of HD chemotherapy (DOX/CDDP/5-FU) was given. The patient had no evidence of recurrent disease during the 6 years after his second A-BMT. Patient 3, with initial multiple pulmonary metastases, has achieved CR with six cycles of conventional dose chemotherapy (cisplatin, doxorubicin, carboplatin, and etoposide) and resection of the liver tumor. The initial lung metastases were completely cleared by neo-adjuvant chemotherapy (three cycles). Despite CR he received HD chemotherapy (doxorubicin, etoposide, carboplatin, 5-FU) with ABMT. He remained in CR for the last follow-up (6 years) (Nishimura et al. 2002).

Although the authors suggest that "the better outcome of our patients indicates that multimodal therapy, including high-dose chemotherapy, may improve the outcome of the patients with metastatic hepatoblastoma," regarding the role of high-dose chemotherapy, the reported cases prove the contrary. Both in the first and second patients, HD chemotherapy could not prevent the development of lung metastases. Both patients illustrate the curative potential of metastectomy in patients with resectable pulmonary lesions. In the third patient, it is impossible to judge the (additional) value of HD chemotherapy, since it has been given in a situation in which the expected (event-free) survival would be high. According to the large cooperative studies of SIOPEL and COG, patients with cleared pulmonary metastases, either with chemotherapy alone or with complete resection, have a realistic chance of cure (Casanova et al. 2009; Katzenstein et al. 2002a; Meyers et al. 2007; Perilongo et al. 2000b, 2004, 2009; Zsíros et al. 2010). In the SIOPEL 3 trial, only 2 of the

26 patients who achieved CR in the lungs and whose liver tumor was resected with partial hepatectomy relapsed (both could be salvaged and were alive at last follow-up) (Casanova et al. 2009, Zsíros et al. 2010). In the light of these results, the favorable outcome of the third patient is not unexpected and does not provide any proof for the additional value of HD chemotherapy.

Niwa reports on a 4-year-old boy who developed a small solitary metastasis (6.5 mm on CT) 9 months after first-line chemotherapy and living-related LTX for stage III HB. After resection of the metastatic lesion, he received an auto-PBSCT with a double-conditioning regimen consisting of melphalan and thiotepa because the prognosis was thought to be poor. Auto PBSCT could be safely performed without any serious regimen-related toxicity or infection. However, transient cessation of tacrolimus during myelosuppression resulted in graft rejection of the liver just after hematological engraftment, but rejection was resolved by tacrolimus and methylprednisolone. The patient was alive and free from disease 2 years after auto-PBSCT without any signs of graft rejection. The authors conclude that HD chemotherapy using this conditioning regimen may be feasible for recurrent HB after liver transplantation in terms of safety and antitumor activity (Niwa et al. 2009; Umeda and Watanabe 2009).

As Perilongo et al. pointed out in their comment, the most important message of this report is that HD chemotherapy seems feasible in patients who underwent previous liver transplantation, although the case also highlights the potential difficulties of concurrent immunosuppression and chemotherapy (Perilongo and Otte 2009). The question whether HD therapy has any additional value in such a situation has, however, not been answered. As mentioned above, the prognosis of patients with single or few resectable lung metastases is more favorable than that of those with multiple or not resectable lung lesions. As shown by many authors, complete surgical resection of (isolated) lung metastasis/relapse is potentially curative and offers a realistic chance of long-term cure, even without additional chemotherapy (Casanova et al. 2009; Katzenstein et al. 2002a; Meyers et al. 2007; Perilongo 2000, 2004, 2009; Zsíros et al. 2010). These data make it questionable whether the intensive regimen with which this child was treated, after complete resection of a small tumor, had any impact on the outcome.

Miyamura reported on a child with stage IV HB whose liver tumor remained unresectable with partial hepatectomy after preoperative chemotherapy. High-dose chemotherapy consisting of carboplatin, ifosfamide, THP-adriamycin, and etoposide with autologous PBSCT was not effective in reducing tumor size (Miyamura et al. 2010).

The reports published so far provide some information on the feasibility of (myelo-ablative) HD chemotherapy in different clinical situations in patients with HB. Due to the limited data and the diversity of the used regimens, the optimal drug (combination) and preconditioning regimen remain unknown. Regarding efficacy, the published results do not suggest a clear (additional) benefit of HD chemotherapy in the treatment of primary or refractory/recurrent HB. On the contrary, some of the published cases demonstrated that HD chemotherapy could not prevent the development of early (second) relapse. In the light of these data and the significant treatment related toxicity, at the present level of knowledge, no indications can be established for the use of HD chemotherapy in the treatment of (recurrent) HB and high-dose treatment is not recommended for the treatment of individual patients. In order to explore the true efficacy and the potential value of HD chemotherapy in HB, controlled clinical trials are needed with careful patient selection.

13.5 Conclusions

Despite the significant improvement in the treatment of HB, approximately in 10–15% of the patients, second-line (salvage) treatment has to be considered at a certain point in an effort to achieve complete tumor eradication and/or cure. An aggressive surgical approach to remove all (residual) recurrent lesions is necessary and justified by the realistic prognosis for patients who achieve a tumor-free status. In most cases, surgical treatment has to be combined with salvage chemotherapy in order to achieve CR or resectability of the tumor. The choice of chemotherapy depends mainly on the previous regimens given. Most patients would have received cisplatin, with significant total cumulative dose, making its (re)use impossible and unreasonable. The use of doxorubicin can be an important option for patients who have not received anthracycline in their previous regimens. There is some evidence for the use of carboplatin + etoposide, but the rate of activity remains unclear. There is a growing body of evidence for the activity of irinotecan in HB. Its toxicity profile makes it very attractive even in heavily pretreated patients and its use should be considered with high priority in these situations. The use of (myeloablative) HD chemotherapy is currently not recommended due to lack of proven activity/benefit and the significant toxicity of the procedure. To improve the prognosis of patients with refractory or recurrent HB, more effective salvage drugs and regimens are needed.

References

Black CT, Cangir M, Choroszy D, Andrassy RJ (1991) Marked response to pre-operative high-dose cis-platinum in children with unresectable hepatoblastoma. J Paed Surg 26:1070–1173

Blaney S et al (2001) A phase I study of Irinotecan in pediatric patients: a pediatric oncology group study. Clin Cancer Res 7(1):32–37

Bleiberg H et al (1996) Characterisation and clinical management of CPT-11 (Irinotecan)-induced adverse events: the European perspective. Eur J Cancer 32A(Suppl 3):S18–S23

Blouin P, Brugières L, Tabone MD, Leverger G, Rubie H, Branchereau S, De Kraker J (2004) Carboplatin–epirubicin regimen for the treatment of hepatoblastoma. Pediatr Blood Cancer 42(2):149–154

Bomgaars LR, Bernstein M, Krailo M et al (2007) Phase II trial of irinotecan in children with refractory solid tumors: a Children's Oncology Group Study. J Clin Oncol 25(29):4622–4627

Brown J, Perilongo G, Shafford E et al (2000) Pretreatment prognostic factors for children with hepatoblastoma – results from the International Society of Paediatric Oncology (SIOP) study SIOPEL-1. Eur J Cancer 36:1418–1425

Cacciavillano WD, Brugières L, Childs M et al (2004) Phase II study of high-dose cyclophosphamide in relapsing and/or resistant hepatoblastoma in children: a study from the SIOPEL group. Eur J Cancer 40(15):2274–2279

Casanova M, Zsiros J, Brock P et al (2009) Metastatic hepatoblastoma – results of the SIOPEL-3 study from the International Childhood Strategy Group – SIOPEL. Pediatr Blood Cancer 53:744

Champion J, Green AA, Pratt CB et al (1982) Cisplatin (DDP) an effective therapy for unresectable or recurrent hepatoblastoma. Proc Am Soc Clin Oncol (ASCO) 1:671

Cosetti M, Wexler LH, Calleja E et al (2002) Irinotecan for pediatric solid tumors: the Memorial Sloan-Kettering experience. Pediatr Hematol Oncol 24(2):101–105

Czauderna P, Otte JB, Aronson DC et al (2005) Guidelines for surgical treatment of hepatoblastoma in the modern era – recommendations from the Childhood Liver Tumour Strategy Group of the International Society of Paediatric Oncology (SIOPEL). Eur J Cancer 41:1031–1036

Czauderna P, Otte JB, Roebuck DJ (2006) Surgical treatment of hepatoblastoma in children. Pediatr Radiol 36(3):187–191

Dall'Igna P, Cecchetto G, Dominici C et al (2001) Carboplatin and doxorubicin (CARDOX) for non-metastatic hepatoblastoma: a discouraging pilot study. Med Pediatr Oncol 36:332–334

De Ioris M, Brugieres L, Zimmermann A, et al (2007) Hepatoblastoma with a low serum alpha-fetoprotein level at diagnosis: The SIOPEL group experience. Eur J Cancer 44; 545-50

Douglass EC, Green AA, Wrenn E, Champion J, Shipp M, Pratt CB (1985) Effective cisplatin (CDDP) based chemotherapy in the treatment of hepatoblastoma. Med Pediatr Oncol 13:187–190

Douglass EC, Finegold M, Reynolds M et al (1993) Cisplatin, vincristine and fluorouracil therapy for hepatoblastoma: a Paediatric Oncology Group Study. J Clin Oncol 11:96–99

Evans AE, Land VJ, Newton WA et al (1982) Combination chemotherapy (vincristine, adriamycin, cyclophosphamide, and 5-fluorouracil) in the treatment of children with malignant hepatoma. Cancer 50:821–826

Feusner JH, Krailo MD, Haas JE et al (1993) Treatment of pulmonary metastases of initial stage I hepatoblastoma in childhood. Rep Children's Cancer Group Cancer 71:859–864

Fuchs J, Wenderoth M, von Schweinitz D et al (1998) Comparative activity of cisplatin, ifosfamide, doxorubicin, carboplatin, and etoposide in heterotransplanted hepatoblastoma. Cancer 83(11):2400–2407

Fuchs J, Bode U, Von Schweinitz D et al (1999) Analysis of treatment efficiency of carboplatin and etoposide in combination with radical surgery in advanced and recurrent childhood hepatoblastoma: a report of the German Cooperative Pediatric Liver Tumor Study HB 89 and HB 94. Klin Padiatr 211:305–309

Fuchs J, Rydzynski J, Von Schweinitz D et al (2002) Pretreatment prognostic factors and treatment results in children with hepatoblastoma: a report from the German Cooperative Pediatric Liver Tumor Study HB 94. Cancer 95:172–182

Furman WL et al (1999) Direct translation of a protracted Irinotecan schedule from a xenograft model to a phase I trial in children. J Clin Oncol 17(6):1815–1824

Haas JE, Feusner JH, Finegold MJ (2000) Small cell undifferentiated histology in hepatoblastoma may be unfavorable. Cancer 92(12):3130–3134

Haberle B, Bode U, von SD (2003) Differentiated treatment protocols for high- and standard-risk hepatoblastoma – an interim report of the German Liver Tumor Study HB99. Klin Padiatr 215:159–165

Haberle B, Schmid I, Bode U et al (2008) High dose chemotherapy does not improve the overall survival of children with hepatoblastoma. Pediatr Blood Cancer 53, DOI 10.1002/pbc

Hara J, Osugi Y, Ohta H et al (1998) Double-conditioning regimens consisting of thiotepa, melphalan and busulfan with stem cell rescue for the treatment of pediatric solid tumors. Bone Marrow Transplant 22:7–12

Hare CB et al (1997) Therapeutic efficacy of the topoisomerase I inhibitor 7-ethyl-10-(4-[1-piperidino]-1-piperidino)-carbonyloxy-camptothecin against pediatric and adult central nervous system tumor xenografts. Cancer Chemother Pharmacol 39(3):187–191

Hecht JR et al (1998) Gastrointestinal toxicity of Irinotecan. Oncology 12(8 Suppl 6):72–78

Ijichi O, Ishikawa S, Shinkoda Y et al (2006) Response of heavily treated and relapsed hepatoblastoma in the transplanted liver to single-agent therapy with irinotecan. Pediatr Transplant 10(5):635–638

Katzenstein HM, London WB, Douglass EC et al (2002a) Treatment of unresectable and metastatic hepatoblastoma: a pediatric oncology group phase II study. J Clin Oncol 20:3438–3444

Katzenstein HM, Rigsby C, Shaw PH (2002b) Novel therapeutic approaches in the treatment of children with hepatoblastoma. J Pediatr Hematol Oncol 24(9):751–755

Langevin AM et al (1998) Phase I trial of 9-aminocamptothecin in children with refractory solid tumors: a Pediatric Oncology Group study. J Clin Oncol 16(7):2494–2499

Lockwood L, Heney D, Giles GR et al (1993) Cisplatin-resistant metastatic hepatoblastoma: complete response to carboplatin, etoposide, and liver transplantation. Med Pediatr Oncol 21:517–520

Malogolowkin MH, Katzenstein H, Krailo MD et al (2006) Intensified platinum therapy is an ineffective strategy for improving outcome in pediatric patients with advanced hepatoblastoma. J Clin Oncol 24:2879–2884

Malogolowkin MH, Katzenstein HM, Krailo M et al (2008) Redefining the role of doxorubicin for the treatment of children with hepatoblastoma. J Clin Oncol 26(14):2379–2383

Matsunaga T, Sasaki F, Ohira M et al (2003) Analysis of treatment outcome for children with recurrent or metastatic hepatoblastoma. Pediatr Surg Int 19:142–146

McCrudden KW, Yokoi A, Thosani A et al (2002) Topotecan is anti-angiogenic in experimental hepatoblastoma. J Pediatr Surg 37(6):857–861

Meyers RL, Katzenstein HM, Krailo M et al (2007) Surgical resection of pulmonary metastatic lesions in children with hepatoblastoma. J Pediatr Surg 42(12):2050–2056

Miyamura T, Chayama K, Yoshida R et al (2010) Successful treatment of unresectable advanced hepatoblastoma: living liver transplantation after surgical removal of lung metastasis. Pediatr Transplant. 2010 Jan 11

Mugishima H, Matsunaga T, Yagi K (2002) Phase I study of irinotecan in pediatric patients with malignant solid tumors. J Pediatr Hematol Oncol 24(2):94–100

Neglia JP, Woods WG (1986) Continuous-infusion doxorubicin in the treatment of primary hepatic malignancies of childhood. Cancer Treat Rep 70(5):655–657

Nishimura S, Sato T, Fujita N, Yamaoka H, Hiyama E, Yokoyama T, Ueda K (2002) High-dose chemotherapy in children with metastatic hepatoblastoma. Pediatr Int 44(3):300–305

Nitschke R, Parkhurst J, Sullivan J et al (1998) Topotecan in pediatric patients with recurrent and progressive solid tumors: a Pediatric Oncology Group phase II study. J Pediatr Hematol Oncol 20(4):315–318

Niwa A, Umeda K, Awaya T et al (2009) Successful autologous peripheral blood stem cell transplantation with a double-conditioning regimen for recurrent hepatoblastoma after liver transplantation. Pediatr Transplant 13(2):259–262

O'Leary J et al (1998) Camptothecins: a review of their development and schedules of administration. Eur J Cancer 34(10):1500–1508

Ortega JA, Krailo MD, Haas JE et al (1991) Effective treatment of unresectable or metastatic hepatoblastoma with cisplatin and continuous infusion doxorubicin chemotherapy: a report from the Childrens Cancer Study Group. J Clin Oncol 9:2167–2176

Ortega JA, Douglass EC, Feusner JH et al (2000) Randomized comparison of cisplatin/vincristine/fluorouracil and cisplatin/continuous infusion doxorubicin for treatment of pediatric hepatoblastoma: a report from the Children's Cancer Group and the Pediatric Oncology Group. J Clin Oncol 18:2665–2675

Otte JB, Pritchard J, Aronson DC et al (2004) Liver transplantation for hepatoblastoma: results from the International Society of Pediatric Oncology (SIOP) study SIOPEL-1 and review of the world experience. Pediatr Blood Cancer 42:74–83

Otte JB, de Ville GJ, Reding R (2005) Liver transplantation for hepatoblastoma: indications and contraindications in the modern era. Pediatr Transplant 9:557–565

Palmer RD, Williams DM (2003) Dramatic response of multiply relapsed hepatoblastoma to irinotecan (CPT-11). Med Pediatr Oncol 41(1):78–80

Pappo AS, Lyden E, Breitfeld P (2007) Two consecutive phase II window trials of irinotecan alone or in combination with vincristine for the treatment of metastatic rhabdomyosarcoma: the Children's Oncology Group. J Clin Oncol 25(4):362–369

Pazdur R et al (1998) Irinotecan: toward clinical end points in drug development. Oncology 12(8 Suppl 6):13–21

Perilongo G, Otte JB (2009) Autologous peripheral blood stem-cell transplantation with a double-conditioning regimen for recurrent hepatoblastoma after liver transplantation – a valid therapeutic option or just too much? Pediatr Transplant 13(2):148–149

Perilongo G, Shafford EA (1999) Liver tumours. Eur J Cancer 35:953–958

Perilongo G, Shafford E, Plaschkes J (2000a) SIOPEL trials using preoperative chemotherapy in hepatoblastoma. Lancet Oncol 1:94–100

Perilongo G, Brown J, Shafford E et al (2000b) Hepatoblastoma presenting with lung metastases: treatment results of the first cooperative, prospective study of the International Society of Paediatric Oncology on childhood liver tumors. Cancer 89:1845–1853

Perilongo G, Shafford E, Maibach R et al (2004) Risk-adapted treatment for childhood hepatoblastoma. Final report of the second study of the International Society of Paediatric Oncology – SIOPEL 2. Eur J Cancer 40:411–421

Perilongo G, Maibach R, Shafford E et al (2009) Cisplatin versus cisplatin plus doxorubicin for standard-risk hepatoblastoma. N Engl J Med 361(17):1662–1670

Pritchard J, Brown J, Shafford E et al (2000) Cisplatin, doxorubicin, and delayed surgery for childhood hepatoblastoma: a successful approach – results of the first prospective study of the International Society of Pediatric Oncology. J Clin Oncol 18:3819–3828

Qayed M, Powell C, Morgan ER et al (2010) Irinotecan as maintenance therapy in high-risk hepatoblastoma. Pediatr Blood Cancer 54(5):761–763

Raymond E, Fabbro M, Boige V et al (2003) Multicentre phase II study and pharmacokinetic analysis of irinotecan in chemotherapy-naïve patients with glioblastoma. Ann Oncol 14(4):603–614

Saliba F et al (1998) Pathophysiology and therapy of Irinotecan-induced delayed-onset diarrhea in patients with advanced colorectal cancer: a prospective assessment. J Clin Oncol 16(8):2745–2751

Sasaki F, Matsunaga T, Iwafuchi M et al (2002) Outcome of hepatoblastoma treated with the JPLT-1 (Japanese Study Group for Pediatric Liver Tumor) Protocol-1: a report from the Japanese Study Group for Pediatric Liver Tumor. J Pediatr Surg 37(6):851–856

Schnater JM, Aronson D, Plaschkes J et al (2002) Surgical view of the treatment of patients with hepatoblastoma. Cancer 94:1111–1120

Semerano M, Brugieres L, Zsiros J et al (2009) Relapses in hepatoblastoma patients: clinical characteristics and outcome: experience of the International Childhood Liver Tumour strategy Group – SIOPEL. Ped Blood Cancer 53:746

Shitara T, Shimada A, Hanada R et al (2006) Irinotecan for children with relapsed solid tumors. Pediatr Hematol Oncol 23(2):103–110

Thompson J et al (1997a) Efficacy of oral Irinotecan against neuroblastoma xenografts. Anticancer Drugs 8(4):313–322

Thompson J et al (1997b) Efficacy of systemic administration of Irinotecan against neuroblastoma xenografts. Clin Cancer Res 3(3):423–431

Turner CD, Gururangan S, Eastwood J et al (2002) Phase II study of irinotecan (CPT-11) in children with high-risk malignant brain tumors: the Duke experience. Neuro Oncol 4(2):102–108

Umeda K, Watanabe K (2009) Autologous peripheral blood stem-cell transplantation with a double-conditioning regimen for recurrent hepatoblastoma after liver transplantation – a valid therapeutic option or just too much? – author reply. Pediatr Transplant 13(6):794–795

Vassal G et al (1996) Therapeutic activity of CPT-11, a DNA-topoisomerase I inhibitor, against peripheral primitive neuroectodermal tumour and neuroblastoma xenografts. Br J Cancer 74(4):537–545

Vassal G, Boland I, Santos A et al (1997) Potent therapeutic activity of irinotecan (CPT-11) and its schedule dependency in medulloblastoma xenografts in nude mice. Int J Cancer 73(1):156–163

Vassal G, Pondarré C, Boland I (1998) Preclinical development of camptothecin derivatives and clinical trials in pediatric oncology. Biochimie 80(3):271–280

Vassal G, Doz F, Frappaz D et al (2003) A phase I study of irinotecan as a 3-week schedule in children with refractory or recurrent solid tumors. J Clin Oncol 21(20):3844–3852

Vassal G, Couanet D, Stockdale E et al (2007) Phase II trial of irinotecan in children with relapsed or refractory rhabdomyosarcoma: a joint study of the French Society of Pediatric Oncology and the United Kingdom Children's Cancer Study Group. J Clin Oncol 25(4):356–361

Vassal G, Giammarile F, Brooks M et al (2008) A phase II study of irinotecan in children with relapsed or refractory neuroblastoma: a European cooperation of the Société Française d'Oncologie Pédiatrique (SFOP) and the United Kingdom Children Cancer Study Group (UKCCSG). Eur J Cancer 44(16):2453–2460

Von Schweinitz D, Hecker H, Schmidt-von Arndt G, Harms D (1987) Prognostic factors and staging system in childhood hepatoblastoma. Intern J Cancer 74:593–599

Von Schweinitz D, Hecker H, Harms D et al (1995) Complete resection before development of drug resistance is essential for survival from advanced hepatoblastoma – a report from the German Cooperative Pediatric Liver Tumor Study HB-89. J Pediatr Surg 30:845–852

Von Schweinitz D, Byrd DJ, Hecker H et al (1997) Efficiency and toxicity of ifosfamide, cisplatin and doxorubicin in the treatment of childhood hepatoblastoma. Eur J Cancer 33:1243–1249

Warmann SW, Fuchs J, Wilkens L et al (2001) Successful therapy of subcutaneously growing human hepatoblastoma xenografts with topotecan. Med Pediatr Oncol 37(5): 449–454

Yoshinari M, Imaizumi M, Hayashi Y et al (1998) Peripheral blood stem cell transplantation for hepatoblastoma with microscopical residue: a therapeutic approach for incompletely resected tumor. Tohoku J Exp Med 184(3):247–254

Zhang J, Cheng C, He CL et al (2008) The expression of Bcl-XL, Bcl-XS and p27Kip1 in topotecan-induced apoptosis in hepatoblastoma HepG2 cell line. Cancer Invest 26(5): 456–463

Zsiros J, Childs M, Brugieres L et al (2009) Irinotecan single-drug treatment for children with refractory or recurrent hepatoblastoma – a phase II trial of the International Childhood Liver Tumour strategy Group – SIOPEL. Pediatr Blood Cancer 53:745

Zsíros J, Maibach R, Shafford E et al (2010) Successful treatment of childhood high-risk hepatoblastoma with dose-intensive multiagent chemotherapy and surgery: final results of the SIOPEL-3HR study. J Clin Oncol 28(15):2584–2590

14 Alternative Approaches for Treatment

Derek J. Roebuck

Contents

D.J. Roebuck
Great Ormond Street Hospital, NHS Trust and Institute of Child Health, Great Ormond Street, London WC1N 3JH, United Kingdom
e-mail: roebud@gosh.nhs.uk

14.1 Introduction

Various nonsurgical regional treatments may be applicable in the treatment of children with liver tumors. Although none is currently used as part of major pediatric liver cancer trials, each has certain advantages and may be considered in selected patients. It remains to be seen whether any of these ideas become a part of standard protocols in the future.

Other interventional radiology techniques relevant to the management of children with liver tumors, including biopsy (Chap. 9) (Bittles and Hoffer 2007; Hoffer 2000), central venous access (Kaye et al. 2000), and biliary drainage and stenting (Roebuck and Stanley 2000; Akinci 2007; Roebuck 2010) are not discussed here. Laparoscopic and open surgical tumor ablation techniques (e.g., cryotherapy) are also not covered.

14.2 Theoretical Aspects of Intraarterial Chemotherapy

The potential advantages of delivering chemotherapy directly to the tumor using an intraarterial (IA) approach have been realized for several decades (Table 14.1) (Chen and Gross 1980). The dual blood supply of the liver makes this site almost uniquely favorable for IA treatment. Normal liver derives most of its supply (about 75–80%) from the portal vein, and only about 20–25% from the hepatic artery. Because primary and metastatic liver tumors derive most of their blood supply from the hepatic artery, IA drugs can be expected to have maximal antitumor effect with minimal damage to the normal liver.

A. Zimmermann et al. (eds.), *Pediatric Liver Tumors*, Pediatric Oncology,
DOI: 10.1007/978-3-642-14504-9_14, © Springer-Verlag Berlin Heidelberg 2011

Table 14.1 Potential advantages of intraarterial (IA) chemotherapy and chemoembolization

Higher concentration of antineoplastic drug in tumor blood vessels
Protection of normal liver (which is supplied mostly by portal venous blood)
Embolic effect
Prolonged "dwell time" of drug
First pass effect (low systemic levels, less toxicity)
Increased extraction of drug by tumor cells
Ischemic injury to tumor
Possible safer modulation of drug resistance
Use of agents in high concentration without causing systemic toxicity

IA chemotherapy is given either by repeated catheterization or via an implanted hepatic artery catheter connected to a subcutaneous port. Although this is feasible in adults, technical problems often arise in children (Golladay et al. 1985), and hepatic artery chemoembolization (HACE) is usually preferred. In this technique, IA chemotherapy is combined with an embolic agent, in order to prolong dwell time of the drugs in the tumor and to add an ischemic effect.

HACE, however, has significant disadvantages. It is expensive and requires angiographic skills and equipment that are not universally available. Perioperative care must be meticulous; general anesthesia (GA) is required and complications are not rare. Because there is very little release of chemotherapeutic agents into the systemic circulation, HACE must be used in conjunction with systemic chemotherapy (Li et al. 2008; Oue et al. 1998). Finally, HACE may need to be repeated several times in each patient.

Because most primary liver tumors of childhood are resectable or can be made resectable with systemic chemotherapy, the indications for HACE are somewhat limited. The most significant indication should be to treat children with tumors that remain unresectable after systemic chemotherapy in an attempt to make them resectable without transplantation (Tashjian et al. 2002; Malogolowkin et al. 2000). The improving results of transplantation, however, have made this indication less important, and no current protocols for hepatoblastoma (HB) include HACE. HACE may also be used as a "bridge" to transplantation in children who cannot be transplanted immediately for any reason (Arcement et al. 2000). A third indication is palliation in children with unresectable primary or secondary liver tumors who are not candidates for transplantation (Cardinal et al. 2009).

Portal vein invasion by tumor is not an absolute contraindication to HACE in children (Pentecost et al. 1993).

Two quite different approaches have been taken with the embolization part of HACE. In one system, the cytostatic drugs are mixed with water-soluble radiographic contrast and an embolic agent (Malogolowkin et al. 2000). Systemic levels of cisplatin and doxorubicin are very low after this type of HACE (Malogolowkin et al. 2000).

The alternative is to use ethiodized oil (Lipiodol) as a carrier (Li et al. 2008; Oue et al. 1998; Czauderna et al. 2006; Han et al. 1999; Nakagawa et al. 1993; Ogita et al. 1987; Sue et al. 1989). Lipiodol was originally designed as a contrast agent, and was used extensively for many years in lymphangiography. It is hypothesized that it is selectively taken up in the tumor, and that it releases the chemotherapeutic agents gradually (Ogita et al. 1987; Sue et al. 1989). Lipiodol also has an embolic effect of its own (Sue et al. 1989). There is very extensive experience with the use of Lipiodol for HACE in adults. When injected into the hepatic artery, Lipiodol is retained in tumor sinusoids (Bhattacharya et al. 1994), and can be detected by computed tomography for at least several weeks and sometimes up to a year (Han et al. 1999). There is evidence from both adult and pediatric patients that the concentration of cisplatin delivered with Lipiodol is much higher in tumor than nontumor liver tissue (Sue et al. 1989; Shibata et al. 1989). The procedure is completed by embolization of the feeding arteries of the tumor to decrease washout of the cytostatic agents (Raoul et al. 1992) and cause tumor ischemia. Gelatin foam (Gelfoam® or Spongostan®) is usually used for this purpose, and appears to be superior to polyvinyl alcohol particles (Geschwind et al. 2003). Coils have also been used (Li et al. 2008), but are not recommended as they make repeated procedures more difficult. Recanalization of the feeding arteries usually occurs by about 2 weeks.

Advantages of the use of Lipiodol include greater worldwide familiarity and availability and ease of injection through small catheters. One disadvantage may be that water-soluble cytostatic agents may wash out of the oily Lipiodol suspension and reach the systemic circulation (Raoul et al. 1992).

In general, both HB and hepatocellular carcinoma (HCC) are treated with cisplatin and doxorubicin. In the SIOPEL 5 protocol, verapamil was added in an attempt to overcome *MDR1*-mediated drug resistance, which is common in HCC (Soini et al. 1996). The overall chemoembolization "cocktail" consisted of cisplatin 6 mg/mL, doxorubicin 3 mg/mL, and verapamil 0.1 mg/mL, in Lipiodol. The volume of Lipiodol used is determined by the maximum diameter of the tumor: a maximum of 0.6–0.7 mL/cm should be used in order to reduce the risk of pulmonary embolism. A maximum volume of 10 mL is recommended (Li et al. 2008; Czauderna et al. 2006; Jiang et al. 2006).

In addition to HB and HCC, HACE has been used for treatment of liver metastases in stage 4S (MS) neuroblastoma (Weintraub et al. 2004) and in patients with epithelioid hemangioendothelioma (Cardinal et al. 2009), fibrolamellar carcinoma (Czauderna et al. 2006; Nakagawa et al. 1993), and embryonal sarcoma (Malogolowkin et al. 2000; Nakagawa et al. 1993).

14.3 Technical Aspects of Hepatic Artery Chemoembolization

The following description is based on the SIOPEL 5 protocol, which is now closed. Intravenous hydration is commenced 3 h before HACE and continued for at least 24 h (Czauderna et al. 2006). Intravenous antibiotics (metronidazole, ceftazidime, and vancomycin), an antiemetic (ondansetron) and an H2-antagonist (ranitidine) are given with induction of GA, and continued for 48 h (Malogolowkin et al. 2000; Czauderna et al. 2006).

Access to the femoral artery is obtained under sterile conditions, using ultrasound-guided puncture (Heran et al. 2010), and a 4-Fr valved vascular sheath is inserted. Careful diagnostic angiography is essential. If there is doubt about portal vein patency, this may be confirmed by delayed angiographic images at this stage. Four-French catheters with 0.97-mm (0.038-in.) lumens are appropriate for most children and young adults. Aortography may show unsuspected collateral supply to the tumor, for example, from the inferior phrenic, subcostal, and intercostal arteries (Fig. 14.1). Angiography of the internal thoracic (internal mammary) arteries should be performed for tumors that extend close to the diaphragm because they often supply the tumor. The diagnostic hepatic angiograms should be evaluated carefully for arteriovenous shunting and to locate the origins of the gastroduodenal and right and left gastric arteries. It may be possible to occlude focal intratumoral arteriovenous shunts with embolization coils, but major diffuse shunting (which is not rare in HCC) may be a contraindication to HACE because of the risk of pulmonary embolization of the Lipiodol suspension.

The guiding principle for HACE should be that the catheter tip should be placed as close to the tumor as possible, to minimize injury to normal liver tissue (Li et al. 2008). The 4-Fr angiographic catheter is advanced to a stable position in the artery supplying the tumor, taking care not to occlude the artery or cause spasm. A microcatheter (3 Fr or smaller) is introduced coaxially through the 4-Fr catheter and advanced to a position where injection of contrast confirms absence of flow to nontarget organs. The HACE suspension is then injected slowly, using fluoroscopic guidance to avoid reflux into nontarget arteries, and confirm the accumulation of Lipiodol in the tumor. If necessary, coil embolization may be used to protect nontarget organs. Examples of this include occlusion of the origin of the gastroduodenal artery to protect the duodenum and pancreas and occlusion of cutaneous branches of the right internal thoracic artery to protect the skin and chest wall. It may be necessary to divide the HACE suspension between two or more arteries (e.g., right and left hepatic branches and right internal thoracic artery) to cover the entire tumor. It is usual to restrict the proportion of the liver treated at any one HACE procedure to 70% (Li et al. 2008; Malogolowkin et al. 2000). When an arterial branch supplies both a significant part of the tumor and also a significant volume of normal liver, flow may be directed into the tumor by intraarterial injection of angiotensin II (0.25 μg/kg) or epinephrine (0.5 μg). These agents cause selective vasoconstriction of nontumor arteries, and maximize delivery of the HACE suspension to the tumor (Shibata et al. 1989; Ensminger and Gyves 1984), although they may also increase systemic levels of the chemotherapeutic drugs (Ensminger and Gyves 1984).

The injection is stopped when complete accumulation in tumor vessels is observed, or if there is retrograde filling of distal portal vein branches (Nakagawa et al. 1993). Following injection of each artery, temporary occlusion with gelatin foam is then performed. The easiest way to do this is to cut a sheet of gelatin foam

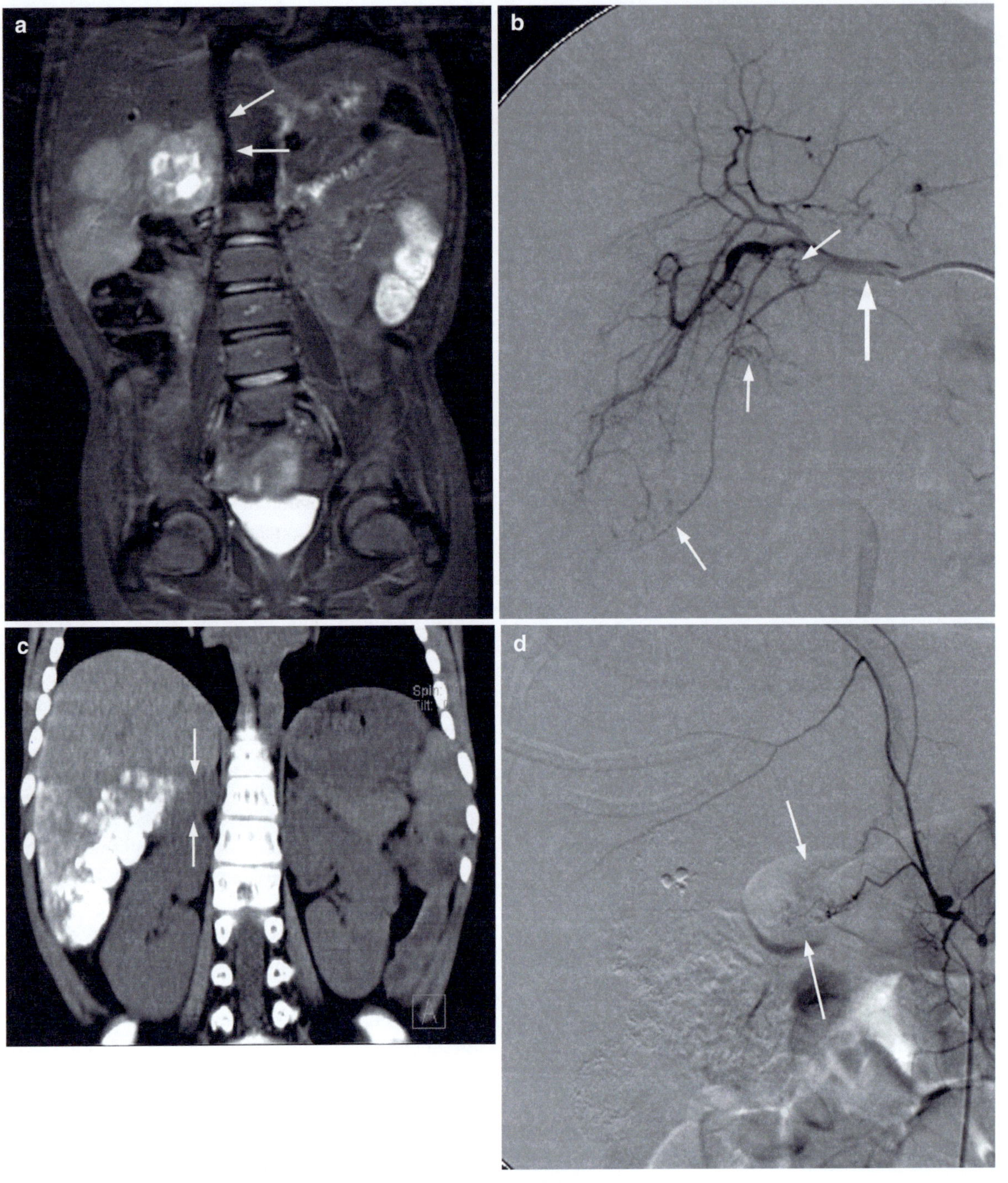

Fig. 14.1 Hepatic artery chemoembolization (HACE) in an 11-year-old male with HCC. (**a**) Coronal short-tau inversion recovery MRI shows a tumor centered on segments 5 and 6. It abuts the inferior vena cava (*arrows*). (**b**) Selective angiography of the right hepatic artery (*large arrow*) reveals pathological tumor vessels (*small arrows*). HACE was performed using doxorubicin, cisplatin, and verapamil, with ethiodized oil (Lipiodol) as a carrier. The treated arteries were then embolized with a slurry of gelatin foam. (**c**) Day 10 CT shows accumulation of Lipiodol in the tumor. Note that the medial part of the tumor (*arrows*) has not taken up Lipiodol, and has therefore presumably not been treated. (**d**) Angiography at the second HACE procedure shows supply to the previously untreated part of the tumor from branches of the right inferior phrenic artery (*arrows*). This was treated in addition to the hepatic artery branches to the tumor

into extremely small pieces (<1 mm), place them in a 2-mL Luer-Lok® syringe, and add water-soluble contrast (e.g., iohexol or iopamidol). The slurry of gelatin and contrast may then be injected under fluoroscopic guidance, until stasis is achieved in the artery. Care should be taken to avoid reflux of the embolic agent into nontarget arteries. Even small particles may clog up microcatheters, and embolization through the 4-Fr catheter may be required. Completion angiography should show substantial devascularization of the tumor.

HACE can be repeated every few weeks if necessary.

14.3.1 Complications

Most children who undergo HACE will develop some degree of postembolization syndrome, with fever and pain (Li et al. 2008; Malogolowkin et al. 2000), and patient- or nurse-controlled analgesia will be appropriate. Anorexia, nausea, and vomiting are all common (Li et al. 2008; Arcement et al. 2000). There may also be transient biochemical abnormalities (elevation of liver enzymes and bilirubin) (Li et al. 2008; Malogolowkin et al. 2000). These may be regarded as anticipated effects rather than complications.

Major complications are unusual, but may be severe (Table 14.2, Fig. 14.2). Tumor lysis syndrome has been described in a patient who was not previously given systemic chemotherapy (Malogolowkin et al. 2000). Fatal complications have been described (Czauderna et al. 2006; Czauderna et al. 2005).

Table 14.2 Reported major complications of hepatic artery chemoembolization

Pancreatitis (Shibata et al. 1989)
Injury to stomach (Arcement et al. 2000) or duodenum (Arcement et al. 2000; Shibata et al. 1989)
Injury to gallbladder or bile ducts (including biloma formation) (Shibata et al. 1989)
Systemic arterial embolization (e.g., injury to skin) (Arora et al. 1999)
Pulmonary embolization via intratumoral arteriovenous shunts (Czauderna et al. 2005)
Septicemia and/or hepatic abscess (Arcement et al. 2000)
Hepatic artery thrombosis (Arcement et al. 2000)
Mucositis (Malogolowkin et al. 2000)
Myelosuppression (Malogolowkin et al. 2000)

14.4 Results of Hepatic Artery Chemoembolization

There is only one published prospective trial of HACE in children (Malogolowkin et al. 2000). Malogolowkin et al. reported six heavily pretreated HB patients and three HCC patients who underwent multiple courses of HACE using cisplatin, doxorubicin, and in some patients, mitomycin. The embolic agent was a preparation of cross-linked bovine collagen fibers (Angiostat®, Regional Therapeutics, Pacific Palisades, CA, USA), which is no longer available. All patients with HB responded, and three underwent subsequent tumor resection, although four of the six later died of disease progression. Two of the three HCC patients were rendered resectable after HACE. One had a complete resection and remained disease-free, while another had microscopic residual disease after delayed resection, received additional postoperative chemotherapy, and succumbed after a 3.5-year remission, due to progression of underlying liver disease (Malogolowkin et al. 2000).

It is difficult to assess the many small retrospective series of HACE in children, partly because of the possibility of publication bias, and partly because the definition of unresectability used is often not clear. A basic summary of published case series is given in Table 14.3.

Oue et al. described eight patients with HB treated by HACE with doxorubicin (or pirarubicin), cisplatin, and Lipiodol (Oue et al. 1998). All patients showed a response, with median tumor shrinkage (product of two diameters method) of 32% and median AFP fall of 96%. Delayed tumor resection was possible in all eight children. Two died later because of lung metastases. Han et al. described HACE with Lipiodol, doxorubicin, and cisplatin in four children with unresectable HB (Han et al. 1999). All tumors became resectable after two HACE procedures. Czauderna et al. reported the Polish experience of HACE in four heavily pretreated children with locally advanced HB and one

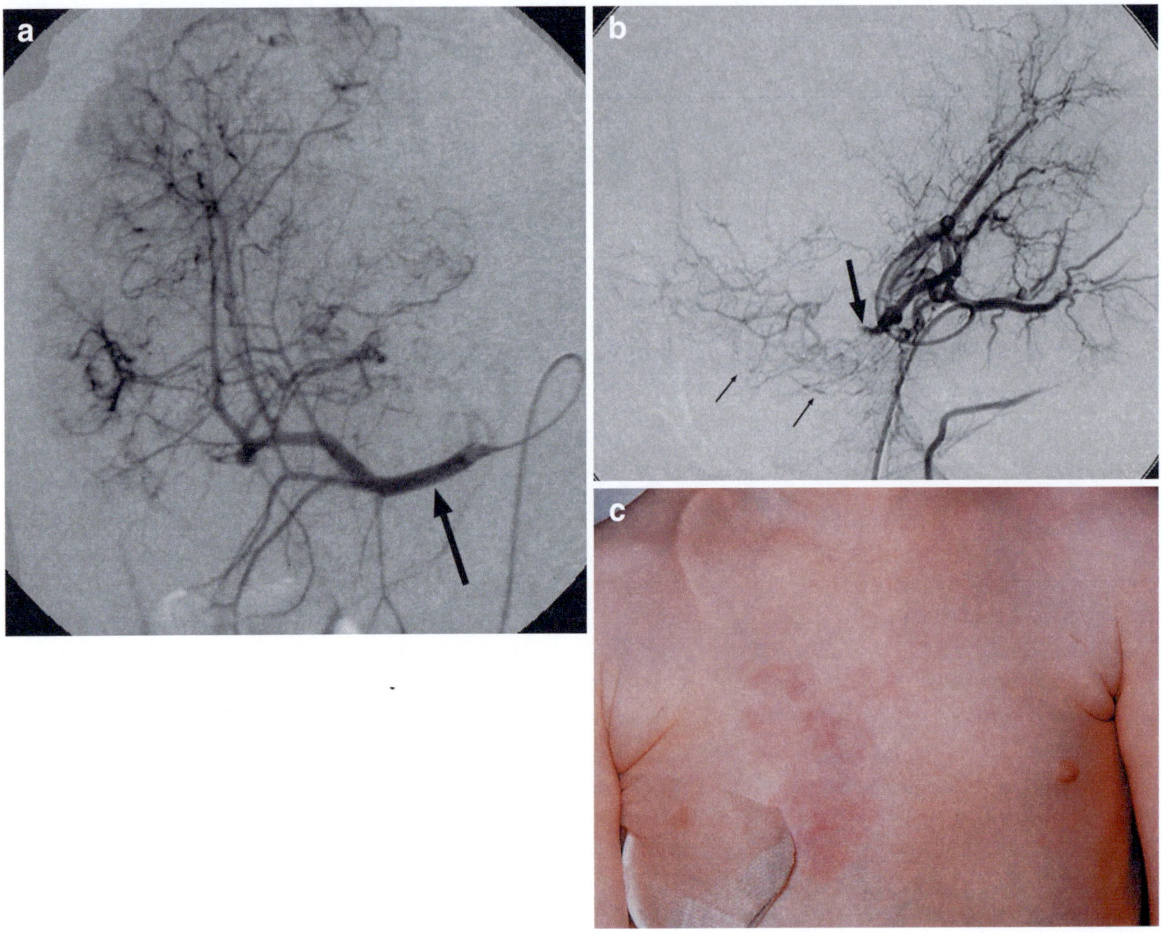

Fig. 14.2 Complications of hepatic artery chemoembolization (HACE) in a 3-year-old male with HB. (**a**) Angiography performed at the time of the first HACE procedure. There is a huge liver tumor with abnormal tumor vasculature, supplied by the right hepatic artery (RHA, *arrow*). (**b**) Angiography at the third HACE procedure (8 weeks later) shows occlusion of the RHA (*large arrow*). The left hepatic artery is patent, and the RHA branches are reconstituted by innumerable tiny extrahepatic collaterals (*small arrows*). (**c**) Skin changes following chemoembolization via the distal right internal thoracic (mammary) artery. There was no detectable reflux into cutaneous branches at the time of the procedure

with fibrolamellar carcinoma, who had shown insufficient response to systemic chemotherapy (Czauderna et al. 2006). In three patients, the mass reduced in size (by 25–33%) and AFP fell by 20–98%. Two patients underwent complete hepatic resection and one had total hepatectomy and liver transplantation. One HB patient died of systemic myelotoxicity after the first HACE procedure. One patient with metastatic HCC did not respond to "SuperPLADO" systemic chemotherapy, but responded significantly to HACE, with regression of pulmonary nodules. However, this patient died after the third HACE procedure following pulmonary Lipiodol embolization.

Arcement described 14 children who underwent IA chemotherapy or HACE as a "bridge" to transplantation (Arcement et al. 2000). Of the eight who underwent HACE, five patients had HB and three HCC. At the time of reporting, four children (including one with HCC) were alive, three following transplantation and one awaiting transplantation.

Overall, it seems that HACE is a promising treatment with a significant but acceptable complication rate.

Table 14.3 Published reports ($n > 1$) of hepatic artery chemoembolization (HACE) in children

First author	HB	HCC	FLC	ES	Pre-Rx	Agents	Carrier	Embolic	Courses
Ogita et al. (1987)	2	0	0	0	0/2	PIR CDDP	Lip		1
Sue et al. (1989)	2	0	0	0	2/2	CDDP 5FU	Lip		1
Nakagawa et al. (1993)	0	1	1	1	3/3	CDDP CARBO DOX	Lip	Gelatin	3–11
Oue et al. (1998)	8	0	0	0	2/8	CDDP DOX PIR	Lip	Gelatin	1
Han et al. (1999)	4	0	0	0	0/4	CDDP DOX	Lip	Gelatin	2
Arcement et al. (2000)	5	3	0	0	5/8	CDDP DOX		Gelatin	2–12
Malogolowkin et al. (2000)	6	3	0	2	10/11	CDDP DOX MMC		Collagen	2–5
Ohtsuka et al. (2004)	7	0	0	0	3/7	PIR	Lip	Gelatin	7
Jiang et al. (2006)	8	0	0	0	0/8	CDDP DOX VCR		Coils	1–3
Czauderna et al. (2006)	4	0	1	0	5/5	CDDP DOX MMC	Lip	Gelatin	1–3
Li et al. (2008)	16	0	0	0	0/16	CDDP DOX	Lip	Gelatin Coils	1–3

HB number of patients with hepatoblastoma, *HCC* number of patients with hepatocellular carcinoma, *FLC* number of patients with fibrolamellar carcinoma, *ES* number of patients with undifferentiated (embryonal) sarcoma, *pre-Rx* number of patients treated with systemic chemotherapy before HACE *PIR* pirarubicin, *CDDP* cisplatin, *5FU* fluorouracil, *CARBO* carboplatin, *DOX* doxorubicin, *MMC* mitomycin, *VCR* vincristine, *Lip* ethiodized oil (Lipiodol), *courses* number of HACE procedures

14.5 Other Transarterial Techniques

Transarterial embolization without chemotherapy may occasionally be useful in children with liver tumors. The most common reason for "bland" embolization is in the management of cardiac failure associated with vascular tumors in neonates and young infants. These are almost always either diffuse or multifocal infantile hemangiomas (Draper et al. 2008; O'Hagan et al. 2004; Kassarjian et al. 2004) or unifocal rapidly involuting congenital hemangiomas (Zenzen et al. 2009). Embolization is usually attempted only when all medical treatments have failed and so it is perhaps not surprising that it is not always successful.

The next most common indication is for emergency treatment of tumor rupture, which has been reported in children with HB (Ueno et al. 2005; Iida et al. 2004; Chan and Tam 1998) and angiosarcoma (Dimashkieh et al. 2004). Bland embolization has also been used to control rapid tumor growth in a baby with liver metastases from stage 4S (MS) neuroblastoma (Boztug et al. 2006).

Radioembolization with yttrium-90 microspheres, also known as selective internal radiation (SIR), allows extremely high radiation doses to be delivered to tumors supplied by the hepatic artery, without the development of severe radiation hepatopathy (Lau et al. 1998). Yttrium-90 is a beta-emitting radionuclide with a half-life of 64 h, which can be irreversibly bound in resin microspheres (approximate diameter 30 μm) at an activity of about 30 Bq per microsphere. The size of the microspheres is calculated to ensure peripheral embolization in the hepatic arterial circulation. It is important that the tumor is selectively irradiated relative to normal liver (to prevent radiation hepatopathy) (Lau et al. 1994), and that arteriovenous shunting in the tumor is low (to prevent radiation pneumonitis) (Leung et al. 1995). For these reasons, simulation with technetium-99m macroaggregated albumin (Leung et al. 1994) must be performed before the injection of the microspheres (Fig. 14.3). In general,

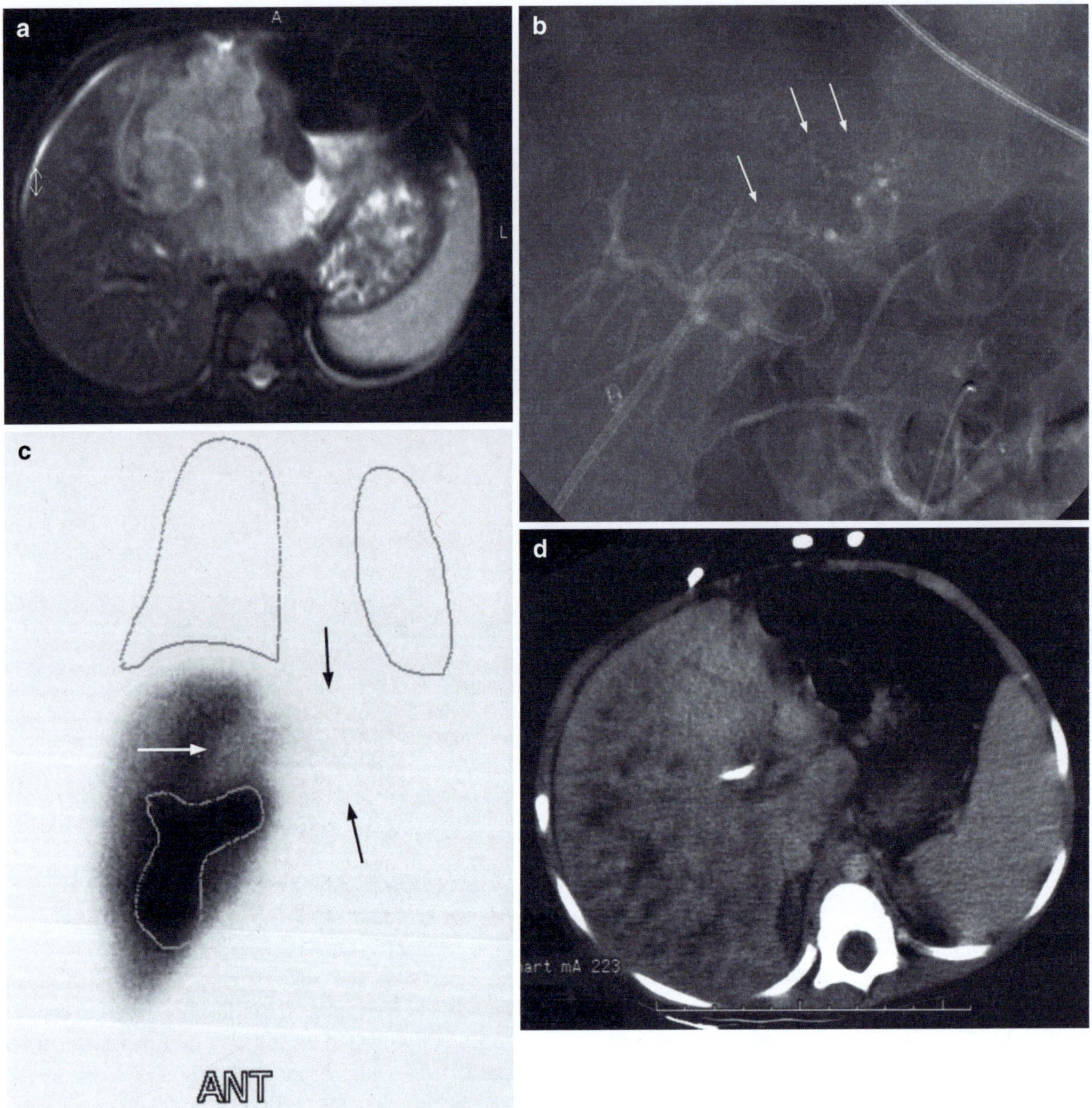

Fig. 14.3 Planning for radioembolization (selective internal radiation) in 22-month-old male with a hepatic sarcoma. (**a**) T2-weighted MR image following systemic chemotherapy shows an unresectable tumor. (**b**) Angiography shows a few abnormal vessels (*arrows*) feeding the tumor, but essentially normal branches of the right hepatic artery. (**c**) Simulation with injection of technetium-99m labeled macro-aggregated albumin (37 MBq), probably into the right hepatic artery, shows normal perfusion of most of the right lobe of the liver, but almost no embolization in the hypovascular tumor (*white arrow*) or left lobe (*black arrows*). There is very little arteriovenous shunting, as shown by almost absent activity in the lungs (calculated shunt = 2.4%). The relatively hypervascular area in the right lobe (outlined) was used in error to calculate the ratio of activity in the tumor to that in normal liver. (**d**) CT performed after radioembolization shows severe radiation hepatopathy in the right lobe of the liver

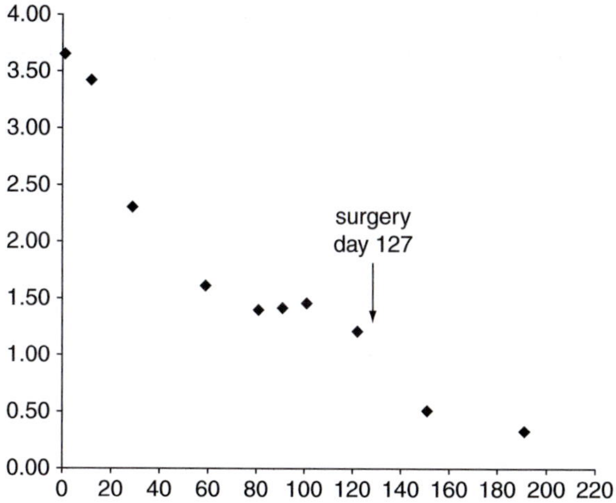

Fig. 14.4 Prolonged response to radioembolization (selective internal radiation) in a 12-year-old female with unresectable HCC. A single procedure induced a fall in serum alpha-fetoprotein (AFP) to almost normal levels, and the tumor became resectable. y-axis: $\log_{10}$AFP[in μg/L]. x-axis: time in days from selective internal radiation

the ratio of activity in the tumor to that in the liver should exceed 2:1, and lung shunting should be less than 13–15% (Lau et al. 1998; Leung et al. 1995). Up to 5 GBq can be given (Lau et al. 1998), depending on the size of the patient.

Experience with SIR in children is very limited (Lau et al. 2004). The main reason why this technique is not more widely used is that specialized equipment and expertise are required for its safe use. It is clear, however, that it may be used to convert unresectable tumors (Lau et al. 2004). This would probably be most applicable to children with unresectable HCC who are not eligible for transplantation (Fig. 14.4).

14.6 Percutaneous Tumor Ablation

The main techniques used for the percutaneous ablation of liver tumors in adults are radiofrequency ablation (RFA), ethanol injection, cryoablation, and laser and microwave ablation. None of these ideas has found widespread use in pediatrics.

For RFA, a special needle (or needles) is placed in the tumor using imaging guidance. Ultrasound is typically used for pediatric liver tumors, and computed tomography for lung metastases. A circuit is completed with grounding pads, usually on the patient's thighs. Thermal necrosis of tumor cells (which occurs at >50°C) is then induced by application of a radiofrequency alternating current (Iannitti 2002). With current equipment, impedance and temperature at the needle tip can be monitored during the procedure.

RFA works best for small liver lesions; complete necrosis can be expected in most lesions <30 mm in diameter. Larger lesions (>100 mm) can be treated with RFA by using multiple needles (Iannitti et al. 2002), but cure is unlikely. Tumors adjacent to major blood vessels are protected by perfusion-mediated tissue cooling. This effect may be mitigated by temporary vascular occlusion, although this is difficult to achieve with percutaneous procedures and is not routinely used.

Hepatic RFA has been used in children to treat metastases (Bittles and Hoffer 2007; Goncalves de Oliveira-Filho et al. 2003), unresectable multiple fibrolamellar carcinoma (Hoffer et al. 2009), and local recurrence of HB (Iannitti et al. 2002; Ye et al. 2008). It would also be a reasonable choice for palliation when other options are not available (Iannitti et al. 2002). Other indications, such as treatment of a very small (e.g., screening-detected) HB, or of a small segment 2 or 3 lesion to allow right trisectionectomy rather than transplantation, are speculative. It has also been suggested that RFA could be used to treat lung metastases in children with HB (Bittles and Hoffer 2007).

Liver abscess is the most important complication of RFA (Iannitti et al. 2002; Schindera et al. 2006). Other adverse effects include segmental infarction (Iannitti et al. 2002), transient liver dysfunction (Hoffer et al. 2009), hemoglobinuria or myoglobinuria (Hoffer et al. 2009), pain (Hoffer et al. 2009), hypoxia (Hoffer et al. 2009), and leukocytosis (Hoffer et al. 2009).

14.7 Portal Vein Embolization

Although the absence of tumor in segments 2 and 3 (or 6 and 7) means that trisectionectomy is technically possible, in some cases, the volume of these segments, which will constitute the remnant liver, is insufficient to support postoperative liver function. In children without underlying liver disease, this is likely when the liver remnant is less than 20–25% of the estimated total liver volume or less than 5 mL/kg of body mass (Liu and Zhu 2009; Truant et al. 2007). In these circumstances, portal vein embolization (PVE) may be used to induce growth of the intended liver remnant prior to surgery.

The mechanism of hypertrophy is complicated and involves various molecules including hepatocyte growth factor (HGF) (Liu and Zhu 2009).

PVE in children typically requires a contralateral approach (Fig. 14.5), because it is usually impossible to puncture the ipsilateral portal vein without transgressing the large primary tumor. It is extremely important not to damage the portal venous supply to the intended liver remnant, so the puncture is performed with ultrasound guidance, and the smallest possible (usually 4 Fr) valved angiographic sheath is used. Portal venography is performed and used as a "road map." Embolization is usually achieved with metal coils, although vascular plugs, ethanol, and cyanoacrylate glue and other agents have also been used, sometimes in combination (Liu and Zhu 2009). Surgery is performed when sufficient hypertrophy of the liver remnant has occurred, typically at 3 weeks (van Gulik et al. 2008).

Complications of PVE are surprisingly uncommon (Liu and Zhu 2009; van Gulik et al. 2008). Although

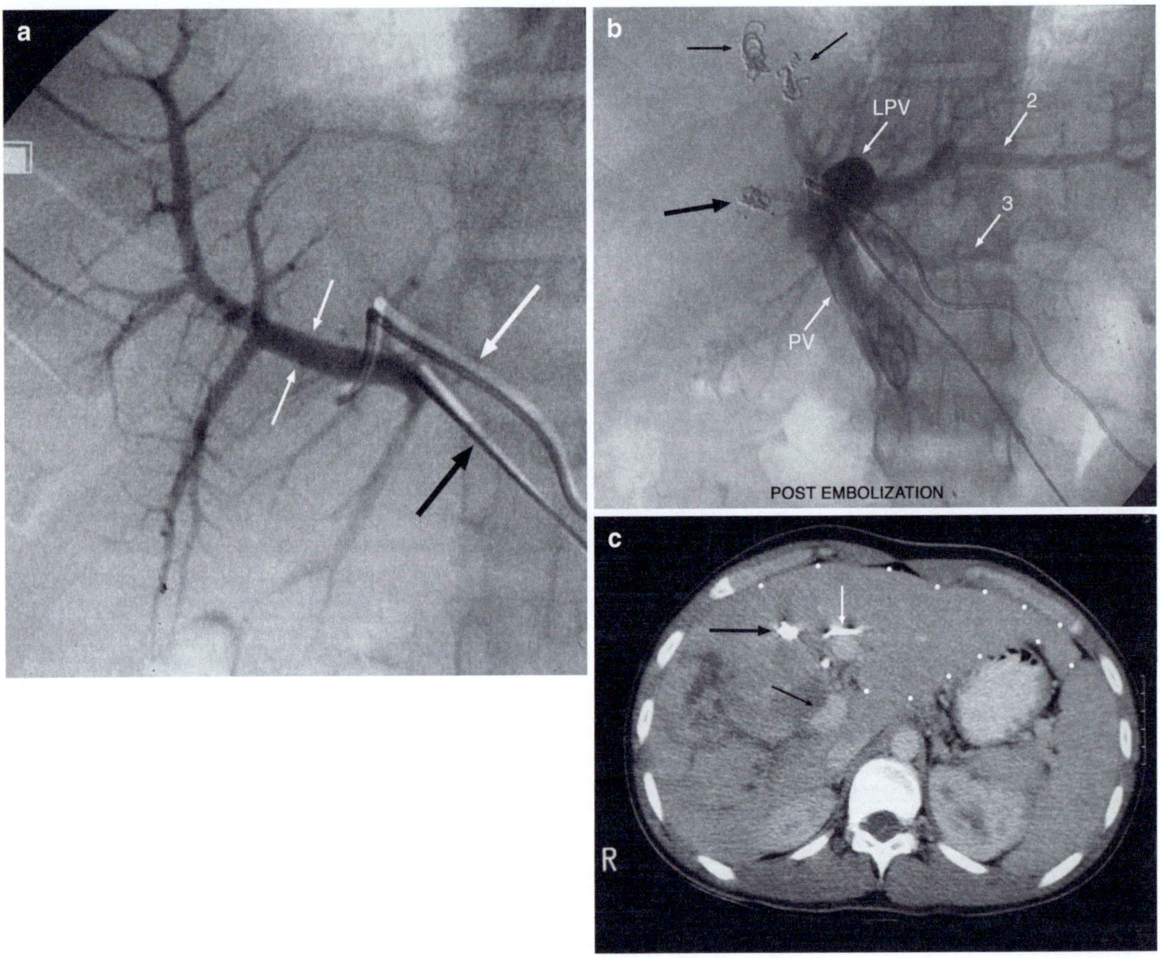

Fig. 14.5 Portal vein embolization (PVE) in a 14-year-old male with hepatocellular carcinoma. (**a**) The left portal vein (LPV) has been punctured under ultrasound guidance. A vascular sheath (*black arrow*) has been advanced to the origin of the right portal vein (RPV, *small white arrows*) and contrast injected to perform a portal venogram. There is also an external biliary drainage catheter (*large white arrow*). (**b**) Metal coils have been used to occlude the RPV (*large black arrow*) and the major vein to segment 4 (*small black arrows*). The main portal vein (PV), the LPV and the branches to segments 2 and 3 remain patent. (**c**) Following PVE, there has been considerable growth of the intended liver remnant, segments 2 and 3 (outlined by *dots*). Coils are present in the largest portal vein branch to segment 4 (*large black arrow*). The tumor abuts but does not encase the right portal vein (*small black arrow*) near its origin. The short white arrow indicates the external biliary drain

there is concern that PVE could lead to increased tumor growth, this has not been proved (de Graaf et al. 2009). Nevertheless, the observation that HB cells proliferate in response to HGF (Von Schweinitz et al. 2000) supports the restriction of this technique to patients in whom it is absolutely necessary (van Gulik et al. 2008).

References

Akinci D, Gumus B, Ozkan OS et al (2007) Percutaneous management of tumoral biliary obstruction in children. Pediatr Radiol 37:975–980

Arcement CM, Towbin RB, Meza MP et al (2000) Intrahepatic chemoembolization in unresectable pediatric liver malignancies. Pediatr Radiol 30:779–785

Arora R, Soulen MC, Haskal ZJ (1999) Cutaneous complications of hepatic chemoembolization via extrahepatic collaterals. J Vasc Interv Radiol 10:1351–1356

Bhattacharya S, Novell JR, Winslet MC et al (1994) Iodized oil in the treatment of hepatocellular carcinoma. Br J Surg 81:1563–1571

Bittles MA, Hoffer FA (2007) Interventional radiology and the care of the pediatric oncology patient. Surg Oncol 16:229–233

Boztug K, Kiely E, Roebuck DJ et al (2006) Successful treatment of MYCN amplified, progressive stage 4S neuroblastoma in a neonate with hepatic artery embolization in addition to multimodality treatment. Pediatr Blood Cancer 46:253–257

Cardinal J, de Vera ME, Marsh JW et al (2009) Treatment of hepatic epithelioid hemangioendothelioma: a single-institution experience with 25 cases. Arch Surg 144:1035–1039

Chan KL, Tam PK (1998) Successful right trisegmentectomy for ruptured hepatoblastoma with preoperative transcatheter arterial embolization. J Pediatr Surg 33:783–786

Chen HS, Gross JF (1980) Intra-arterial infusion of anticancer drugs: theoretic aspects of drug delivery and review of responses. Cancer Treat Rep 64:31–40

Czauderna P, Zbrzezniak G, Narozanski W et al (2005) Pulmonary embolism: a fatal complication of arterial chemoembolization for advanced hepatocellular carcinoma. J Pediatr Surg 40:1647–1650

Czauderna P, Zbrzezniak G, Narozanski W et al (2006) Preliminary experience with arterial chemoembolization for hepatoblastoma and hepatocellular carcinoma in children. Pediatr Blood Cancer 46:825–828

de Graaf W, van den Esschert JW, van Lienden KP et al (2009) Induction of tumor growth after preoperative portal vein embolization: is it a real problem? Ann Surg Oncol 16:423–430

Dimashkieh HH, Mo JQ, Wyatt-Ashmead J et al (2004) Pediatric hepatic angiosarcoma: case report and review of the literature. Pediatr Dev Pathol 7:527–532

Draper H, Diamond IR, Temple M et al (2008) Multimodal management of endangering hepatic hemangioma: impact on transplant avoidance: a descriptive case series. J Pediatr Surg 43:120–125, discussion 126

Ensminger WD, Gyves JW (1984) Regional cancer chemotherapy. Cancer Treat Rep 68:101–115

Geschwind JFH, Ramsey DE, Cleffken B et al (2003) Transcatheter arterial chemoembolization of liver tumors: effects of chemoembolization protocol on injectable volume of chemotherapy and subsequent arterial patency. Cardiovasc Intervent Radiol 26:111–117

Golladay ES, Mollitt DL, Osteen PK et al (1985) Conversion to resectability by intra-arterial infusion chemotherapy after failure of systemic chemotherapy. J Pediatr Surg 20:715–717

Goncalves de Oliveira-Filho A, Lopes Miranda M, Leonelli Diz F et al (2003) Use of radiofrequency for ablation of unresectable hepatic metastasis in desmoplastic small round cell tumor. Med Pediatr Oncol 41:476–477

Han YM, Park HH, Lee JM et al (1999) Effectiveness of preoperative transarterial chemoembolization in presumed inoperable hepatoblastoma. J Vasc Interv Radiol 10:1275–1280

Heran MK, Marshalleck F, Temple M et al (2010) Joint quality improvement guidelines for pediatric arterial access and arteriography: from the Societies of Interventional Radiology and Pediatric Radiology. Pediatr Radiol 40:237–250

Hoffer FA (2000) Liver biopsy methods for pediatric oncology patients. Pediatr Radiol 30:481–488

Hoffer FA, Daw NC, Xiong X et al (2009) A phase 1/pilot study of radiofrequency ablation for the treatment of recurrent pediatric solid tumors. Cancer 115:1328–1337

Iannitti DA, Dupuy DE, Mayo-Smith WW et al (2002) Hepatic radiofrequency ablation. Arch Surg 137:422–426, discussion 427

Iida T, Suenaga M, Takeuchi Y et al (2004) Successful resection of a ruptured hepatoblastoma prior to chemotherapy: report of a case. Surg Today 34:710–714

Jiang XW, Li JH, Hu XL et al (2006) Combined treatment of hepatoblastoma with transcatheter arterial chemoembolization and surgery. Pediatr Hematol Oncol 23:1–9

Kassarjian A, Zurakowski D, Dubois J et al (2004) Infantile hepatic hemangiomas: clinical and imaging findings and their correlation with therapy. AJR Am J Roentgenol 182:785–795

Kaye R, Sane SS, Towbin RB (2000) Pediatric intervention: an update – part II. J Vasc Interv Radiol 11:807–822

Lau WY, Leung TW, Ho S et al (1994) Diagnostic pharmacoscintigraphy with hepatic intra-arterial technetium-99m macroaggregated albumin in the determination of tumour to non-tumour uptake ratio in hepatocellular carcinoma. Br J Radiol 67:136–139

Lau WY, Ho S, Leung TW et al (1998) Selective internal radiation therapy for nonresectable hepatocellular carcinoma with intraarterial infusion of 90yttrium microspheres. Int J Radiat Oncol Biol Phys 40:583–592

Lau WY, Ho SK, Yu SC et al (2004) Salvage surgery following downstaging of unresectable hepatocellular carcinoma. Ann Surg 240:299–305

Leung WT, Lau WY, Ho SK et al (1994) Measuring lung shunting in hepatocellular carcinoma with intrahepatic-arterial technetium-99m macroaggregated albumin. J Nucl Med 35:70–73

Leung TW, Lau WY, Ho SK et al (1995) Radiation pneumonitis after selective internal radiation treatment with intraarterial 90yttrium-microspheres for inoperable hepatic tumors. Int J Radiat Oncol Biol Phys 33:919–924

Li JP, Chu JP, Yang JY et al (2008) Preoperative transcatheter selective arterial chemoembolization in treatment of unresectable hepatoblastoma in infants and children. Cardiovasc Intervent Radiol 31:1117–1123

Liu H, Zhu S (2009) Present status and future perspectives of preoperative portal vein embolization. Am J Surg 197:686–690

Malogolowkin MH, Stanley P, Steele DA et al (2000) Feasibility and toxicity of chemoembolization for children with liver tumors. J Clin Oncol 18:1279–1284

Nakagawa N, Cornelius AS, Kao SC et al (1993) Transcatheter oily chemoembolization for unresectable malignant liver tumors in children. J Vasc Interv Radiol 4:353–358

O'Hagan AH, Irvine AD, Sands A et al (2004) Miliary neonatal hemangiomatosis with fulminant heart failure and cardiac septal hypertrophy in two infants. Pediatr Dermatol 21:469–472

Ogita S, Tokiwa K, Taniguchi H et al (1987) Intraarterial chemotherapy with lipid contrast medium for hepatic malignancies in infants. Cancer 60:2886–2890

Ohtsuka Y, Matsunaga T, Yoshida H et al (2004) Optimal strategy of preoperative transcatheter arterial chemoembolization for hepatoblastoma. Surg Today 34:127–133

Oue T, Fukuzawa M, Kusafuka T et al (1998) Transcatheter arterial chemoembolization in the treatment of hepatoblastoma. J Pediatr Surg 33:1771–1775

Pentecost MJ, Daniels JR, Teitelbaum GP et al (1993) Hepatic chemoembolization: safety with portal vein thrombosis. J Vasc Interv Radiol 4:347–351

Raoul JL, Heresbach D, Bretagne JF et al (1992) Chemoembolization of hepatocellular carcinomas. A study of the biodistribution and pharmacokinetics of doxorubicin. Cancer 70:585–590

Roebuck DJ (2010) Gastrointestinal intervention in children. Pediatr Radiol (in press)

Roebuck DJ, Stanley P (2000) External and internal-external biliary drainage in children with malignant obstructive jaundice. Pediatr Radiol 30:659–664

Schindera ST, Nelson RC, DeLong DM et al (2006) Intrahepatic tumor recurrence after partial hepatectomy: value of percutaneous radiofrequency ablation. J Vasc Interv Radiol 17:1631–1637

Shibata J, Fujiyama S, Sato T et al (1989) Hepatic arterial injection chemotherapy with cisplatin suspended in an oily lymphographic agent for hepatocellular carcinoma. Cancer 64:1586–1594

Soini Y, Virkajarvi N, Raunio H et al (1996) Expression of P-glycoprotein in hepatocellular carcinoma: a potential marker of prognosis. J Clin Pathol 49:470–473

Sue K, Ikeda K, Nakagawara A et al (1989) Intrahepatic arterial injections of cisplatin-phosphatidylcholine-Lipiodol suspension in two unresectable hepatoblastoma cases. Med Pediatr Oncol 17:496–500

Tashjian DB, Moriarty KP, Courtney RA et al (2002) Preoperative chemoembolization for unresectable hepatoblastoma. Pediatr Surg Int 18:187–189

Truant S, Oberlin O, Sergent G et al (2007) Remnant liver volume to body weight ratio > or =0.5%: A new cut-off to estimate postoperative risks after extended resection in noncirrhotic liver. J Am Coll Surg 204:22–33

Ueno S, Hirakawa H, Yokoyama S et al (2005) Treatment of infantile hepatoblastoma and related complications. Tokai J Exp Clin Med 30:203–209

van Gulik TM, van den Esschert JW, de Graaf W et al (2008) Controversies in the use of portal vein embolization. Dig Surg 25:436–444

Von Schweinitz D, Faundez A, Teichmann B et al (2000) Hepatocyte growth-factor-scatter factor can stimulate postoperative tumor-cell proliferation in childhood hepatoblastoma. Int J Cancer 85:151–159

Weintraub M, Bloom AI, Gross E et al (2004) Successful treatment of progressive stage 4s hepatic neuroblastoma in a neonate with intra-arterial chemoembolization. Pediatr Blood Cancer 43:148–151

Ye J, Shu Q, Li M et al (2008) Percutaneous radiofrequency ablation for treatment of hepatoblastoma recurrence. Pediatr Radiol 38:1021–1023

Zenzen W, Perez-Atayde AR, Elisofon SA et al (2009) Hepatic failure in a rapidly involuting congenital hemangioma of the liver: failure of embolotherapy. Pediatr Radiol 39: 1118–1123

Supportive Therapy and Toxicity

15

Penelope Brock and Gill Levitt

Contents

15.1 Introduction

The supportive care for children with liver tumors has improved considerably since the first children started being cured of primary liver cancer through multimodality means in the last quarter of the twentieth century. Aggressive supportive care including safer blood products, central intravenous catheters, improved nutritional support, appropriate antiemetic therapy, better use of broad-spectrum antibiotics, and more effective antifungal therapy has improved outcome considerably. The pediatric surgeon also plays an integral part in ensuring the safe passage of immunologically impaired patients through the additional stress of surgery (Corbally 1993). New technology in lung and liver surgery, as well as newer immunotherapy agents post liver transplant, has also improved outcome but will be discussed elsewhere. Primary liver cancer affects children at a young median age including neonates. It is essential to support these very young children appropriately throughout their treatment in order to gain the highest cure rates. International treatment protocols addressing supportive care, as well as guidelines on how to best administer chemotherapy, have improved cure rates worldwide. Strategies which take into account local health care provision in deciding on the most appropriate treatment approach for an individual child and where ever possible transferring the child to a specialized pediatric oncology/liver center have also improved outcomes.

15.2 Supportive Care

15.2.1 Safer Blood Products

In most countries, safe blood products are available, and if strict transfusion policies are followed, children requiring blood products, either during chemotherapy

P. Brock (✉) and G. Levitt
Department Paediatric Oncology, Great Ormond Street Hospital, NHS Trust and Institute of Child Health, Great Ormond Street, London WC1N 3JH, United Kingdom
e-mail: brockp@gosh.nhs.uk; levitg@gosh.nhs.uk

A. Zimmermann et al. (eds.), *Pediatric Liver Tumors*, Pediatric Oncology,
DOI: 10.1007/978-3-642-14504-9_15, © Springer-Verlag Berlin Heidelberg 2011

or at the time of surgery, should not experience acute or life-threatening side effects. Children should be treated in centers where access to safe blood products is available. The practice of blood product administration in children's cancer centers, however, still varies widely, even in a single country (Nathan and Selwood 2006). If safe blood products cannot be assured, then treatment with cisplatin monotherapy should be the initial chemotherapy regimen of choice for all stages of disease, introducing doxorubicin only if the therapeutic response is inadequate. Anatomical surgical resection should be planned with extreme care concerning hemostasis and predeposit autologous plasma donation (PAPD) considered, particularly in the older child (Ishizawa et al. 2009).

15.2.2 Central Intravenous Catheters

Most young children benefit and have minimal complications from an indwelling catheter placed under general anesthetic (Hockenbury et al. 1989). Long-term venous access devices such as silastic Hickman catheters can be placed under local anesthesia by open cut down procedure, but this practice is usually reserved for the older child (Shukla et al. 2002). The indwelling device can be placed at the same time as the initial biopsy if serum markers are raised and the imaging is typical of liver cancer, or prior to the start of treatment once the histopathological diagnosis is certain. It is possible to administer chemotherapy through peripheral lines, but these need to be rigorously controlled and changed if not optimal, prior to each dose. This is particularly important when administering anthracyclines, as they cause severe local extravasation damage.

15.2.3 Improved Nutritional Support and Antiemetic Therapy

Many children present in a poor nutritional state and experience a degree of anorexia together with nausea and vomiting during chemotherapy. In resource-challenged nations, malnutrition at diagnosis is a frequent occurrence and is known to increase the risk of infection, profound neutropenia, toxic death, and major surgical mortality (Israëls et al. 2009a). This challenge has been addressed during the preoperative chemotherapy phase in children with Wilms tumor in Malawi. In this setting, the authors showed that introducing a locally made peanut butter-based food supplement not only reduced toxic morbidity and mortality but also increased tumor response to preoperative chemotherapy (Israëls et al. 2009b). Enteral feeding has also been shown to lower mortality from infection post allogeneic stemcell transplantation and improve 100 day overall survival (OS) (Seguy et al. 2006).

Optimal feeding therefore orally, by nasogastric tube, or total parenteral nutrition, prior to and during chemotherapy, is important in combination with the optimal use of antiemetic combinations. It has also been shown that enteral feeding should be encouraged even when chemotherapy-induced mucositis is present. Amino-acid transport, as measured by leucine uptake in the intestine, is not impaired even under these circumstances (de Koning et al. 2007).

The introduction of the serotonin 5-HT_3 receptor antagonists into pediatric practice, commonly known as "setrons," in the 1990s generally improved the quality of life during chemotherapy and reduced acute cisplatin emesis (Hewitt et al. 1993). The probable mechanism for prevention of acute chemotherapy-induced nausea and vomiting is antagonism of 5-HT_3 binding sites in the peripheral and central nervous system. Increasing the loading dose of ondansetron from 5 to 10 mg/m^2, however, did not improve antiemetic control in a randomized double blind controlled trial in children (Brock et al. 1996).

Delayed emesis occurring after the first 24 h, particularly from cisplatin, is insufficiently controlled by "setrons" alone. However, the addition of dexamethasone to ondansetron did improve the control of cisplatin-induced nausea and vomiting (CINV) in a randomized controlled trial (Alverez et al. 1995), and the addition of corticosteroid to "setrons" has since become established practice.

The physiology of the different serotonin (5-HT) receptor subtypes in relation to emesis (Hasler 1999) has shown that the 5-HT_3 antagonists are not only useful in preventing emesis from cancer chemotherapy but also in preventing postoperative nausea.

In countries where the cost of "setrons" is prohibitive or where side effects such as migraine headaches occur (Khan 2002), combinations of other antiemetic medications can be effective too. A useful review of the evidence base for both known and novel emerging antiemetic therapeutic interventions in children was written by Depuis and Nathan (2010).

It is beneficial to prevent nausea and vomiting early during the first cycle of treatment to prevent anticipated vomiting which improves the quality of life during subsequent cycles (Stockhurst et al. 2000). Anticipatory vomiting is a classical conditioned response, which although well recognized is best prevented as once established it cannot be easily controlled.

15.2.4 Management of Infection and Prophylaxis

In neutropenic patients, broad-spectrum antibiotics should be used promptly if fever develops or the child becomes septic until blood and other cultures are reported negative after 48–72 h. If cultures become positive, then antibiotic therapy should be adapted according to the organisms known or tested sensitivities. Where possible, aminoglycosides should be avoided in children receiving platinum chemotherapy, and monotherapy may be as effective as combined treatment (Pereira et al. 2009). The approach to the treatment of febrile neutropenia has evolved considerably over the years (Meckler and Lindemulder 2009). In some settings, it may be effective and safe to allow early hospital discharge (Härtel et al. 2007). In children with indwelling central lines, staphylococcal epidermidis colonization is frequent and can be difficult to eradicate. Prolonged antibiotic treatment increases the risk of fungal infection. It may be more appropriate to remove the central line and replace it 72 h later rather than to continue long-term antibiotic cover.

Fungal infections rarely develop during the treatment of hepatoblastoma (HB) as the period of neutropenia is relatively short. However, in high-risk disease or hepatocellular carcinoma (HCC), where immunosuppression may be prolonged, a liposomal form of amphotericin should be introduced in cases of persistent febrile neutropenia nonresponsive to broad-spectrum antibiotics. The clinical features of invasive fungal infections may be difficult to distinguish from relapsing disease as the locations are the liver, lung, and brain, (Kobayashi et al. 2008) and the pattern of candidemia may be different in neonates and children from that in adults (Blyth et al. 2009).

The prophylactic use of cotrimoxazole has become standard practice to prevent pneumocystis carinii pneumonitis in children who experience prolonged neutropenia. When administering cisplatin monotherapy, if the neutrophil count remains above 1×10^9/L, then cotrimoxazole prophylaxis is not essential. It is, however, best prescribed in children requiring multiagent chemotherapy up to 2–3 months after count recovery.

15.3 Toxicity

A clearer understanding of the working of chemotherapy and the effect of dose and administration can reduce side effects. The number of chemotherapy agents used in the treatment of liver cancer is relatively limited.

15.3.1 Platinum-Containing Agents

15.3.1.1 Administration

Cisplatin should be administered in an intravenous infusion of 6 h or more. It causes less renal toxicity if given in a solution with an optimal amount of chloride ions. It should also be given with electrolytes to prevent acute electrolyte disturbances. This is particularly important in the very young (Brock et al. 1992). Some regimens have a pre- and post-hydration phase which can last up to 24 h after the cisplatin infusion. The aim of the longer-term pre- and post-hydration is to reduce the long-term permanent renal and audiological toxicity.

Carboplatin should be administered over 1 h or more, but does not require extrahydration.

15.3.1.2 Acute Toxicity

Nausea and Vomiting

This occurs after both cisplatin and carboplatin, but cisplatin is the most highly emetogenic agent. Antiemetics are essential and should be continued for 2–3 days after the platinum infusion. After cisplatin, relative anorexia occurs for about 1 week. Young children receiving regular cisplatin require additional nutritional support. This can be oral, usually nasogastric and given at home provided the parents are taught how to care for a nasogastric tube. Nursing support in the community should be available. The use of percutaneous gastrostomies or PEGs are rarely indicated in these children as treatment is relatively short.

Allergic Reactions

These can occur after carboplatin, rarely after cisplatin. These reactions tend to present during the infusion or shortly afterward. Most commonly, a rash or cough is an early sign, breathing difficulties may develop, and full-blown anaphylaxis is possible. If allergic symptoms occur, then the treatment should be stopped and antihistamines given intravenously as well as steroids, if necessary. The carboplatin infusion can be tried again on a subsequent day after premedication with antihistamines, if given more slowly over a longer infusion time. If this is not tolerated, however, alternative treatment should be sought. Carboplatin allergy tends to occur after a number of months of treatment and is therefore not a common problem in liver cancer treatment.

Bone Marrow Toxicity

Carboplatin suppresses bone marrow production of all peripheral blood cells. The full blood count needs to be monitored regularly every few days and there is an increased risk of infection when the neutrophil count gets below 1×10^9/L. Carboplatin regimens are therefore usually count dependant being given every 3–4 weeks on count recovery. Cisplatin can, however, be administered independent of the result of the peripheral count. Both platinum agents can cause gradual anemia; however, the need for red cell blood transfusions is more common when children are treated with carboplatin than with cisplatin.

15.3.1.3 Late Toxicity

Renal Toxicity

Cisplatin nephrotoxicity occurs both at the level of the glomerule and the proximal tubule. This damage results in both a reduction of the glomerular filtration rate (GFR) as well as low serum magnesium levels from proximal tubular damage and reduced magnesium reuptake. Ionized cisplatin is more toxic and decreasing the ratio of ionized versus non-ionized cisplatin in the glomerular filtrate, by increasing the chloride content of the administrated fluid, is beneficial. There would appear to be a distinct mechanism of cisplatin toxicity in actively dividing tumor cells versus the normally quiescent renal proximal tubular epithelial cells. It has been found that gamma-glutamyl transpeptidase plays a role in cisplatin nephrotoxicity and that the proximal tubular cells have the ability to metabolize cisplatin to a nephrotoxin. There is also evidence that apoptosis is a major mechanism underlying cisplatin-induced renal cell injury (Hanigan and Devarajan 2003). The damage measured at the end of treatment in young children may improve to a certain extent in the first year or two in young children, but becomes chronic after that (Brock et al. 1991). Both GFR and serum magnesium should be measured regularly throughout treatment and at intervals after treatment if abnormal. If the GFR, corrected for surface area, is below the normal lower limit for age, then long-term follow up of the patient is advised. It is wise to supplement low levels of serum magnesium as it has been shown to increase the risk of osteoporosis if left untreated. Low serum magnesium may affect long-term bone metabolism (Rude et al. 2009). It is unusual for a child to develop renal toxicity when treated with carboplatin alone, unless it is used at myeloablative doses. However, in combination with cisplatin, renal toxicity increases.

Hearing Loss

Cisplatin hearing loss is genetically determined, permanent, bilateral, dose dependant with significantly increased severity in young children. The typical pattern of high-frequency loss was first noted when high-dose cisplatin was used in young children with neuroblastoma at 200 mg/m^2 per dose (Brock and Bellman 1991; Fig. 15.1). The typical fall off affects consonants more than vowels which can severely affect speech and learning particularly in the young (Fig. 15.2).

The reported incidence of cisplatin ototoxicity in children ranges from 26% to over 90% with the

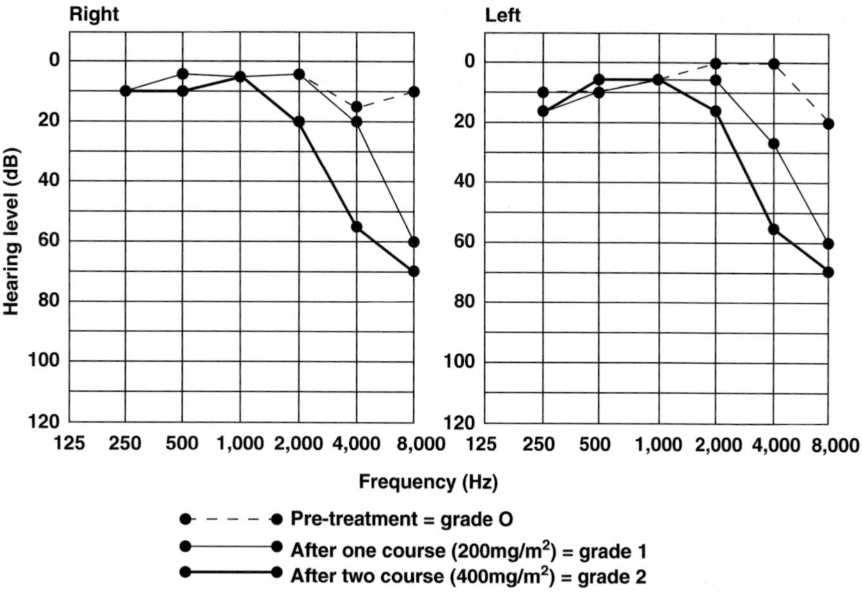

Fig. 15.1 Typical progression of high-frequency hearing impairment during high-dose cisplatin therapy

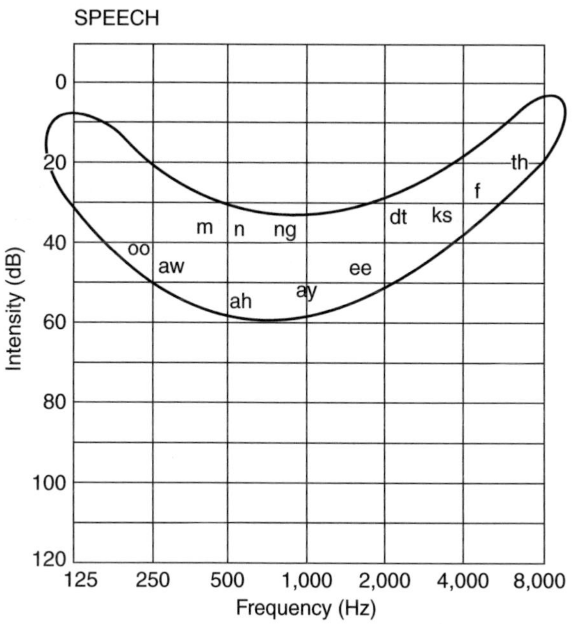

Fig. 15.2 Speech frequencies superimposed on an audiogram. The letters correspond to phonemes. High-frequency hearing loss renders some consonants inaudible and speech incomprehensible

variation influenced by treatment and patient-related factors (Ilveskoski et al. 1998). Younger children are more affected than older children or adults (Li et al. 2004). In an excellent review of cisplatin ototoxicity, recent understanding of how the damage has been found to affect learning and social integration particularly in the young is highlighted (Gilmer Knight et al. 2005).

Cisplatin damages the outer hair cells of the cochlea starting with the higher frequencies. The level of hearing loss measured a few weeks after the end of treatment is usually permanent. Functional measures of hearing are the most appropriate but need to be age adapted. It is not easy to measure hearing during treatment particularly if the child is unwell. Pure-tone audiometry is the gold standard but play audiometry and visual reinforced audiometry are useful in young children (Brock et al. 1992). Because children tire easily, a different order to testing hearing thresholds of children on cisplatin is necessary. It is essential to start by measuring the higher frequencies 8,000, 4,000, 2,000 Hz then 1,000 Hz before testing 500 and 250 Hz. The first frequency of the normal audiogram to be affected will be 8,000 Hz. In a research setting, extended high-frequency audiometry can be a useful predictor of platinum hearing loss (Knight et al. 2007).

Other nonbehavioral methods can be used to give an idea of the effect of treatment. The most useful of the nonbehavioral methods is distortion product otoacoustic emissions which can be easily carried out and can be particularly useful for monitoring during treatment in young children, particularly if they are sick and unable to co-operate well (Zorowka et al. 1993; Allen et al. 1998; Dhooge et al. 2006; Coradini 2007).

A grading system particularly designed to compare hearing loss from cisplatin, between children treated on the same treatment protocol and on different treatment protocols, became known as the Brock grading. Ototoxicity was assessed in children treated with cisplatin (60–100 mg/m^2 per course), who were at least 2 years from stopping treatment. The median age at diagnosis was 2 years 2 months (range 1 month to 13.5 years). On the basis of hearing assessment by pure-tone audiometry, a practical grading system of hearing loss from 0 to 4 was designed. Moderate to severe high-frequency hearing loss (grade 2–4) was found in half the children and ten required appropriate hearing aids. The risk of developing ototoxicity increased significantly with cumulative cisplatin dose ($p = 0.027$), although there was considerable individual susceptibility. Serial follow-up testing, to a median of 4 years after completion of cisplatin treatment, showed no recovery of hearing in any of these children. The authors advised careful monitoring of young children by a consultant audiological physician throughout treatment with cisplatin, particularly when doses of 400 mg/m^2 or over were reached. The design of this system was based on the analysis of the audiograms from 41 children (82 ears), who had developed high-frequency hearing loss. The slope of these audiograms, over the impaired hearing frequencies, averaged 45 dB per octave. At a given frequency, where hearing loss was less than 40 dB, it was rare to see worse impairment at a lower frequency. In 72 of 82 ears which developed high-frequency hearing loss (HFHL), at a given frequency, hearing remained at or better than 15 dB at all lower frequencies. In 10 of 82 ears, hearing threshold levels were 20 dB in 5 and 25 dB in 5 at one octave below; hearing was normal at the remaining lower frequencies. In the knowledge that hearing would be normal or minimally affected at frequencies below this, 40 dB was chosen as the cut-off level. The hearing loss was graded according to the frequency at which this cut-off level was reached (Table 15.1). Hearing loss was consistently bilateral, so the results obtained from the "better" ear were those used to define the grade (Brock et al. 1991).

Table 15.1 Brock classification of cisplatin-induced bilateral high-frequency hearing loss[a]

Bilateral hearing loss	Grade	Description
≤40 dB at all frequencies	0	Minimal
>40 dB at 8,000 Hz and above	1	Mild
>40 dB at 4,000 Hz and above	2	Moderate
>40 dB at 2,000 Hz and above	3	Marked
>40 dB at 1,000 Hz and above	4	Severe

[a] The results used are obtained by pure-tone audiometry, from the "better" ear.

The Brock grading system has been used in SIOPEL studies to assess the ototoxicity of different regimens since the 1990s, using institutional results. In the most recent publications of the SIOPEL 3 standard risk study, approximately, 30% of children had Brock grade 1–4 hearing loss (Perilongo et al. 2009). However, when the standard risk ototoxicity results of SIOPEL 2 and 3 were pooled, including data only from countries with an audiology reporting rate of over 60% of patients, a larger proportion of patients were shown to have Brock grade 1–4 hearing loss (R. Maibach, 2007, personal communication). The alternating cisplatin/carboplatin and doxorubicin dose dense regimen used in the high-risk SIOPEL 2 and 3 studies is more ototoxic confirming findings reported in other pediatric cancers where combined cisplatin/carboplatin regimens are used (Kushner et al. 2006). As in all international clinical trials, getting full compliance with complete audiological testing in all patients remains a challenge. Attempts to reduce ototoxicity have so far failed. Unfortunately, the introduction of amifostine did not reduce platinum toxicity in HB patients in an American study (Katzenstein et al. 2009). The SIOPEL 6 trial, in standard risk HB, is testing the otoprotectant sodium thiosulfate (STS) in a randomized Phase III setting in the hope of reducing cisplatin ototoxicity, at the same time as improving compliance and introducing central review of audiological test results.

If high-frequency hearing loss is impairing speech and learning (grade 2 or more) then hearing aids will be necessary. Digital hearing aids should be preferred. They do not completely correct hearing, but improve learning and speech development. In many cases, after treatment for liver tumors, hearing loss is minimal or mild but learning is facilitated when the family and teacher understand the pattern of hearing loss and help the child to compensate. Children should be seated at the front and to the side of the class and the teacher should turn to face them when turning toward the class. Provided the child can see the teacher he/she will learn to distinguish sounds and language and spontaneously learn to lip read. Family, friends, and teachers need to speak clearly to the child without shouting. Shouting increases the lower frequency sounds as well as the higher frequency sounds which are already difficult to hear. Reducing background noise is always helpful (Helt-Cameron and Allen 2009).

It is unusual for a child to develop high-frequency hearing loss when treated with carboplatin alone, unless it is used at myeloablative doses. However, in combination with cisplatin, ototoxicity increases.

Neurological Toxicity

Neurological toxicity is very rare in children, although it is the dose-limiting factor in the adult population, particularly the elderly. Carboplatin does not cause neurotoxicity.

15.3.2 Doxorubicin

15.3.2.1 Administration

This should be administered in a glucose solution as a slow intravenous infusion of 1 h or more. In some treatment protocols, long-term infusion has been advocated over 24–48 h with the aim of reducing cardiotoxicity. More recently, cardioprotectants have been used together with short-term infusions. However, the long-term effects of using cardioprotectants in children are still awaited. Longer-term infusions are known to increase the risk of mucositis which in turn increases the risk of infection.

15.3.2.2 Acute Toxicity

Nausea and Vomiting

Emesis is marked as with cisplatin. Should extravasation occur locally, the infusion should be stopped immediately when pain is experienced and the area abundantly flushed subcutaneously with saline. Some skin areas may require skin grafting if a third-degree burn develops. Mucositis can be severe particularly with longer infusion times. Mouth care is important but cannot prevent mucositis. At the first signs of pain, adequate pain medication should be given. In many cases, morphine or morphine derivatives are necessary as well as nutritional support.

Bone Marrow Toxicity

The pancytopenia produced by standard dose anthracyclines is similar to that of carboplatin. Time to full blood count recovery is approximately 21 days. Granulocyte colony stimulating factor, G-CSF, can be useful in reducing days in hospital due to infection.

Mucositis

The longer the anthracycline infusion the more marked the mucositis will be. This can be extremely painful and require opiate support.

15.3.2.3 Late Toxicity

Cardiotoxicity

Anthracyclines are an effective modality in the treatment of HB. Unfortunately, their efficacy comes at a cost. It has been known since their initial use in the 1970s that they can cause early and late onset cardiac failure due to the direct effect on the cardiac myocytes (Van hoff et al. 1979).

Pathologically, anthracyclines cause Z band disruption, vacuolation, and myocyte death with replacement fibrosis but no inflammatory changes, differentiating the cause from myocarditis (Billingham and Masek 1993). The anticancer effects of anthracyclines are mediated primarily through inhibition of DNA synthesis, transcription, and replication, but they also generate oxygen-derived free radicals, using iron as a co-factor and the mitochondrial respiratory chain. These free radicals cause direct damage to proteins, lipids, and DNA. The cardiac myocytes appear to have a poorly functioning oxygen-free radical scavenging enzyme system, compared with other tissues and this may explain the preferential toxicity of anthracyclines for cardiac muscle.

Damage occurs at the time of the insult but may be clinically significant only after many years. Studies have suggested that the cumulative incidence of cardiac failure shows no plateau even at 30 years posttreatment (Mulrooney et al. 2009; Pein et al. 2004). The myocardium heals by replacing the myocytes by fibrosis and remodeling rather than regrowth. Previously it was thought that the total number of myocytes was static after birth, but recent studies suggest that there is a low rate of turnover. However, cardiac myocytes do not increase in overall numbers after the postnatal period and in fact, there is a low level loss year on year (Nadal-Ginard et al. 2003). Adaptation occurs in the young by remodelling, using the capacity to increase myocyte volume and therefore often delaying the onset of clinical symptoms, or in severe cases, early onset cardiac failure may improve initially.

There are no specific studies on the incidence of cardiotoxicity in HB patients, but publications of clinical trials mention cardiotoxicity occurring in patients. In addition, a UK population-based study evaluating the requirement for cardiac transplantation in childhood cancer survivors identified two HB patients requiring heart transplantation, in a group of 43, over a 20 year period (Levitt et al. 2009).

Mortality and morbidity studies, performed on survivors of all types of childhood cancer, highlight an increased relative risk of cardiac disease after anthracycline administration (Tukenova et al. 2009; Mertens et al. 2008; Mulrooney et al. 2009). Tukenova reported a fourfold higher risk of cardiac deaths, compared to the general population, when treated with a cumulative dose of anthracyclines of 360 mg/m^2 in a cohort diagnosed before 1986. This was similar to the Childhood Cancer Survivor Study (CCSS) which reported a 3.1 relative risk for doses of 401 mg/m^2 or more. The recent report on cardiac morbidity highlighted the increased risk of cardiac failure after anthracycline exposure, in excess of 250 mg/m^2 (Mulrooney et al. 2009).

Kremer et al. conducted a systematic review of the frequency of and risk factors for subclinical and clinical cardiomyopathy after anthracycline treatment (Kremer et al. 2002a, b). An incidence of cardiac decompensation of 0–16% was reported with an increased incidence for subclinical damage of 0–57% with evidence of progression to the clinical state.

Cumulative dose is the most important risk factor linked to increasing duration from the end of treatment (Sorensen et al. 2003). All doses have been implicated, but studies suggest that doses above 250–350 mg/m^2 represent an increased risk of deteriorating cardiac disease over a 10–30 year period (Pein et al. 2004; Mulrooney et al. 2009; Tukenova et al. 2009). Other risk factors include young age, an important risk factor for liver tumor patients who tend to be under 2 years at diagnosis. In some studies, females appear to be more at risk compared to males, although not universally identified (Silber et al. 1993; Lipshultz et al. 1995; Sorensen et al. 2003).

Initially, patients with liver tumors were treated with bolus doses of anthracyclines. The two heart transplant patients, mentioned above, received their anthracyclines as bolus doses. Subsequently, 48 h infusion or cover with dexrazoxane has been used to protect against cardiac damage. Interestingly, this method of administration of anthracyclines has been shown to be relevant in adult studies, although no clear difference has been identified in children; however, this is probably due to the rarity of randomized studies (Van Dalen et al. 2009). The use of a cardioprotectant such as dexrazoxane has been shown in adult and pediatric randomized studies to be effective in reducing the incidence of cardiac events (Van Dalen et al. 2008; Bryant et al. 2007). Dexrazone's action is to reduce the oxygen-free radicals available to cause damage to the cardiac myocytes by iron chelation. Concerns have been raised about a potentially increased risk of second cancers, but these were in studies of patients with Hodgkins lymphoma (Tebbi et al. 2010) and in patients with high-risk acute lymphoblastic leukemia (Salzer et al. 2010). The concern for the relative risk of dexrazones producing second cancers has to be weighed against the solid evidence of the risk of anthracycline-induced cardiotoxicity in the very young (Lipshultz et al. 2007).

It is vital to appreciate the risk of progressive cardiomyopathy in liver tumor survivors who have received anthracyclines and to monitor them carefully over many years. The method of choice is noninvasive 3D echocardiogram performed serially to give information of progressive cardiac impairment. Care must be taken with interpretation due to the effect of anthracyclines on septal motion which can make accurate assessment of the fractional shortening difficult. Various long-term follow-up guidelines (SIGN 2004; COG 2004; Skinner et al. 2005) suggest 3–5 yearly ultrasound assessments if the end of treatment echocardiogram is normal. If abnormal (FS < 28%) then referral to a cardiologist is advisable. Female patients who become pregnant should receive cardiac monitoring throughout pregnancy as there are anecdotal reports of decompensation during pregnancy. However, a small study of 53 females did not identify an increased incidence of cardiac failure during pregnancy (Van Dalen et al. 2006). The use of "anti failure" drugs is established for clinical cardiac dysfunction, but there is still ongoing debate as to their use in the subclinical situation.

15.3.3 *Vincristine*

15.3.3.1 Administration

This is given as a slow (5–10 min) bolus intravenous injection into a free flowing vein. It causes superficial extravasation wounds.

15.3.3.2 Side Effects

The most frequent is constipation and all parents should be taught about constipation and laxatives should be prescribed for all children receiving vincristine.

Another important side effect is pain which is often located around the jaw and can impair eating. Paracetamol is often sufficient for pain relief but sometimes gabapentin can be useful. Loss of tendon reflexes, clumsy gait, and reduced dorsiflexion of the foot are all temporary side effects. However, if active dorsiflexion is lost, this can lead to foot drop and side stepping if not surveyed sufficiently and the vincristine dose is not reduced or temporarily stopped. Fortunately, this is rarely a problem in young children. It is possible that the therapeutic index could be improved (Moore and Pinkerton 2009).

Other side effects include ileus and seizures. Prolonged use can produce thinning of the thenar and hypothenar eminence of the hands, again not common in children with liver tumors.

15.4 Conclusion

The majority of children being treated for the most common primary liver cancer, HB, with multimodal treatment can be cured. However, this comes with a medical cost. Children susceptible to the late effects of therapy will have potential permanent late effects which in the case of platinum toxicity, if present in the year after treatment, will require life-long attention. These include the renal and audiological damage. The cardiac effects from anthracyclines may not be apparent at the end of treatment, and therefore, long-term follow-up of patients with echocardiograms is necessary.

References

Allen GC, Tiu C, Koike K, Ritchey AK, Kurs-Lasky M, Wax MK (1998) Transient-evoked otoacoustic emissions in children after cisplatin chemotherapy. Otolaryngol Head Neck Surg 118(5):584–588

Alvarez O, Freeman A, Bedros A, Call SK, Volsch J, Kalbermatter O, Halverson J, Convy L, Cook L, Mick K et al (1995) Randomized double-blind crossover ondansetron–dexamethasone versus ondansetron-placebo study for the treatment of chemotherapy-induced nausea and vomiting in pediatric patients with malignancies. J Pediatr Hematol Oncol 17(2):145–150

Billingham ME, Masek MA (1993) The pathology of anthracycline cardiotoxicity in children, adolescents and adults. In: Bricker JT, Green DM, D'Angio GJ (eds) Cardiac toxicity after anthracycline treatment for childhood cancer. Wiley-Liss, New York, pp 17–24

Blyth CC, Chen SC, Slavin MA, Serena C, Nguyen Q, Marriott D, Ellis D, Meyer W, Sorrell TC, Australian Candidemia Study (2009) Not just little adults: candidemia epidemiology, molecular characterization, and antifungal susceptibility in neonatal and pediatric patients. Pediatrics 123(5):1360–1368

Brock P, Bellman S (1991) Ototoxicity of cisplatinum. Br J Cancer 63(1):159–160

Brock PR, Koliouskas DE, Barratt TM, Yeomans E, Pritchard J (1991a) Partial reversibility of cisplatin nephrotoxicity in children. J Pediatr 118(4 (Pt 1)):531–534

Brock PR, Bellman SC, Yeomans EC et al (1991b) Cisplatin ototoxicity in children: a practical grading system. Med Pediatr Oncol 19:295–300

Brock PR, Yeomans EC, Bellman SC, Pritchard J (1992) Cisplatin therapy in infants: short and long-term morbidity. Br J Cancer Suppl 18:S36–S40

Brock P, Brichard B, Rechnitzer C, Langeveld NE, Lanning M, Söderhäll S, Laurent C (1996) An increased loading dose of ondansetron: a north european, double-blind randomised study in children, comparing 5 mg/m^2 with 10 mg/m^2. Eur J Cancer 32A(10):1744–1748

Bryant J, Picot J, Levitt G, Sullivan I, Baxter L, Clegg A (2007) Clinical and cost effectiveness of cardioprotection against the toxic effects of anthracyclines given to children with cancer: a systematic review. Br J Cancer 96(2):226–230

Children's Oncology Group (2004) Long-term follow-up guidelines for survivors of childhood, adolescent, and young adult cancers. www.survivorshipguidelines.org

Coradini PP, Cigana L, Selistre SG, Rosito LS, Brunetto AL (2007) Ototoxicity from cisplatin therapy in childhood cancer. J Pediatr Hematol Oncol 29(6):355–360

Corbally MT (1993) Supportive care of the paediatric cancer patient. Semin Surg Oncol 9(6):461–466

de Koning BA, van der Schoor SR, Wattimena DL, de Laat PC, Pieters R, van Goudoever JB (2007) Chemotherapy does not influence intestinal amino acid uptake in children. Pediatr Res 62(2):195–199

Dhooge I, Dhooge C, Geukens S, De Clerck B, De Vel E, Vinck BM (2006) Distortion product otoacoustic emissions: an objective technique for the screening of hearing loss in children treated with platin derivatives. Int J Audiol 45(6): 337–343

Dupuis LL, Nathan PC (2010) Optimizing emetic control in children receiving antineoplastic therapy: beyond the guidelines. Paediatr Drugs 12(1):51–61

Gilmer Knight KR, Kraemer DF, Neuwelt EA (2005) Ototoxicity in children receiving platinum chemotherapy: underestimating a commonly occurring toxicity that may impact academic and social development. SIOPEL Publ JCO 23(34): 8588–8596

Hanigan MH, Devarajan P (2003) Cisplatin nephrotoxicity: molecular mechanisms. Cancer Ther 1:47–61

Härtel C, Deuster M, Lehrnbecher T, Schultz C (2007) Current approaches for risk stratification of infectious complications in pediatric oncology. Pediatr Blood Cancer 49(6):767–773, Review

Hasler WL (1999) Serotonin receptor physiology: relation to emesis. Dig Dis Sci 44(8 Suppl):108S–113S, Review

Helt-Cameron J, Allen PJ (2009) Cisplatin ototoxicity in children: implications for primary care providers. Pediatr Nurs 35(2):121–127, Review

Hewitt M, McQuade B, Stevens R (1993) The efficacy and safety of ondansetron in the prophylaxis of cancer-chemotherapy induced nausea and vomiting in children. Clin Oncol (R Coll Radiol) 5(1):11–14

Hockenberry MJ, Schultz WH, Bennett B, Bryant R, Falletta JM (1989) Experience with minimal complications in implanted catheters in children. Am J Pediatr Hematol Oncol 11(3): 295–299

Ilveskoski I, Saarinen UM, Wiklund T, Perkkio M et al (1998) Ototoxicity in children with malignant brain tumors treated with the "8 in 1" chemotherapy protocol. Med Pediatr Oncol 27:26–31

Ishizawa T, Hasegawa K, Tsuno NH, Tanaka M, Mise Y, Aoki T, Imamura H, Beck Y, Sugawara Y, Makuuchi M, Takahashi K, Kokudo N (2009) Predeposit autologous plasma donation in liver resection for hepatocellular carcinoma: toward allogenic blood-free operations. J Am Coll Surg 209(2): 206–214, Epub 2009 May 1

Israëls T, van de Wetering MD, Hesseling P, van Geloven N, Caron HN, Molyneux EM (2009a) Malnutrition and neutropenia in children treated for Burkitt lymphoma in Malawi. Pediatr Blood Cancer 53(1):47–52

Israëls T, Borgstein E, Jamali M, de Kraker J, Caron HN, Molyneux EM (2009b) Acute malnutrition is common in Malawian patients with a Wilms tumour: a role for peanut butter. Pediatr Blood Cancer 53(7):1221–1226

Katzenstein HM, Chang KW, Krailo M, Chen Z, Finegold MJ, Rowland J, Reynolds M, Pappo A, London WB, Malogolowkin M, Children's Oncology Group (2009) Amifostine does not prevent platinum-induced hearing loss associated with the treatment of children with hepatoblastoma: a report of the Intergroup Hepatoblastoma Study P9645 as a part of the Children's Oncology Group. Cancer 115(24):5828–5835

Khan RB (2002) Migraine-type headaches in children receiving chemotherapy and ondansetron. J Child Neurol 17(11): 857–858

Knight KR, Kraemer DF, Winter C, Neuwelt EA (2007) Early changes in auditory function as a result of platinum chemotherapy: use of extended high-frequency audiometry and evoked distortion product otoacoustic emissions. J Clin Oncol 25(10):1190–1195

Kobayashi R, Kaneda M, Sato T, Ichikawa M, Suzuki D, Ariga T (2008) The clinical feature of invasive fungal infection in pediatric patients with hematologic and malignant diseases: a 10-year analysis at a single institution at Japan. J Pediatr Hematol Oncol 30(12):886–890

Kremer LC, van Dalen EC, Offringa M, Voûte PA (2002a) Frequency and risk factors of anthracycline-induced clinical heart failure in children: a systematic review. Ann Oncol 13(4):503–512, Review

Kremer LC, van der Pal HJ, Offringa M, van Dalen EC, Voute PA (2002b) Frequency and risk factors of subclinical cardiotoxicity after anthracycline therapy in children: a systematic review. Ann Oncol 13(6):819–829

Kushner BH, Budnick A, Kramer K, Modak S, Cheung NK (2006) Ototoxicity from high-dose use of platinum compounds in patients with neuroblastoma. Cancer 107(2): 417–422

Levitt G, Anazodo A, Burch M, Bunch K (2009) Cardiac or cardiopulmonary transplantation in childhood cancer survivors: an increasing need? Eur J Cancer 45(17):3027–3034

Li Y, Womer RB, Silber JH (2004) Predicting ototoxicity in children: influence of age and the cumulative dose. Eur J Cancer 40(16):2445–2451

Lipshultz SE, Lipsitz SR, Mone SM et al (1995) Female sex and higher drug dose as risk factors for late cardiotoxic effects of doxorubicin therapy for childhood cancer. N Engl J Med 332:1738–1743

Lipshultz SE, Lipsitz SR, Orav EJ (2007) Dexrazoxane-associated risk for secondary malignancies in pediatric Hodgkin's disease: a claim without compelling evidence. J Clin Oncol 25(21):3179, Author reply 3180

Meckler G, Lindemulder S (2009) Fever and neutropenia in pediatric patients with cancer. Emerg Med Clin North Am 27(3):525–544

Mertens AC, Liu Q, Neglia JP, Wasilewski K, Leisenring W, Armstrong GT, Robison LL, Yasui Y (2008) Cause-specific late mortality among 5-year survivors of childhood cancer: the Childhood Cancer Survivor Study. J Natl Cancer Inst 100(19):1368–1379

Moore A, Pinkerton R (2009) Vincristine: can its therapeutic index be enhanced? Pediatr Blood Cancer 53(7):1180–1187, Review

Mulrooney DA, Yeazel MW, Kawashima T, Mertens AC, Mitby P, Stovall M, Donaldson SS, Green DM, Sklar CA, Robison LL, Leisenring WM (2009) Cardiac outcomes in a cohort of adult survivors of childhood and adolescent cancer: retrospective analysis of the Childhood Cancer Survivor Study cohort. BMJ 339:b4606

Nadal-Ginard B, Kajstura J, Leri A, Anversa P (2003) Myocyte death, growth, and regeneration in cardiac hypertrophy and failure. Circ Res 92(2):139–150

Nathan M, Selwood K, Clinical Practice Group of the RCN Paediatric Oncology Nurses Forum (2006) The use of blood products in paediatric oncology units in the UK. Paediatr Nurs 18(7):14–17

Pein F, Sakiroglu O, Dahan M et al (2004) Cardiac abnormalities 15 years and more after adriamycin therapy in 229 childhood survivors of a solid tumour at the Instit Gustave Roussy. Br J Cancer 91:37–44

Pereira CA, Petrilli AS, Carlesse FA, Luisi FA, da Silva KV, de Martino Lee ML (2009) Cefepime monotherapy is as effective as ceftriaxone plus amikacin in pediatric patients with cancer and high-risk febrile neutropenia in a randomized comparison. J Microbiol Immunol Infect 42(2):141–147

Perilongo G, Maibach R, Shafford E, Brugieres L, Brock P, Morland B, de Camargo B, Zsiros J, Roebuck D, Zimmermann A, Aronson D, Childs M, Widing E, Laithier V, Plaschkes J, Pritchard J, Scopinaro M, MacKinlay G, Czauderna P (2009) Cisplatin versus cisplatin plus doxorubicin for standard-risk hepatoblastoma. N Engl J Med 361(17):1662–1670

Rude RK, Singer FR, Gruber HE (2009) Skeletal and hormonal effects of magnesium deficiency. J Am Coll Nutr 28(2):131–141, Review

Salzer WL, Devidas M, Carroll WL et al (2010) Long-term results of the pediatric oncology group studies for childhood acute lymphoblastic leukemia. 1984–2001: A report from the children's oncology group leukemia 24:355–370

Seguy D, Berthon C, Micol JB, Darré S, Dalle JH, Neuville S, Bauters F, Jouet JP, Yakoub Agha I (2006) Enteral feeding and early outcomes of patients undergoing allogeneic stem cell transplantation following myeloablative conditioning. Transplantation 82(6):835–839

SIGN (2004) Long term follow up of survivors of childhood cancer. A national clinical guideline. www.sign.ac.uk/pdf/sign76.pdf

Silber JH, Jakacki RI, Larsen RL, Goldwein JW, Barber G (1993) Increased risk of cardiac dysfunction after anthracyclines in girls. Med Pediatr Oncol 21:477–479

Skinner R, Levitt G, Wallace WH (2005) Therapy based LTFU Practice Statement UKCCSG. www.ukccsg.org.uk/public/followup

Sorensen K, Levitt GA, Bull C, Dorup I, Sullivan ID (2003) Late anthracycline cardiotoxicity after childhood cancer: a prospective longitudinal study. Cancer 97:1991–1998

Stockhorst U, Spennes-Saleh S, Körholz D, Göbel U, Schneider ME, Steingrüber HJ, Klosterhalfen S (2000) Anticipatory symptoms and anticipatory immune responses in pediatric cancer patients receiving chemotherapy: features of a classically conditioned response? Brain Behav Immun 14(3):198–218

Tebbi CK, London WB, Friedman D, Villaluna D, De Alarcon PA, Constine LS, Mendenhall NP, Sposto R, Chauvenet A, Schwartz CL (2007) Dexrazoxane-associated risk for acute myeloid leukemia/myelodysplastic syndrome and other secondary malignancies in pediatric Hodgkin's disease. J Clin Oncol 25(5):493–500

Tukenova M, Guibout C, Oberlin O et al (2009) Long-term overall and cardiovascular mortality following childhood cancer: the role of cancer treatment. BMJ 339:b4691

van Dalen EC, van der Pal HJ, van den Bos C, Kok WE, Caron HN, Kremer LC (2006) Clinical heart failure during pregnancy and delivery in a cohort of female childhood cancer survivors treated with anthracyclines. Eur J Cancer 42(15):2549–2553

van Dalen EC, Caron HN, Dickinson HO, Kremer LC (2008) Cardioprotective interventions for cancer patients receiving anthracyclines. Cochrane Database Syst Rev 2:CD003917

van Dalen EC, van der Pal HJ, Caron HN, Kremer LC (2009) Different dosage schedules for reducing cardiotoxicity in cancer patients receiving anthracycline chemotherapy. Cochrane Database Syst Rev 4:CD005008

Von Hoff DD, Layard MW, Basa P et al (1979) Risk factors for doxorubicin-induced congestive heart failure. Ann Intern Med 91:710–717

Zorowka PG, Schmitt HJ, Gutjahr P (1993) Evoked otoacoustic emissions and pure tone threshold audiometry in patients receiving cisplatinum therapy. Int J Pediatr Otorhinolaryngol 25(1–3):73–80

Challenges and Opportunities of International Therapeutic Trials

16

Rudolf Maibach

Contents

R. Maibach
IBCSG Coordinating Center, Effingerstrasse 40, CH-3008 Berne, Switzerland
e-mail: rudolf.maibach@ibcsg.org

16.1 Introduction

Clinical trials provide the best means to test and establish new treatments. Childhood liver cancer is no exception to this rule. However, the rarity of the disease poses a special challenge because it severely limits the number of trials that can be conducted. Any decision for a new trial sets the direction for a prolonged period. Such decisions therefore need to be taken with great circumspection in order to maximize the benefit derived from the research. Precious time may be lost otherwise.

International collaboration for the conduct of multicenter trials has been organized in the past by SIOPEL, the International Childhood Liver Tumor Strategy Group. This successful research has yielded excellent results, and the outcome was improved greatly by the introduction of effective presurgery chemotherapy, a staging system useful for treatment stratification, surgical guidelines, and careful monitoring of adverse events. Part of the improvement in treatment results can certainly also be attributed to the enhanced communication among investigators assembled in a collaborative group.

The environment for clinical research has greatly evolved. It takes more than a group of friends and a consensus about a therapeutic approach to start clinical research. The legal requirements for the conduct of trials have changed completely in the past few years and the researchers need to comply with a complicated set of rules not only in their work with their patients but above all in their interaction with supervisory agencies at the regulatory level. This is a major challenge, especially for academic clinical research. It may, however, also constitute an opportunity to reorganize and improve.

A. Zimmermann et al. (eds.), *Pediatric Liver Tumors*, Pediatric Oncology,
DOI: 10.1007/978-3-642-14504-9_16, © Springer-Verlag Berlin Heidelberg 2011

The way forward in the development of improved treatment strategies in childhood liver cancer is not very different from other malignant diseases in which surgery plays a central role. Clinical trials are needed to reach firm evidence on the efficacy and feasibility. The challenge is to quickly reach a good recruitment rate to complete studies in reasonable time. Many parameters contribute to the relative attractiveness of a trial, and these need to be considered with circumspection. A maximum of information should be derived from the limited number of patients. For the investigators, it is crucial not to be burdened with any task, which is not strictly necessary to attain the objectives of the trial. The correct staging and prognostic stratification at diagnosis is a good example for an essential requirement. It must also be clear that a central review of histology and (in advanced disease) imaging is mandatory. In addition, the collection of biological material constitutes a unique opportunity to obtain a maximum of information on the tumor and the host. The combination of standardized clinical documentation and determination of biological markers in a central laboratory has proven successful in other diseases, and will certainly do so in childhood liver cancer as well.

16.2 Challenges

16.2.1 Clinical Trials in Very Rare Diseases

Extremely rare diseases may be perceived as less rewarding to study, both for the academic investigator and the medicines producer. Building a career on clinical research in childhood liver tumors may take a disproportionate time. The development of special medicines for the treatment of hepatoblastoma (HB) or childhood hepatocellular carcinoma (HCC) may be unrealistic, but even the rigid proof of efficacy in childhood cancer for substances already in use for adults is time-consuming, and moderate improvements with respect to standard treatment may not be statistically provable at all. There is a set of considerations on the safety and welfare of the trial subject, which is accepted universally, and must be respected. Can they be relaxed in very rare diseases? The established principles governing the generating of firm evidence should not be softened hastily when confronted with a rare disease. Yet indiscriminately applied strict rules on the planning and conduct of therapeutic trials have led to bureaucratic impediments for rare childhood diseases, which are clearly counterproductive. The price to be paid by the patients, their families, and society as a whole is too high when new academic trials are not run because financial and work burden hurdles cannot be overcome by the medical community. The implementation of the Clinical Trials Directive in the European Union in 2005 directly delayed the implementation of new SIOPEL trials by 1–2 years due to the obligation to obtain regulatory approval. While member states developed their own adaptation of the regulation, often counter-acting the harmonization planned by the Directive, academic researchers were facing additional hurdles in the activation process without any trial-related funding available.

16.2.2 Staging Systems

Correct staging is crucial to determine the therapeutic approach. Currently, two staging systems are in use. The Children's Oncology Group (COG) uses a postoperative staging for operable patients (Ortega et al. 2000). The SIOPEL group has always used an anatomic diagnostic staging for stratification of patients in view of treatment decisions (Roebuck et al. 2007). This difference complicates the comparison of treatment results obtained by the respective groups. Staging is the first step in taking care of a patient, and the treatment strategy will be chosen based on a classification into prognostic categories. The intergroup conduct of common clinical trials requires the use of the same staging system. The PRETEXT system lends itself well and is increasingly used throughout the world (Chap. 7). A retrospective evaluation of data from the Intergroup CCG/POG study INT-0098 on diagnostic imaging, histology, and AFP level as prognostic factors is readily available as diagnosis of a hepatoblastoma has shown the relative merits of PRETEXT and the COG staging system (Meyers et al. 2009). This encouraging report will lead to more widespread use of the PRETEXT system.

16.3 Trial Designs

16.3.1 The Hypothesis Dictates the Trial Design

Trials with small sample sizes are ideal in the early phase of developing a therapeutic approach. There are several single arm phase II designs, which are widely used. Two-stage designs have a built-in interim evaluation after the inclusion and evaluation of patients in stage 1, allowing an early look at the efficacy endpoint with predefined criteria for early stopping in case of lower than expected efficacy (Simon 1989). A multinomial design can take into account more than a simple success or failure in the endpoint. In a single arm trial for relapsed hepatoblastoma patients, SIOPEL uses a two-stage design based on the simultaneous assessment of both response and early progression in the patients. Accrual is stopped after stage 1 if the required number of responses is not attained or the rate of early progression is elevated. Otherwise, recruitment continues up to the total planned sample size (Zee et al. 1999).

Phase II trials usually lack a control arm, and will only deliver a preliminary estimation for efficacy and tolerability, which will be heavily influenced by patient selection. They are therefore only useful to give an indication whether the tested substance is worth being studied in more detail. The classical randomized phase III trial for the comparison of two or more treatment arms gives much more definite answers about the value of a new therapeutic approach. In an extremely rare disease such as childhood liver cancer, a phase III is very difficult to conduct due to the elevated sample size needed to obtain adequate statistical power. One might be tempted to use a randomized phase II design to reduce the required sample size. There is, however, an important distinction between the hypotheses to be tested: a phase III is typically used to test the superiority of one treatment over another in a head-to-head comparison, whereas a randomized phase II must be seen as two or more single-arm trials run in parallel and yielding preliminary efficacy results, like estimates of a success or event rate (Simon et al. 1985). The result of a randomized phase II trial may be used to select the most promising of two or more new substances for further study, but does not allow a definitive conclusion about superiority.

The SIOPEL 3 trial for HB encompassed two trial runs in parallel, a randomized study for standard-risk HB (SR-HB) and a single-arm study for high-risk HB (HR-HB). HR-HB aimed to improve the success rate (here: the rate of complete resection after preoperative chemotherapy) over the one observed in the SIOPEL 1 study, which had introduced for the first time the cisplatin–doxorubicin regimen. The comparison with a historical control was chosen because it was felt that the group would be unable to accrue a sufficient number of patients for a randomized comparison. The use of historical controls is, however, debatable, and the risk of a stage-shift and external factors evolving over time and influencing the outcome is high, especially in a rare disease: The historical controls from SIOPEL 1 were treated between 1990 and 1994, HR-HB recruited patients between 1998 and 2004; institutions joining the group during HR-HB were less experienced than the long-term participants of SIOPEL1; a stage downshift from higher to lesser risk may have counterbalanced an increase of efficacy (Zsiros et al. 2010).

The SR-HB part of SIOPEL 3 was designed to test the hypothesis that preoperative chemotherapy with cisplatin alone was not less efficacious than the cisplatin–doxorubicin combination introduced in SIOPEL 1. This was a very ambitious goal in view of the limited recruitment rate of about 35 per year, because noninferiority designs usually call for elevated sample sizes. A compromise was made by choosing a relatively high noninferiority margin of 10% difference in rates of complete resection. A reduction of the success rate by this amount would hardly be clinically acceptable. This margin was, however, useful for the group-sequential interim monitoring designed to stop the trial early in case of emerging evidence of inferiority, limiting the risk that too many patients would be treated with an inferior chemotherapy. Yearly interim analyses were submitted to an Independent Data Monitoring Committee, and the trial was not stopped early because the results were reassuring (Perilongo et al. 2009). The trial has shown that the difference in resection rates was much less than 10% and that cisplatin monotherapy for standard-risk patients yields excellent short- and long-term results and lower acute toxicity rates, while avoiding the potential late sequelae of anthracyclines.

16.3.2 Biomolecular Investigations

Biological properties of both tumor and host play an important role in the natural course of the disease and in the success of therapeutic interventions (Chap. 3). At the time when a new trial protocol is being developed, known biomarkers may already be used to stratify patients. The determination of these markers may take place at the treating institution or centrally at one laboratory for all sites participating in the trial. The second option is logistically very challenging since results must be available within very few days in order to reach a decision on the treatment of a newly diagnosed patient. Therefore, fresh frozen or paraffin-embedded biopsy material is usually assessed and stored locally. Central review can be done later without time pressure and is important to give feedback to local sites about the accurateness of their results, thus providing an incentive to adjust the quality where necessary. Such exchange of expert advice is particularly valuable for very rare diseases. Beyond the decision-making use for the patient, such material may, however, also become extremely valuable for the next generation of patients at a later stage. New treatment targets may be identified years after the treatment of the patient has been completed. Such new findings will not benefit the patient who has donated the material, but will help assign treatment for future patients who are susceptible to benefit. Only centralized material can be assayed relatively quickly. Central banking is a hallmark for a modern clinical trial, and should be clearly mentioned both in the protocol and in the patient information. The availability of the standardized clinical documentation of the treatment and follow-up for patients who have participated in trials renders the material even more precious and allows conclusions, which may not be obtainable from simple case series. The tumor bank of SIOPEL demonstrates the feasibility of central banking (Chap. 5).

16.3.3 Case Report Forms

It is crucial that the cooperative group coordinating the trial prepares a clearly readable protocol and case report forms (CRFs), which capture the essential information without going into unnecessary details. CRF design is a science in its own right. Nevertheless, some principles are repeated here:

- Great care has to be used to make sure that *primary and secondary endpoints* are captured correctly and completely.
- The *schedule and scope of examinations* should adhere to generally accepted standards and should not impose unwarranted burdens on the patient or the investigator.
- Reporting of certain adverse events can only be considered complete for *targeted events*; unspecific questions asking for “any other” adverse events should only be used if they are necessary in the clinical context and can add to the understanding of the case history of single patients. Summary reporting will have to refrain from calculating rates for such events since they are likely to be underreported.
- The “end-users” need to be involved in the design phase of the CRF, because they will be working with the collected information: chairperson, safety officer, medical reviewer, data manager, and last but not the least, the statistician.
- The data collection should be restricted to the necessary minimum, asking for too many details is counterproductive and may reduce the overall data quality.

16.4 Trial Conduct

16.4.1 Why Bother to Treat Patients in Clinical Trials?

Many factors are critical for the successful conduct of a clinical trial and need to be considered carefully. A rare type of cancer in children poses an even greater challenge. Participating sites may not see a HB case for many months or even years. Yet they should be ready not only to treat the patient according to the protocol but also to enroll the patient into the trial and to document treatment and outcome. The investigator needs to take many preparatory steps (preparation of patient information and consent form, ethics committee submission, health authority submission, essential documents according to GCP) well in advance and without guarantee that she will have to treat patients who are eligible for inclusion into a certain trial.

The investigator may therefore face the dilemma of making a choice and concentrate on the activation of trials in his particular area of interest or expertise, or the disease category in which the majority of patients are seen. In this respect, liver cancer protocols are not in the pole position in the race for early activation. Yet the option of keeping the protocol in the drawer and only opening it once a patient is diagnosed with this particular disease is not a valid alternative either. Off-protocol use of protocol treatment may mean that an experimental therapy is applied without proper support and documentation. Apart from violating the rules of Good Clinical Practice (GCP), it excludes the treating physician from the often indispensable access to peers who have developed the therapy and are most knowledgeable about it. Furthermore, the experience of the particular patient is lost to the scientific community, a loss that is particularly high in a very rare disease.

16.4.2 Complete Documentation of All Included Patients

Often, trial protocols state that the analyses will be done according to intention to treat (ITT). The meaning of ITT will be covered in the next section. This principle has important consequences for the local investigator: the clinical course of the patient will need to be documented completely, regardless of any deviations from protocol treatment, including complete stop of the trial treatment. The investigator has two commitments, which need to be reconciled. He has to treat the patient according to his best knowledge, including deviations from protocol treatment if clinically indicated. But equally important, the patient (or legal representative) has agreed to participate in scientific research and therefore has declared the will to be completely documented, and may not be "withdrawn from protocol," except if she has withdrawn consent to any further documentation. In case of treatment being stopped, a patient may only be considered as having "stopped protocol treatment", but will remain in the protocol, and the documentation of long-term outcome needs to continue.

16.4.3 Interim Monitoring

During the conduct of the trial, the sponsor has the obligation to monitor several aspects, which are all crucial for the safety of the patient and for the success of the trial:

- Actual recruitment rates are compared to rates anticipated in the protocol to determine if the trial will complete recruitment within reasonable time.
- The documentation on case report forms has to be available almost in real time, to ensure that no important developments and trends in both outcome and toxicity are missed.
- Patient safety needs to be continually verified by monitoring adverse events, especially suspected unexpected serious adverse reactions (SUSARs), which are subjected to expedited reporting to regulatory authorities.
- If the primary endpoint of the trial is a measure of efficacy, benefit and sometimes futility need to be assessed at points predetermined in the protocol.

The sponsor of the trial must compile interim reports covering the above-mentioned issues. There is a potential for the sponsor to be biased in favor of the experimental therapy tested in the trial. Its conclusions from an interim report need to be critically reviewed by experts with no vested interest in the trial results. An independent body, usually called Independent Data Monitoring Committee (IDMC) or Data and Safety Monitoring Committee (DSMC) should therefore be in place to review interim and final reports. The IDMC must be knowledgeable with respect to the disease and its standard treatment, and has to consider not only the interim results but also any other important findings from other sources such as recent publications, which may have appeared after the trial was started. It is the responsibility of the IDMC to formulate recommendations, while the sponsor (or a Trial Steering Committee) is responsible for deciding and taking actions. The guidelines governing the role of the IDMC determine the periodicity of its meetings.

Interim evaluations are usually outlined in the protocol. Modern randomized phase III trials comprise formal monitoring of the primary efficacy endpoint. Sequential or group-sequential designs include rules on early stopping based on statistical reasoning on the likelihood of interim results. They serve to check if the data collected so far are in line with the hypothesis formulated in the protocol. Early stopping may be indicated in case of a higher than expected effect size. In this case, it may be unethical to continue to expose a portion of the patients to an inferior treatment. The randomization may also have to be stopped for futility, i.e., in case it appears highly unlikely that the trial will ever yield a significant difference between treatment arms. For both scenarios, stopping rules should be prospectively formulated and based on statistical considerations. Safety concerns may also lead to early stopping or a major revision of the protocol. Such findings are sometimes unexpected and therefore lend themselves much less for a prospective formulation of a precise rule. In such cases, the expertise assembled in the IDMC weighs in to judge the situation.

16.5 Presentation and Interpretation of Results

16.5.1 Intention to Treat Analysis

As mentioned in Sect. 16.4.2, clinical trials generally plan an evaluation according to ITT. This means that patients are counted in the analysis as they were included, independent of any deviation from the protocol during their treatment. The principle of doing an ITT evaluation is based on the fundamental rationale that only ITT will avoid the introduction of an undue selection bias into the analysis. As an example, patients who had to stop trial treatment early due to lack of tolerability must be counted in the denominator of the rate of success, even though they never had a chance to respond to the treatment. The effect size estimation will show a reduced success rate reflecting that some patients cannot tolerate the treatment. The ITT result can therefore be interpreted as describing what is to be expected at the time the treatment decision is taken, and not post hoc, after elimination of the "bad players."

Noncompliance with protocol treatment may bias the results in both directions, since patients may receive overtreatment in some and undertreatment in other cases. The investigator may have had an excellent reason for such deviations and indeed does have to change the regimen if this is needed in the best interest of the patient. The protocol may describe an ideal situation, and clinical practice may look substantially different. Still, deviations should only occur for good reasons, and consulting with the trial coordinator may be appropriate to avoid unnecessary noncompliance.

In randomized trials, the situation becomes more complicated. In addition to the above-mentioned problems, inadvertent application of the wrong randomization treatment will lead to dilution of ITT results. For a two-arm trial, a simple calculation shows that effect sizes of 50% in arm A and 60% in arm B will change to 51% and 59% in both arms if 10% of patients are treated in the opposite arm. This can be described as a deviation toward the null hypothesis of no difference. A trial designed to detect the difference from 50% to 60% with a power of 80% will have its power reduced to 61% in the ITT analysis by such an amount of noncompliance. Should noncompliant patients therefore be excluded from the analysis? The answer is no: Any exclusion of patients from an analysis may raise the suspicion that these patients are removed arbitrarily because they influence the results in the direction opposite to what the investigator would like to achieve. Only ITT will prevent such undue influence in the results. Moreover, a certain degree of deviation from the ideal situation assumed in the protocol is inevitable and reflects clinical reality. However, the trial team may add a per protocol analysis (PP), which only includes patients who have been treated according to randomization (ICH Harmonised Tripartite Guideline 1999). If the results of ITT and PP lead to different conclusions, then this has to be discussed carefully when the results are published. Such a procedure was adopted for SIOPEL 3 SR-HB (Perilongo et al. 2009). This was a noninferiority trial where the deviation toward no difference is seen as particularly problematic, because a sufficient amount of noncompliance will by its very nature lead to a result of noninferiority: Due to the dilution effect, the results of the two treatment arms will approach each other, suggesting noninferiority even in case of a real underlying difference. An extension of the CONSORT statement gives recommendations on how to present the results of such trials (Piaggio et al. 2006).

16.6 Opportunities

Several cooperative groups have built up a solid reputation for their long-standing investigations into childhood liver cancer, notably the Children's Oncology Group, a merger of the former POG, CCG, IRS, and NWTS; the International Childhood Liver Cancer Strategy Group SIOPEL; the German Society for Pediatric Oncology-Hematology GPOH; and the Japanese Study Group for Pediatric Liver Tumor JPLT. All these groups conduct their own innovative investigational program. Because of the very low incidence of HB and HCC, their potential to recruit patients into clinical trials is limited. Most of their trials are therefore phase I and II single arm, whereas randomized trials are the exception. Only by a combined effort could they conduct a sizeable phase III trial in a reasonable time. This appears like a very attractive option, but it can be discussed in good faith if this would be worth the huge effort of coordination: the legal framework differs between countries and much more so between continents, requirements like pharmacovigilance or protection of confidentiality constitute practical as well as cultural differences, which would have to be taken into account. SIOPEL with its membership spread over five continents has shown that this can be achieved, but experiences increasing difficulty to cope with this formidable task.

A sound competition between research groups for ideas and treatment concepts is an important factor as well in the quest for a cure for the disease. The upfront surgery approach for early-stage disease advocated by COG and the neoadjuvant concept of SIOPEL have both proven their value. The small world of childhood liver tumor specialists know each other well and the communication has greatly increased in the past years. This has only just started to transform into a cooperation. COG and SIOPEL have decided to start a project with the acronym CHIC (Childhood Hepatic tumors International Collaboration). The goal is to define a basic set of variables, which will allow merging of data from previously conducted clinical trials. This will allow retrospective analyses especially for fine-tuning the prognostic stratification in view of developing therapeutic strategies, and to identify prognostic factors at diagnosis independent of the initial therapeutic approach. For such data to be really valuable, they need to be available on a per patient basis, not as summary statistics. The challenge is to find a common data set despite the different structure and content of existing databases. Once CHIC will have proven its usefulness, it will serve as a basis for a closer coordination of research agendas and perhaps also for common clinical trials, where appropriate.

References

ICH Harmonised Tripartite Guideline (1999) Statistical principles for clinical trials. International Conference on Harmonisation E9 Expert Working Group. Stat Med 18(15):1905–1942

Meyers RL, Rowland JR, Krailo M, Chen Z, Katzenstein HM, Malogolowkin MH (2009) Predictive power of pretreatment prognostic factors in children with hepatoblastoma: a report from the children's oncology group. Pediatr Blood Cancer 53(6):1016–1022

Ortega JA, Douglass EC, Feusner JH et al (2000) Randomized comparison of cisplatin/vincristine/fluorouracil and cisplatin/continuous infusion doxorubicin for treatment of pediatric hepatoblastoma: a report from the Children's Cancer Group and the Pediatric Oncology Group. J Clin Oncol 18:2665–2675

Perilongo G, Maibach R, Shafford E, Brugieres L, Brock P, Morland B, de Camargo B, Zsiros J, Roebuck D, Zimmermann A, Aronson D, Childs M, Widing E, Laithier V, Plaschkes J, Pritchard J, Scopinaro M, Mackinlay G, Czauderna P (2009) Cisplatin versus Cisplatin plus doxorubicin for standard-risk hepatoblastoma. N Engl J Med 361(17):1662–1670

Piaggio G, Elbourne DE, Altman DG, Pocock SJ, Evans SJE (2006) Reporting of non-inferiority and equivalence randomized trials. An extension of the CONSORT statement. JAMA 295:1152–1160

Roebuck DJ et al (2007) PRETEXT: a revised staging system for primary malignant liver tumours of childhood developed by the SIOPEL group. Pediatr Radiol 37:123–132

Simon R (1989) Optimal two-stage designs for phase II clinical trials. Control Clin Trials 10(1):1–10

Simon R, Wittes RE, Ellenberg SS (1985) Randomized phase II clinical trials. Cancer Treat Rep 69(12):1375–1381

Zee B et al (1999) Multinomial phase II cancer trials incorporating response and early progression. J Biopharma Stat 9:351–363

Zsíros J, Maibach R, Shafford E et al (2010) Successful treatment of childhood high-risk hepatoblastoma with dose-intensive multiagent chemotherapy and surgery: final results of the SIOPEL-3HR study. J Clin Oncol 20:28(15):2584–2590

Tumors Other than Hepatoblastoma and Hepatocellular Carcinoma

17

Gianni Bisogno and Arthur Zimmermann

Contents

G. Bisogno (✉)
Hematology Oncology Division, Department of Pediatrics, Clinica di Oncoematologia,
Via Giustiniani 3, I-35100 Padova, Italy
e-mail: gianni.bisogno@unipd.it

A. Zimmermann
Institute of Pathology of the University, Murtenstrasse 31, CH-3010 Berne, Switzerland
e-mail: zimmerma@patho.unibe.ch

17.1 Introduction

Apart from hepatoblastoma (HB) and hepatocarcinoma, other rare hepatic neoplasms can occur in the pediatric age group (Table 17.1). Clinically, the most relevant group is mesenchymal tumors, comprising 9–15% of primary malignant liver tumors. They include undifferentiated (embryonal) sarcoma, malignant rhabdoid tumor, hepatobiliary rhabdomyosarcoma, and tumors showing perivascular epithelioid cell differentiation (PEComas).

Vascular tumors typically arise in the liver. Most of them are benign, but infantile hemangioendothelioma, typical of very young children, and the very aggressive angiosarcoma are often difficult to manage, especially when unresectable.

Exceptionally, other tumors such as lymphoma or germ cell tumors arise primarily in the liver and should be considered in the differential diagnosis of space-occupying liver lesions in the presence of normal levels of alpha-fetoprotein.

Finally, mesenchymal hamartoma, a benign cystic tumor, must also be taken into consideration because of its potential transformation in undifferentiated sarcoma.

17.2 Undifferentiated (Embryonal) Sarcoma of the Liver

17.2.1 Introduction

Different terms such as malignant mesenchymoma, embryonal sarcoma, and fibromyxosarcoma have been unified under the term, undifferentiated

A. Zimmermann et al. (eds.), *Pediatric Liver Tumors*, Pediatric Oncology,
DOI: 10.1007/978-3-642-14504-9_17, © Springer-Verlag Berlin Heidelberg 2011

Table 17.1 Rare hepatic tumors in pediatric age

Mesenchimal tumors
- Undifferentiated (embryonal) sarcoma
- Rhabdomyosarcoma
- Rhabdoid tumor
- Other sarcoma (i.e. PEComa, Leyomiosarcoma)
Vascular tumor
- Angiosarcoma
- Hemangioendotelioma
Other primary liver tumor
- Germ cell tumor
- Lymphoma
Border line tumor
- Mesenchymal hamartoma

(embryonal) sarcoma of the liver (USL) (Stocker and Ishak 1978). USL is considered a neoplasm typical of pediatric age with a peak between 5 and 10 years. No sex predilection has been reported. The distinct age group, a normal level of serum alpha-fetoprotein and the radiological appearance of the tumor usually alert the clinician to consider USL in the differential diagnosis of a liver mass. USL is an aggressive neoplasm and initial studies uniformly reported a poor outcome (Perilongo et al. 1987; Horowitz et al. 1987). More recently, an increasing number of long-term survivors have been observed after complete surgical excision with or without postoperative chemotherapy (Walker et al. 1992; Bisogno et al. 2002).

17.2.2 Epidemiology and Etiology

Due to the rarity of USL, population-based studies are lacking. According to different series of liver tumors, USL accounts for 6–15% of cases.

The etiology is unclear. USL may show rearrangements of chromosomal band 19q13.4, including the translocation t(11;19) (q13;q13.4). The breakpoint at 19q13.4 occurs at a locus referred to as mesenchymal hamartoma of the liver breakpoint 1, or MHLB1. As outlined below, conversion of mesenchymal hamartoma to USL has been documented (O'Sullivan et al. 2001). USL may be part of the Li-Fraumeni syndrome (Lack et al. 1991) and sporadic cases of USL arising in an irradiated liver have been reported (Bisogno et al. 2002).

17.2.3 Clinical Presentation and Diagnosis

The clinical features of mesenchymal tumors compared to the more common HB and hepatocarcinoma are shown in Table 17.2. The child with USL usually presents with an abdominal mass that may be accompanied by pain and, in some cases, by systemic symptoms such as fever, weight loss, or vomiting. Although symptoms are not distinctive, normal levels of alpha-fetoprotein and older age may help suspect that we are not dealing with a classic liver tumor. Leukocytosis may also be present (Emre and McKenna 2004). In some cases, symptoms associated with tumor rupture, such as pain and abdominal bleeding, become evident. USL may spread outside the liver invading the nearby organs, and disseminate along hematogenous routes. Distant metastases are frequently found in lungs and bones, and in rare cases in brain and skin. A particular feature of USL is the presence of multiple lesions affecting most parts of both liver lobes.

The diagnostic work up is not different from that adopted for other liver tumors. Ultrasound (US) followed by CT scan and/or MRI are important to understand the lesion characteristics and plan initial surgery. A discrepancy between the US and CT appearance is considered typical of USL. US evaluation demonstrates a large multiseptated solid mass. Contrast-enhanced CT scan shows a large, markedly hypodense and predominantly cystic mass with minimal enhancement, often limited by a peripheral rim. On MRI, the tumor is heterogeneous with high signal intensity on T2WI and low on T1WI. A peripheral enhancement of the surrounding pseudocapsule, representing compressed liver tissue, and septa are evident on early-enhanced MRI, while neoplastic nodules may became enhanced on delayed imaging (Jha et al. 2009). It was shown that USL demonstrates intense F-18 FDG uptake suggesting that PET/CT can be a useful imaging modality for the evaluation of the primary liver lesion and distant metastasis.

Table 17.2 Clinical presentation of the different pediatric liver tumors

	Hepatoblastoma	Hepatocarcinoma	Undifferentiated sarcoma	Angiosarcoma	Rhabdomyosarcoma
Age	0–3	5–18	5–10	3	2–5
Sex	M>F	M>F	M=F	F>M	M>F
Symptoms	Abdominal mass	Abdominal mass, fever weight loss	Abdominal mass	Abdominal mass	Abdominal mass, jaundice
Markers	Alfa-fetoprotein	Alfa-fetoprotein	none	none	none
Possible preexisting lesion		Tyrosinemia cirrhosis	Mesenchimal hamartoma	hemangioendotelioma	

No recognized tumor staging for USL exists. The tumor is often classified according to the result of initial surgery and further treatment is decided accordingly.

17.2.4 Pathology

Macroscopically, USL are commonly large masses at presentation, measuring up to 35 cm in diameter. Peripheral parts of the lesions are usually solid, whereas the tumor center is often occupied by a cyst or multiple cystic spaces, hemorrhage, and necrosis. Histologically, USL consists of a loose and sometimes myxoid mesenchyme of variable cellularity (Fig. 17.1a). The main cell types consist of spindle cells, stellate cells, and highly polymorphous cells (Fig. 17.1b). Part of the large and giant cells contains multiple eosinophilic globular inclusions, a feature typical for USL (Fig. 17.1c). These inclusions are PAS-positive (Fig. 17.1d) and consist of stored glycoproteins. USL can invade the portal tracts and is then situated around bile ducts (Fig. 17.1e). But also far from portal tracts, USL contains entrapped, damaged, and sometimes dilated bile ducts (Fig. 17.1f).

17.2.5 Treatment

17.2.5.1 Therapy of Non-ruptured Solitary Hepatic Lesions with or Without Metastases

In the old series, treatment was based mainly on tumor resection with radiotherapy and chemotherapy only occasionally employed. Chances of cure relied heavily on radical resection being obtained. In the original report published by Stocker and Ishak, only 6 of 31 cases reported were alive with no evidence of disease (Stocker and Ishak 1978). Subsequent studies confirmed a poor prognosis (Perilongo et al. 1987; Horowitz et al. 1987). A literature review spanning 1950 to 1988 reported only 37% of patients to be alive (Leuschner et al. 1990). It is only in the late 1980s that the first evidence of long-term survivors after multi-agent chemotherapy was reported (Ware et al. 1988; Newman et al. 1989). Since evidence of tumor volume reduction following preoperative chemotherapy has been demonstrated (Urban et al. 1993; Kadomatsu et al. 1992; Bisogno et al. 2002), chemotherapy is now routinely used in the treatment of USL. There are no known prognostic factors but patients with persistently unresectable tumor, multifocal lesions, and tumor rupture have been associated with a poorer prognosis (Bisogno et al. 2002; Uchiyama et al. 2001).

The initial surgical approach must be carefully planned with the help of radiological investigations. When a complete tumor resection is unlikely to be achieved, surgery should not be aggressive and be limited to a biopsy to establish the diagnosis. An open biopsy is usually required. The cystic nature of the lesions and the presence of necrotic material, with neoplastic cells only present in the septa, often preclude a final diagnosis when fine needle aspiration or tru cut biopsy are used.

Multi-agent chemotherapy has produced varying degrees of tumor volume reduction in more than 60% of patients (Bisogno et al. 2002; Horowitz et al. 1987) in the most representative series. Chemosensitivity of USL has also been demonstrated by the histological examination of the post-chemotherapy resected lesions where total or subtotal (more than 95%) tumor necrosis was documented (Urban et al. 1993; Moon et al. 1995;

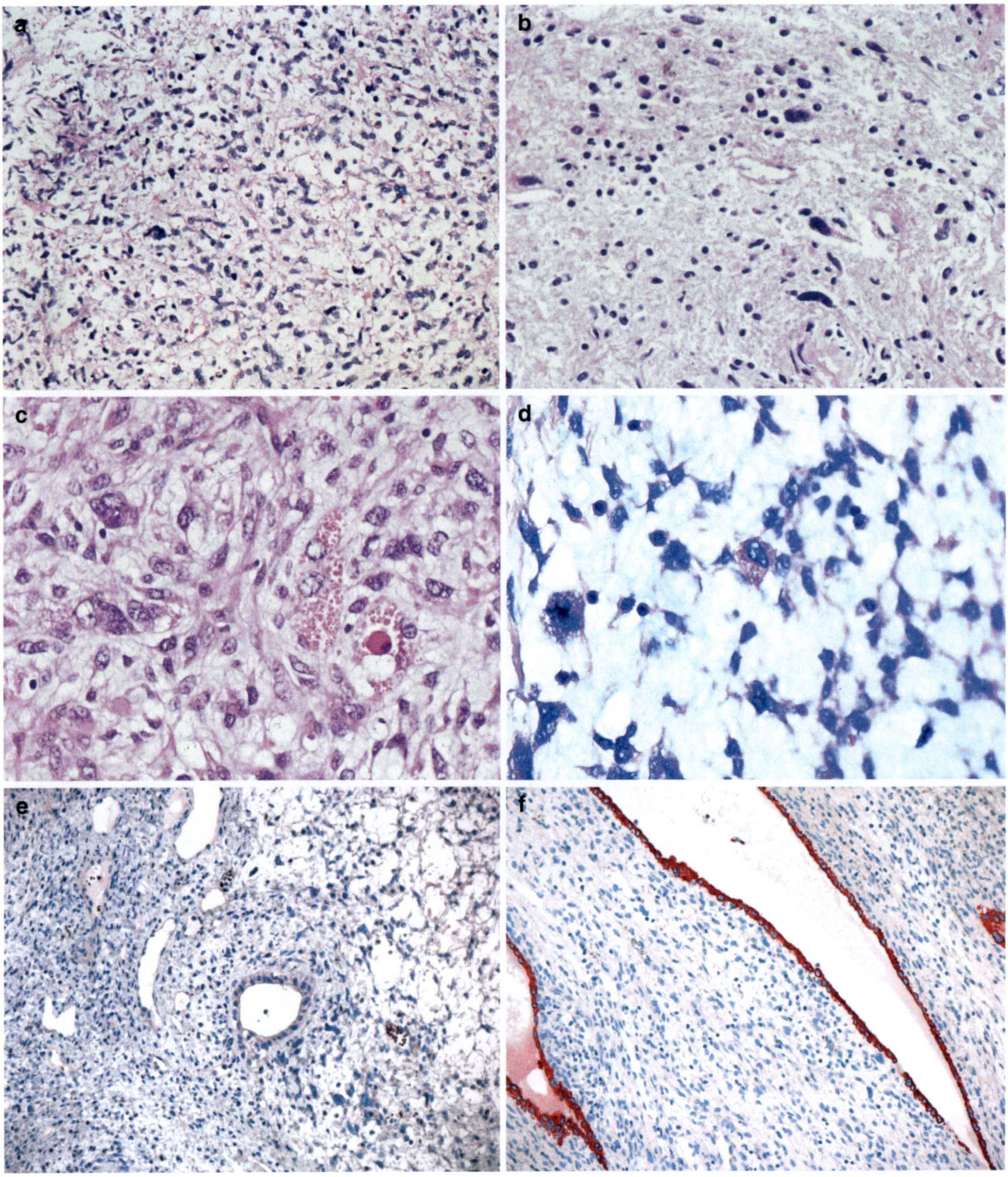

Fig. 17.1 (**a**) Undifferentiated (embryonal) sarcoma (USL). Note the loose mesenchymal tissue consisting of spindle and stellate cells (hematoxylin and eosin stain). (**b**) At higher magnification, pleomorphic giant cells typical for USL are seen (hematoxylin and eosin stain). (**c**) In this part of USL there are few giant cells containing eosinophilic globular inclusions, a characteristic feature of this tumor (hematoxylin and eosin stain). (**d**) The inclusions shown in C are PAS-positive. Note the stellate character of some of the tumor cells (PAS stain). (**e**) Neoplastic tissue of USL tends to grow around preexisting bile ducts, forming a neoplastic tissue sheath (hematoxylin and eosin stain). (**f**) The bile ducts located within the tumor tissue are sometimes markedly dilated (cytokeratin-19 immunostain)

Bisogno et al. 2002). In some of these cases, tumor reduction was minimal in size due to the cysts not shrinking after chemotherapy. The use of chemotherapy in the adjuvant setting is more debatable. Occasional patients cured with surgery alone have been reported (Walker et al. 1992), but the majority of studies report disappointing results (Lack et al. 1991; Aoyama et al. 1991), so that chemotherapy should also be considered in case of radical tumor resection or in case of microscopic residuals. The chemotherapy regimens used against USL are usually based on the experience derived from the treatment of sarcoma (Table 17.3). Ultimately, it is quite difficult to decide which drugs included in the polychemotherapy regimens employed are the most effective. Alkylating-based regimens with or without anthracyclines have shown to be effective (Urban et al. 1993; Bisogno et al. 2002). The IVA (ifosfamide, vincristine, actinomycin-D) or VAIA (IVA plus adriamycin) combinations are currently used in most European countries. The combination of CDDP and ADR also seems effective, even for ruptured tumors (Uchiyama et al. 2001).

Radiotherapy has been utilized in children with USL, especially when surgical margins were not tumor-free or the tumor invaded the nearby organs such as diaphragm or inferior vena cava. However, there is no evidence of its activity and hepatic toxicity may be a dose limiting factor (Horowitz et al. 1987; Bisogno et al. 2002). Despite the effectiveness of chemotherapy, there is no evidence that chemotherapy alone or in combination with radiotherapy can cure these patients.

In conclusion, when tumors are resectable at diagnosis, patients should be treated with complete resection and postoperative chemotherapy. When tumors are unresectable at diagnosis, chemotherapy should be administered before surgery. If complete resection is difficult, even after chemotherapy, and there is no regional

Table 17.3 Summary of the most recently published series on USL

	No. of pts	Age (years)	Treatment (no. of pts)	Type of CT	Outcome
Leuschner et al. (1990)	9	4–19	5 S only (5) 3 S+CT (3) One unknown (1)	Not specified	Four alive (Two after S only)
Lack et al. (1991)	16	2–21	S only (5) S+RT (2) S+CT (7) S+CT+RT (2)	Different combinations	Two alive NED (No pts after S only)
Aoyama et al. (1991)	8	2–13	S only (1) S+CT (5) Embolization (1) Unknown (1)	Different combinations	No pts alive NED reported
Walker (1992)	4	7–29	S only 2 S+Ct in 2	VAC	Three alive NED (Two pts after S only)
Kadomatsu et al. (1992)	3	4–11	S+CT	VACAd/VAdCP	Two alive NED
Urban et al. (1993)	4	6–13	S+CT (3) S+CT+RT (1)	VAIAd/PIAdV	Four alive NED
Webber et al. (1999)	7	2–12	S+Ct (7)	Different combinations of Ad C E I P FU V	Four alive NED
Kim et al. (2002)	6	7–13	S+CT (6)	VAC	Five alive NED
Bisogno et al. (2002)	17	4–16	S+CT (15) S+Ct+RT (2)	VACAd/VAIAd	Twelve alive NED
Nicol (2007)	20	0–21	S+CT (14) S+CT+RT (6)	VAC±I±E	Eighteen alive
Okajima et al. (2009)	3	10–15	S+CT (3)	VAdrC P E	Three alive NED

S surgery, *CT* chemotherapy, *RT* radiotherapy, *NED* no evidence of disease; drugs: *V* vincristine, *A* actinomycin-D, *C* cyclophosphamide, *I* ifosfamide, *Ad* Adriamicin, *P* cisplatin, *E* etoposide, *FU* fluorouracil extrahepatic spread, liver transplantion may be considered (Okajima et al. 2009).

17.2.5.2 Therapy in Case of Tumor Rupture

Tumor rupture may occur at diagnosis or during surgical procedures. In a review of published reports, tumor rupture has been found in 6.5% of patients (Uchiyama et al. 2001). At diagnosis patients may present with severe abdominal pain and bleeding with a risk of hypovolemic shock. When tumor cell dissemination in the abdominal cavity has occurred, surgical complete resection is impossible. An analysis of 14 patients with tumor rupture treated with surgery and chemotherapy showed that only 6 were alive without evidence of recurrence (Ida et al 2009). Relapse occurred mainly in the abdominal cavity. This shows that chemotherapy may control the tumor dissemination in a substantial number of patients but not in all. The use of whole abdominal irradiation, often used in other disseminated soft tissue sarcoma, has not been reported.

17.2.5.3 Therapy of Multifocal Tumors

USL may initially present with multiple lesions involving most of the liver lobes, making the tumor unresectable. Chemotherapy may be useful but a high risk of relapse exists. In a series of 17 patients, 2 presented with multiple hepatic lesions and both died following a local relapse, even though they showed a good response to initial chemotherapy and subsequent surgery showed no tumor in the resected specimen (Bisogno et al. 2002). One more patient with multifocal USL has been described with the same poor outcome (Walker et al. 1992). In this situation, liver transplantation might be considered after an extensive search for regional or distant metastases, but limited experience exists.

17.2.5.4 Relapsing Tumor

Local or distant relapse may occur even after apparently complete tumor resection. When a liver recurrence is evident, surgery and second-line chemotherapy may be proposed again. A combination of platinum derivatives associated with etoposide has been used with controversial results (Bisogno et al. 2002; Kelly et al. 2009). A complete tumor resection remains the goal of treatment and liver transplantation is a potential treatment option for localized recurrent USL relapse as recently described (Kelly et al. 2009).

In conclusion, the most recent studies suggest that the prognosis of USL has improved over time for a concurrence of factors. Progress in diagnostic tools has contributed to better define the tumor extension and help plan surgery. A better supportive therapy has allowed reducing the postoperative mortality and complications. Finally, use of a defined multimodal treatment including surgery and effective, sarcoma-like chemotherapy has increased the number of resectable tumors and has sterilized possible circulating or residual cells. An international collaboration, similar to the one achieved for other liver tumor, is desirable to better understand the biology of USL and further improve the results.

17.3 Hepatobiliary Rhabdomyosarcoma

17.3.1 Introduction

Rhabdomyosarcoma (RMS) is the most common pediatric soft tissue sarcoma and can virtually arise in any part of the body including the liver. It originates from the biliary tree and less frequently from the gallbladder, cystic duct, and ampulla of Vater (Spunt et al. 2000; Perera et al. 2009). It is a very rare tumor and only 25 patients (0.5%) with biliary RMS have been identified among the 4,291 cases registered in the Intergroup Rhabdomyosarcoma Studies I to IV. Median age at presentation was 3.4 years, significantly lower than other patients with RMS (Spunt et al. 2000).

Hepatobiliary RMS in childhood is typical of the embryonal or botryoid subtypes that present, in general, a better prognosis than the alveolar subtype. It may spread outside the liver to involve the duodenum, diaphragm, and mesenteric lymph nodes. Metastases to the liver parenchyma, peritoneum, bone, and lungs have been described (Spunt et al. 2000; Lack et al. 1991).

17.3.2 Clinical Presentation and Diagnosis

The common presenting symptom is obstructive jaundice associated with abdominal pain, vomiting, fever,

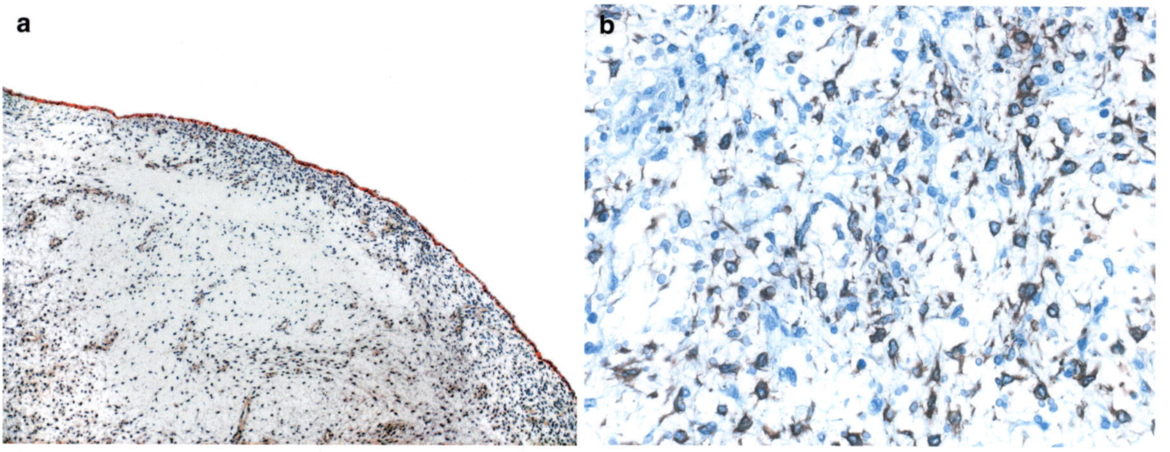

Fig. 17.2 Hepatobiliary rhabdomyosarcoma. (**a**) Rhabdomyosarcoma (embryonal type) protruding into a bile duct lumen (the botryoid growth pattern). The biliary epithelium is flattened owing to atrophy (in *red*). Note the hypercellular band underneath the epithelium, the so-called cambium (cytokeratin-19 immunostain). (**b**) The stellate tumor cells express a myocyte lineage marker, desmin (in *brown*) (desmin immunostain)

and poor appetite (Table 17.2). Laboratory investigations demonstrate moderate to marked conjugated hyperbilirubinemia, with mild elevations of transaminase levels (Spunt et al. 2000). This may help distinguish it from infectious hepatitis that is often the initial suspect.

US and CT scan are helpful to document that biliary obstruction is caused by solid tumor masses that may bulge into the biliary tract cavities, forming the typical grape-like aspect known from other mucosal surfaces (hence the name, botryoid) and variegated filling defects at imaging. MRI offers a more accurate assessment of the extent and number of lesions and their relationship to the hepatic vasculature. A low intensity signal is evident on T1-weighted images with intense but inhomogeneous contrast enhancement, while on T2-weighted images the tumor appears hyperintense. MR cholangiography has also been used to study the extent of biliary tract involvement (Roebuct et al. 1998). Diagnosis is not always simple and the dilatation of the extrahepatic biliary tree has caused confusion with choledochal cyst in some cases (Tireli et al. 2005). An exploratory laparotomy with biopsy is usually required to establish the diagnosis.

17.3.3 Pathology

Macroscopically, the growth of hepatobiliary RMS mainly involves medium-to large-sized bile ducts, with formation of soft and sometimes transparent tumor masses bulging into the lumens. Histologically, the tumor reveals the loose pattern typical for embryonal RMS, with often inconspicuous-looking stellate cells. Underneath the biliary epithelium, the cellularity may be higher (the so-called cambium; Fig. 17.2a). Immunohistochemically, the cells are reactive for muscle lineage markers, that is, desmin (Fig. 17.2b), myogenin, and MyoD.

17.3.4 Treatment

Since the tumor may remain localized to the bile ducts, resection of even very large tumors with biliary reconstruction may be possible. Reduction of tumor bulking was correlated with prognosis in early reports (Martinez et al. 1982). However, a complete tumor resection is unlikely to be achieved, so aggressive surgery at diagnosis is discouraged (Spunt et al. 2000).

The tumor is staged and treatment with chemotherapy and radiotherapy is given according to the protocols for RMS. Vincristine, dactinomycin, and cyclophosphamide or ifosfamide, have proven to be effective in reducing the tumor mass. This may allow a delayed conservative surgery with the intent to resect the tumor and leave the biliary tree structurally and functionally intact. Radiotherapy in the range 40–50 Gy is recommended according to the residual disease and response to chemotherapy.

Treatment of hepatobiliary RMS poses peculiar problems related to biliary tract obstruction. A stent placement is recommended to restore the biliary flow. External drainages have also been used, but they are associated with an increased risk of complications such as ascending cholangitis and peritonitis that may be fatal. In the presence of cholestasis chemotherapeutic agents, such as doxorubicin and vincristine, should be used with caution. Bilirubin elevation should not be considered, however, as a contraindication to the administration of chemotherapy and is determinant to reduce the mass compression to the biliary tract (Spunt et al. 2000).

The prognosis of biliary RMS has improved over time, and by use of modern multidisciplinary strategies the 5-year survival for patients with nonmetastatic disease approached 80%. In case of metastatic disease the prognosis remains very poor (Spunt et al. 2000).

17.4 Malignant Rhabdoid Tumor of the Liver

Extracranial malignant rhabdoid tumors (MRT), like their CNS counterparts, are rare, highly aggressive, and frequently lethal tumors of childhood. MRT has been reported widely at most anatomical sites in the body and very few cases have been described arising from the liver. Biological and morphologic aspects of these lesions are discussed in Chap. 8.

MRT is characterized by resistance to chemotherapy. So, when the tumor is unresectable, prognosis is dismal although sporadical case reports document potential for cure with multimodal therapy (Ravindra et al. 2002).

17.5 Angiosarcoma of the Liver

17.5.1 Introduction

Hepatic angiosarcoma (HAS) is extremely rare in pediatric age. It is a highly aggressive vascular tumor composed of malignant spindle cells of endothelial origin. A female predominance and mean age of presentation of 3.7 year have been reported (Noronha and Gonzalez-Crussi 1984). Pediatric HAS has been regarded as a distinct entity from the HAS seen in adults, which is most common in males and presents a peak incidence in the sixth and seventh decades (Ishak et al. 1999). Causes of HAS in children are unknown. In adults, exposure to environmental toxins (vinylchloride, arsenic) or drugs (anabolic steroids, synthetic estrogens) have been correlated to HAS, but only one pediatric case has been reported after arsenic exposure (Falk et al. 1981). Several case reports have described HAS arising in infantile hemangioendothelioma (Selby et al. 1992) and children with multiple cutaneous hemangiomas have presented with hepatic lesions later found to be HAS (Nord et al. 2006).

17.5.2 Clinical Presentation and Diagnosis

In children, HAS usually presents with a rapidly enlarging abdominal mass, and by the time they are diagnosed, the lesion is often very large, may involve both liver lobes or be multifocal rendering the tumor unresectable. Other signs and symptoms include jaundice, abdominal pain, fever, and dyspnea (Emre and McKenna 2004). Metastatic dissemination is common, frequently to the lung, but also to lymph nodes, pleura, bone, and adrenal glands (Selby et al. 1992).

Ultrasound demonstrates a mixture of hyperechoic and hypoechoic regions that correspond to hemorrhage and necrosis. On unenhanced CT scans, the tumor shows multiple hypodense areas with vague borders. With contrast, the CT scan resembles a hemangioma, with peripheral filling followed by centripetal opacification of the lesion and subsequent puddling of the contrast throughout the tumor (Peterson et al. 2000).

17.5.3 Pathology

Macroscopically, adult-type HAS occurring in the liver of children is solitary or multiple tumor nodules that typically show a hemorrhagic aspect, mainly on the cut surface. Massive angioinvasion may be evident at gross examination. Histologically, the lesions often consist of spindled cells arranged in bundles, but slit-like vascular spaces lined by atypical endothelial cells with hob-nail features may also be noted. Mitotic activity is variable but may be prominent. The neoplastic cells express endothelial lineage markers (Factor VIII-associated antigen and CD31). A distinct type of presentation is that following a diagnosis of infantile hemangioendothelioma type II, thought to be a sarcomatous change in a formerly benign lesion (see below).

17.5.4 Treatment

The mortality rate for pediatric HAS is high, and death usually occurs within the first 2 years from diagnosis (Selby et al. 1992). Complete resection is thought to be curative, but it is often impossible at diagnosis due to the tumor burden. There are anecdotal reports on the effectiveness of intensive chemotherapy in reducing the tumor volume making a delayed radical resection possible (Gunawardena et al. 1997).

The growth pattern and the treatment results have led to consider liver transplantation, but the experience so far accumulated, although mainly on adult patients, is not encouraging, because relapse and death occurred within a year of transplantation in most cases (Hoti and Adam 2008).

The search for new and more effective drugs has been hampered by the rarity of the tumor. Among antineoplastic drugs paclitaxel has gained interest because tumor responses have been recently described. A retrospective analysis of 32 patients treated in EORTC Centers with paclitaxel as single agent reported a response rate of 62%. It is to be noted that no angiosarcoma located in the liver were present in this series and the response rate (78%) appeared superior for angiosarcoma of the face and scalp (Schlemmer et al. 2008).

A more limited but meaningful effect of paclitaxel have been reported in a prospective phase II study enrolling 30 patients with metastatic or relapsed angiosarcoma, including 9 with liver tumor. Paclitaxel was administered weekly to increase the dose intensity. Five patients had an objective response and three of them with locally advanced disease were amenable to surgery, with two complete histologic responses and long disease-free survival (17 and 19 months) (Penel et al. 2008).

Promising reports documenting a response to antiangiogenetic agents or tyrosine kinase inhibitors have been recently published. Evidence of a complete pathologic response has been reported in two patients with angiosarcoma of the nose treated preoperatively with bevacizumab and concurrent radiotherapy (Koontz et al. 2008)

Sorafenib has been found active in a phase II trial including 37 patients with metastatic angiosarcoma. Five patients experienced partial or complete tumor shrinkage for a response rate of 14% (Maki et al. 2009). Sunitinib may also be effective (Yoo et al. 2009), while imatinib was inactive in 16 angiosarcoma patients as part of a phase II study (Chugh et al. 2009). Since these recent experiences included only adult patients, information on pediatric HAS is lacking.

17.6 Other Hepatic Vascular Tumors

17.6.1 Infantile Hepatic Hemangioendothelioma

The term infantile hepatic hemangioendothelioma (IHHE) has traditionally been used to describe different neoplasms of vascular origin with different histologic patterns and clinical behavior. In 1971, Dehner and Ishak proposed the subclassification of IHHE into two histologic groups. (a) Type 1 IHHE, the more common subtype, is composed of capillary-sized vessels lined by a single layer of somewhat plump but bland endothelial cells with rare mitotic figures (Fig. 17.3a and b). (b) Type 2 IHHE is composed of vessels with more pleomorphic endothelial cells and is often difficult to distinguish from HAS. In fact, some authors now consider type 2 IHHE as a distinct form of pediatric low-grade angiosarcoma. IHHE accounts for up to 12% of all pediatric liver tumors. In 80% of the cases, the tumor presents in the first 6 postnatal months. Girls are more frequently affected than boys (female-to-male = 1.5 to 2:1) (Selby et al 1994). IHHE may cause significant high-flow vascular shunts resulting in cardiac failure in about 25% of the patients with large tumors. Some cases of IHHE are associated with hypothyroidism as a result of activity of type 3 iodothyronine deiodinase in the tumor, and few patients have been shown to have elevated serum alfa-fetoprotein, causing difficulties in differential diagnosis. Aspects of diagnosis and treatment of IHHE are dealt with in the chapter on Liver Transplantation.

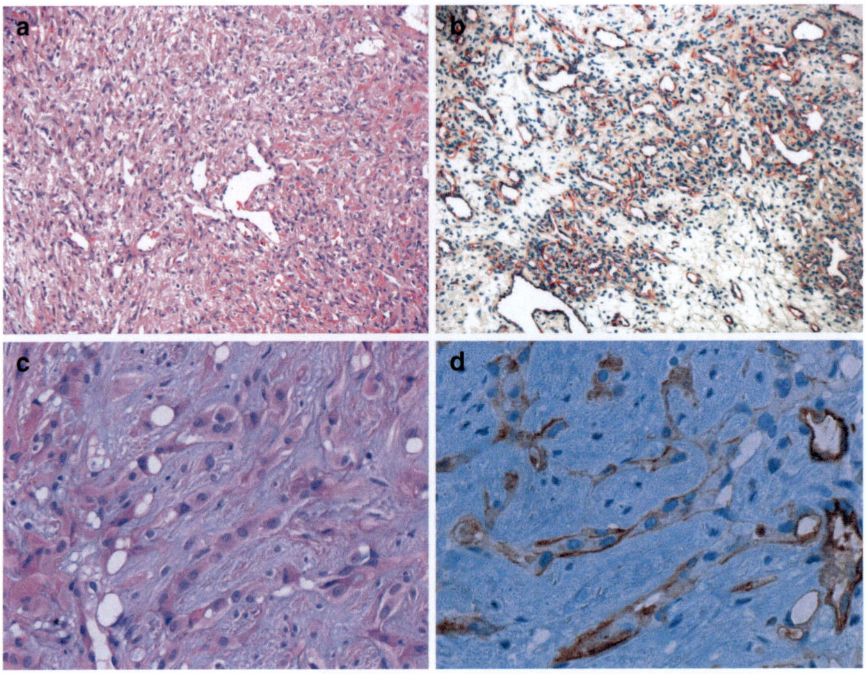

Fig. 17.3 Vascular tumors. (**a**) Infantile hepatic hemangioendothelioma (IHHE). Most of the vascular channels are narrow or slit-like (hematoxylin and eosin stain). (**b**) The endothelial lining of the vascular channels in IHHE are reactive for an endothelial marker (in *red*; CD31 immunostain). (**c**) Hepatic epithelioid hemangioendothelioma (HEHE). Note the strands of epithelioid cells within a stroma. The cells are typically vacuolated (hematoxylin and eosin stain). (**d**) The cells of HEHE are positive for CD31 (in *brown*; CD31 immunostain)

17.6.2 Epithelioid Hemangioendothelioma of the Liver

Epithelioid hemangioendothelioma is a slow-growing vascular tumor, which consist of endothelial cells that morphologically resemble epithelial cells. Being mainly a tumor of adult patients, pediatric cases are rare and usually involved children in the age group 12–14 years. Epithelioid hemangioendothelioma may show a distinct growth pattern with sometimes several nodules showing umbilication at the capsular surface. Histologically, medium sized to large cells with characteristic vacuoles form cords that surround slit-like spaces (Fig. 17.3a). Irrespective of their epithelioid morphology, the cells express endothelial lineage markers (Fig. 17.3b). The treatment of these lesions is discussed in the chapter on Liver Transplantation.

17.7 Mesenchymal Hamartoma

17.7.1 Introduction

Mesenchymal hamartoma of the liver (MHL) is a benign tumor that typically presents in the first 3 years of life (85%) as a large multicystic liver mass. It is the second most common benign hepatic tumor of childhood. Males are slightly more affected (Stringer and Alizai 2005). MHL has traditionally been regarded as a benign tumor-like malformation characterized by a disorganized but limited proliferation of mature cells (Fig. 17.4). However, recent evidence of karyotype abnormalities have suggested a mesenchymal clonal genetic defect (Bove et al. 1998) supporting a neoplastic nature. MHL may be associated with a disorder of the placenta, mesenchymal stem villus hyperplasia.

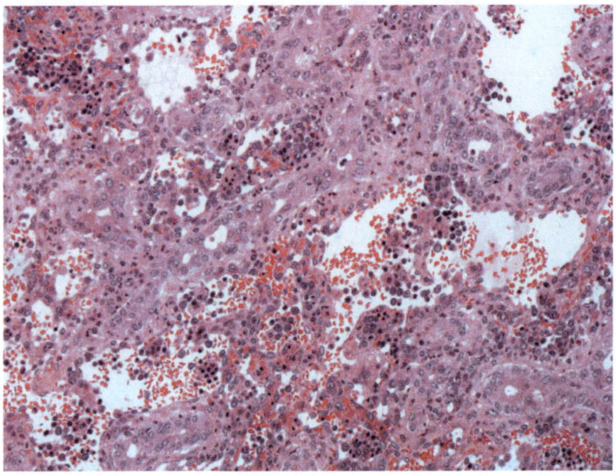

Fig. 17.4 Mesenchymal hamartoma of the liver. The tumor exhibits a complex mixture of vascular channels, small bile ducts, and mesenchymal cells. Within the vascular spaces, hematopoietic foci are seen (hematoxylin and eosin stain)

17.7.2 Clinical Presentation and Diagnosis

MHL may be an incidental finding in an otherwise healthy child or can present with abdominal distension and/or an upper abdominal mass. The tumor has also been detected by prenatal ultrasound where it can cause severe hydrops (Dickinson et al. 1999; Laberge et al. 2005). Imaging investigations demonstrate a multiloculated cystic lesion with a variable amount of solid tissue that may be predominant in some cases when cysts are very small (Koumanidou et al. 1999; Mansour et al. 2005). On contrast CT the solid component, septa and a peripheral rim may be enhanced similar to more aggressive tumors. On MRI a low signal intensity on T1-weighted sequences, but a variable signal intensity on T2-weighted is reported. MHL constitutes a challenging lesion in many aspects concerning diagnosis and risk of malignancy. MHL must be distinguished from parasitic and congenital cysts, and other liver tumors. It is noteworthy that the serum alfafetoprotein concentration may be moderately elevated, and some children have therefore been inappropriately treated for HB (Boman et al. 2004). More demanding is the differential diagnosis with USL, which shares a similar radiologic aspect, but usually affects older children.

A small but proven risk of malignant transformation from MHL to USL has been reported. USL can develop within a preexisting MHL or occur several years after an incomplete excision of the MHL (O'Sullivan et al. 2001; Corbally and Spitz 1992). A possible common origin of these two lesions is supported by similar features on radiology, histology, and cytogenetic abnormalities (see above), where an aberration involving the chromosome 19q13 region has been found in cells from an MHL complicated by UES (O'Sullivan et al. 2001).

17.7.3 Treatment

Although few cases of spontaneous regression have been reported, a complete resection of the lesion with tumor-free margins is reputed necessary to avoid relapse and malignant transformation (Stringer and Alizai 2005). In rare cases, where MHL were deemed unresectable, other surgical techniques including incomplete resection, marsupialization of the cysts, and liver transplantation have been employed. However, high rates of relapse or postsurgical complications have been reported (Meinders et al. 1998; Tepetes et al. 1995). In a few cases chemotherapy has been administered with controversial results: in one case vincristine was ineffective (Silber et al. 1970), while cyclophosphamide and hydrocortisone caused a shrinkage of a highly vascular MHL (Alkalay et al. 1985). Finally radiotherapy was used for a large MHL wrapped around the inferior vena cava with evidence of a smaller and more sclerotic lesion at operation 10 weeks later (Srouji et al. 1978).

17.8 Conclusion

Among primary hepatic mesenchymal tumors, a distinct subset shares with HBs the patient's young age at presentation and certain imaging features. This chiefly applies to hemangioendotheliomas and mesenchymal hamartoma, which therefore demand a special diagnostic workup to avoid misdiagnosis and subsequent overtreatment. Monitoring of serum alpha-fetoprotein (AFP) is usually helpful, but one has to bear in mind that, on the one hand, mesenchymal tumors may cause AFP elevation and, on the other hand, certain subtypes of HB exhibit low or normal serum AFP levels. Part of hepatic mesenchymal tumors involve both liver lobes and can now successfully be treated by liver transplantation. For highly aggressive lesions such as undifferentiated sarcoma, novel chemotherapy strategies will more and more improve the formerly dismal outcome. The rapidly advancing knowledge of molecular features occurring in mesenchymal tumors may hopefully serve to develop more tumor-specific or even individualized therapies in the future.

References

Alkalay AL, Puri AR, Pomerance JJ, Kallus M, Gans SL, Hurvitz CH, Farber SJ, Sloninsky L (1985) Mesenchymal hamartoma of the liver responsive to cyclophosphamide therapy: therapeutic approach. J Pediatr Surg 20(2): 125–128

Aoyama C, Hachitanda Y, Sato JK, Said JW, Shimada H (1991) Undifferentiated (embryonal) sarcoma of the liver. A tumor of uncertain histogenesis showing divergent differentiation. Am J Surg Pathol 15(7):615–624

Bisogno G, Pilz T, Perilongo G, Ferrari A, Harms D, Ninfo V, Treuner J, Carli M (2002) Undifferentiated sarcoma of the liver in childhood: a curable disease. Cancer 94(1): 252–257

Boman F, Bossard C, Fabre M et al (2004) Mesenchymal hamartomas of the liver may be associated with increased serum alpha fetoprotein concentrations and mimic hepatoblastomas. Eur J Pediatr Surg 14:63–66

Bove KE, Blough RI, Soukup S (1998) Third report of t(19q)(13.4) in mesenchymal hamartoma of the liver with comments on link to embryonal sarcoma. Pediatr Dev Pathol 1:438–442

Chugh R, Wathen JK, Maki RG, Benjamin RS, Patel SR, Meyers PA, Priebat DA, Reinke DK, Thomas DG, Keohan ML, Samuels BL, Baker LH (2009) Phase II multicenter trial of imatinib in 10 histologic subtypes of sarcoma using a bayesian hierarchical statistical model. J Clin Oncol 27(19):3148–3153

Corbally MT, Spitz L (1992) Malignant potential of mesenchymal hamartoma: an unrecognised risk. Pediatr Surg Int 7:321–322

Dickinson JE, Knowles S, Phillips JM (1999) Prenatal diagnosis of hepatic mesenchymal hamartoma. Prenat Diagn 19:81–84

Emre S, McKenna GJ (2004) Liver tumors in children. Pediatr Transpl 8:632–638

Falk H, Herbert JT, Edmonds L, Heath CW Jr, Thomas LB, Popper H (1981) Review of four cases of childhood hepatic angiosarcoma-elevated environmental arsenic exposure in one case. Cancer 47:382–391

Gunawardena SW, Trautwein LM, Finegold MJ et al (1997) Hepatic angiosarcoma in a child: successful therapy with surgery and adjuvant chemotherapy. Med Pediatr Oncol 28:139–143

Horowitz ME, Etcubanas E, Webber BL, Kun LE, Rao BN, Vogel RJ et al (1987) Hepatic undifferentiated (embryonal) sarcoma and rhabdomyosarcoma in children. Cancer 59:396–402

Hoti E, Adam R (2008) Liver transplantation for primary and metastatic liver cancers. Transpl Int 21(12):1107–1117

Ida S, Okajima H, Hayashida S, Takeichi T, Asonuma K, Baba H, Inomata Y (2009) Undifferentiated sarcoma of the liver. Am J Surg.198:e7-9

Ishak KG, Goodman ZD, Stocker JT (1999) Tumors of the liver and intrahepatic bile ducts (atlas of tumor pathology). Armed Forces Institute of Pathology, Washington, pp 293–307

Jha P, Chawla SC, Tavri S, Patel C, Gooding C, Daldrup-Link H (2009) Pediatric liver tumors – a pictorial review. Eur Radiol 19(1):209–219

Kadomatsu K, Nakagawara A, Zaizen Y, Nagoshi M, Tsuneyoshi M, Fukushige T et al (1992) Undifferentiated (embryonal) sarcoma of the liver: report of three cases. Surg Today 22:451–455

Kelly MJ, Martin L, Alonso M, Altura RA (2009) Liver transplant for relapsed undifferentiated embryonal sarcoma in a young child. J Pediatr Surg 44(12):e1–e3

Kim DY, Kim KH, Jung SE, Lee SC, Park KW, Kim WK (2002) Undifferentiated (embryonal) sarcoma of the liver: combination treatment by surgery and chemotherapy. J Pediatr Surg 37(10):1419–1423

Koontz BF, Miles EF, Rubio MA, Madden JF, Fisher SR, Scher RL, Brizel DM (2008) Preoperative radiotherapy and bevacizumab for angiosarcoma of the head and neck: two case studies. Head Neck 30(2):262–266

Koumanidou C, Vakaki M, Papadaki M et al (1999) New sonographic appearance of hepatic mesenchymal hamartoma in childhood. J Clin Ultrasound 27:164–167

Laberge JM, Patenaude Y, Desilets V et al (2005) Large hepatic mesenchymal hamartoma leading to mid-trimester fetal demise. Fetal Diagn Ther 20:141–145

Lack EE, Schloo BL, Azumi N, Travis WD, Grier HE, Kozakewich HP (1991) Undifferentiated (embryonal) sarcoma of the liver. Clinical and pathologic study of 16 cases with emphasis on immunohistochemical features. Am J Surg Pathol 15(1):1–16

Leuschner I, Schmidt D, Harms D (1990) Undifferentiated sarcoma of the liver in childhood: morphology, flow cytometry, and literature review. Hum Pathol 21(1):68–76

Maki RG, D'Adamo DR, Keohan ML, Saulle M, Schuetze SM, Undevia SD, Livingston MB, Cooney MM, Hensley ML, Mita MM, Takimoto CH, Kraft AS, Elias AD, Brockstein B, Blachère NE, Edgar MA, Schwartz LH, Qin LX, Antonescu CR, Schwartz GK (2009) Phase II study of sorafenib in patients with metastatic or recurrent sarcomas. J Clin Oncol 27(19):3133–3140

Mansour A, Qandeel M, Sughayer M et al (2005) Solid (stromal predominance) hepatic mesenchymal hamartoma. Pediatr Radiol 35:349–350

Martinez-FLA, Haase GM, Koep LJ et al (1982) Rhabdomyosarcoma of the biliary tree: the case for aggressive surgery. J Pediatr Surg 17:508–511

Meinders AJ, Simons MP, Heij HA et al (1998) Mesenchymal hamartoma of the liver: failed management by marsupialization. J Pediatr Gastroenterol Nutr 26:353–355

Moon WK, Kim WS, Choi BI, Kim IO, Yeon KM, Han MC (1995) Undifferentiated embryonal sarcoma of the liver treated with chemotherapy: CT imaging in four patients. Abdom Imaging 20:133–137

Newman KD, Schisgall R, Reaman G, Guzzetta PC (1989) Malignant mesenchymoma of the liver in children. J Pediatr Surg 24:781–783

Nicol K, Savell V, Moore J, Teot L, Spunt SL, Qualman S (2007) Distinguishing undifferentiated embryonal sarcoma of the liver from biliary tract rhabdomyosarcoma: a Children's Oncology Group study. Pediatr Dev Pathol 10:89–97

Nord KM, Kandel J, Lefkowitch JH, Lobritto SJ, Morel KD, North PE, Garzon MC (2006) Multiple cutaneous infantile hemangiomas associated with hepatic angiosarcoma: case report and review of the literature. Pediatrics 118(3): e907–e913

Noronha R, Gonzalez-Crussi F (1984) Hepatic angiosarcoma in childhood. Am J Surg Pathol 8:863–871

O'Sullivan MJ, Swanson PE, Knoll J, Taboada EM, Dehner LP (2001) Undifferentiated embryonal sarcoma with unusual features arising within mesenchymal hamartoma of the liver: report of a case and review of the literature. Pediatr Dev Pathol 4(5):482–489

Okajima H, Ohya Y, Lee KJ, Yamamoto H, Asonuma K, Nagaoki Y, Ohama K, Korogi M, Anan T, Hashiyama M, Endo F, Iyama K, Inomata Y (2009) Management of undifferentiated sarcoma of the liver including living donor liver transplantation as a backup procedure. J Pediatr Surg 44(2):e33–e38

Penel N, Bui BN, Bay JO, Cupissol D, Ray-Coquard I, Piperno-Neumann S, Kerbrat P, Fournier C, Taieb S, Jimenez M, Isambert N, Peyrade F, Chevreau C, Bompas E, Brain EG, Blay JY (2008) Phase II trial of weekly paclitaxel for unresectable angiosarcoma: the ANGIOTAX Study. J Clin Oncol 26(32):5269–5274

Perera MT, McKiernan PJ, Brundler MA, Hobin DA, Mayer DA, Mirza DF, Sharif K (2009) Embryonal rhabdomyosarcoma of the ampulla of vater in early childhood: report of a case and review of literature. J Pediatr Surg 44(2):e9–e11

Perilongo G, Carli M, Sainati L, Cecchetto G, Mancini A, Cordero di Montezemolo L et al (1987) Undifferentiated (embryonal) sarcoma of the liver in childhood: results of a retrospective Italian study. Tumori 73:213–217

Peterson MS, Baron RL, Rankin SC (2000) Hepatic angiosarcoma: findings on multiphasic contrast-enhanced helical CT do not mimic hepatic hemangioma. AJR Am J Roentgenol 175:165–170

Ravindra KV, Cullinane C, Lewis IJ et al (2002) Long-term survival after spontaneous rupture of a malignant rhabdoid tumor of the liver. J Pediatr Surg 37:1488–1490

Roebuck DJ, Yang WT, Lam WW et al (1998) Hepatobiliary rhabdomyosarcoma in children: diagnostic radiology. Pediatr Radiol 28:101–108

Schlemmer M, Reichardt P, Verweij J, Hartmann JT, Judson I, Thyss A, Hogendoorn PC, Marreaud S, Van Glabbeke M, Blay JY (2008) Paclitaxel in patients with advanced angiosarcomas of soft tissue: a retrospective study of the EORTC soft tissue and bone sarcoma group. Eur J Cancer 44(16): 2433–2436

Selby DM, Stocker JT, Ishak KG (1992) Angiosarcoma of the liver in childhood. A clinicopathologic and follow-up study of 10 cases. Pediatr Pathol 12:485–498

Selby DM, Stocker JT, Waclawiw MA et al (1994) Infantile hemangioendothelioma of the liver. Hepatology 20:39–45

Silber DL, Soper RT, Kent TH (1970) Life-threatening mesenchymal hamartoma of the liver. J Pediatr Surg 5:471–472

Spunt SL, Lobe TE, Pappo AS et al (2000) Aggressive surgery is unwarranted for biliary tract rhabdomyosarcoma. J Pediatr Surg 35:309–316

Srouji MN, Chatten J, Schulman WM et al (1978) Mesenchymal hamartoma of the liver in infants. Cancer 42:2483–2489

Stocker JT, Ishak KG (1978) Undifferentiated (embryonal) sarcoma of the liver. Cancer 42:336–348

Stringer MD, Alizai NK (2005) Mesenchymal hamartoma of the liver: a systematic review. J Pediatr Surg 40(11): 1681–1690

Tepetes K, Selby R, Webb M et al (1995) Orthotopic liver transplantation for benign hepatic neoplasms. Arch Surg 130: 153–156

Tireli GA, Sander S, Dervisoglu S, Demirali O, Unal M (2005) Embryonal rhabdomyosarcoma of the common bile duct mimicking choledochal cyst. J Hepatobiliary Pancreat Surg 12(3):263–265

Uchiyama M, Iwafuchi M, Yagi M, Iinuma Y, Kanada S, Yamazaki S, Ohtaki M, Shirai Y (2001) Treatment of ruptured undifferentiated sarcoma of the liver in children: a report of two cases and review of the literature. J Hepatobiliary Pancreat Surg 8:87–91

Urban CE, Mache CJ, Schwinger W, Pakisch B, Ranner G, Riccabona M, Schimpl G, Brandesky G, Messner H, Pobegen W et al (1993) Undifferentiated (embryonal) sarcoma of the liver in childhood. Successful combined-modality therapy in four patients. Cancer 72(8):2511–2516

Walker NI, Horn MJ, Strong RW, Lynch SV, Cohen J, Ong TH, Harris OD (1992) Undifferentiated (embryonal) sarcoma of the liver. Pathologic findings and long-term survival after complete surgical resection. Cancer 69(1):52–59

Ware R, Friedman HS, Filston HC, Chaffee S, Kurtzberg J, Kinney TR, Falletta JM (1988) Childhood hepatic mesenchymoma: successful treatment with surgery and multiple-agent chemotherapy. Med Pediatr Oncol 16(1):62–65

Webber EM, Morrison KB, Pritchard SL, Sorensen PH (1999) Undifferentiated embryonal sarcoma of the liver: results of clinical management in one center. J Pediatr Surg 34(11): 1641–1644

Yoo C, Kim JE, Yoon SK, Kim SC, Ahn JH, Kim TW, Suh C, Lee JL (2009) Angiosarcoma of the retroperitoneum: report on a patient treated with sunitinib. Sarcoma 2009: 360875

18 Future Prospective

Giorgio Perilongo and Arthur Zimmermann

As documented in some of the chapters, in the last 3 decades, remarkable success has been achieved in the cure of hepatoblastoma (HB); in the late seventies the 5-year overall survival of children affected by this rare neoplasm was 30%; now it has more than doubled (Perilongo et al. 2009). Thus, at the beginning of this century, it can be stated that multidisciplinary approaches including conventional systemic chemotherapy has allowed the cure of more than two-third of the children diagnosed with hepatoblastoma. Remarkable refinements in the diagnostic capabilities, mainly related to the introduction of magnetic resonance images in daily clinical practice, in the surgical approach, in a more extensive and rational, use of orthotopic liver transplantation, in the supportive measures, in the use of systemic chemotherapy, and in tailoring treatment according to more and more individualized risk profiles are the facts that must be accounted to explain these gratifying results. However, it is a common assumption that to make further progress, that is, to cure those children affected by tumors, which are not amenable to any kind of radical surgery (including orthotopic liver transplantation), which are metastatic, do not respond to chemotherapy, recur, or present with low alpha-fetoprotein, different avenues must be envisaged.

G. Perilongo (✉)
Department of Pediatrics "Salus Pueri", University-Hospital of Padua, Via Giustiniani 3, 35128, Padua, Italy
e-mail: giorgio.perilongo@unipd.it

A. Zimmermann
Institute of Pathology of the University, Murtenstrasse 31, 3010 Berne, Switzerland
zimmerma@patho.unibe.ch

Biologically driven therapies are presently dominating the scenario of modern clinical research on human tumors; some initial significant benefits of these innovative agents on the cure of selected neoplasms, have been already firmly documented. In brief, only a better understanding of the intimate mechanisms of cancerogenesis would open new effective therapeutic frontiers. How are problems for HB to be addressed?

The hypothesis that HB derives from derangements of the genetic mechanisms regulating normal hepatic organogenesis is pretty well consolidated. Thus, for HB also embryologists and cancer biologists are expected to feed each others' research in order to find the molecular pathways shifting liver cell lineages from normality to malignancy, from normal ontogenesis to oncogenesis (Si-Tayeb et al. 2010; Wandzioch and Zaret 2009). The complexity of the mechanisms regulating hepatic organogenesis makes the task quite challenging but the direction is right. Actually solid hypotheses have already linked the different histologic subtypes of HB to specific stages of the arrest of normal hepatic organogenesis (Zimmermann 2005). The final targets are to identify which developmental, signaling, and transcriptional pathways are mainly affected, at which level, according to which mechanisms and, if more than one is involved, how they interplay among themselves.

For other childhood embryonal tumors, some insights into these intimate genetic mechanisms, which regulate normal organogenesis and, if altered, bring about tumor development, are already available. These insights have been developed by combining the findings derived from the fields of epidemiology, embryology, and cancer cell biology. For embryonal tumors, the hints for these types of studies have been derived from investigation into those rare cancer family syndromes predisposing to cancer growth. From this prospective,

A. Zimmermann et al. (eds.), *Pediatric Liver Tumors*, Pediatric Oncology,
DOI: 10.1007/978-3-642-14504-9_18, © Springer-Verlag Berlin Heidelberg 2011

the most notable example is the investigation into the Gorlin syndrome and the risk of developing medulloblastoma. Patients affected by Gorlin syndrome, a rare hereditary condition otherwise known as nevoid basal cell carcinoma (NBCC) syndrome, among various somatic abnormalities, have a higher tendency than the normal population to develop medulloblastoma (Lo Muzio 2008). The Gorlin syndrome has been associated with the PTCH gene (9q22.31) loss of function. The PTCH gene encodes a receptor for the signal peptide sonic hedgehog (SHH), which when linked to the PTCH receptors activates the Hedgehog pathway, a major developmental pathway in many organisms, from insects to mammals (Wong and Reiter 2008). Studies into normal cerebellum development have shown that Purkinje cells through soluble molecules ("signal peptides") – SHH – stimulate proliferation of external granular layer cells during cerebellum development through its receptor complex made up of the PTCH and Smoothened (SMO) proteins (Lee et al. 2010). Engineered mice heterozygous for mutated PTCH mimic several aspects of Gorlin's syndrome, including the propensity to develop both NBCC and to have an excessive proliferation of the granule cell precursor population at the surface of the cerebellum (Pazzaglia 2006), which are believed to represent the first step in tumor development. Both in vitro and in vivo models have shown that Cyclopamine (and its analogs), a modulator of the PTCH/SMO receptor activity, is capable of arresting the growth of cells bearing a constitutive PTCH gene loss of function (Enguita-Germán et al. 2010). Actually, cyclopamine analogues are presently entering human experimentation. All this has been cited as a successful example of how combining the results of research of those rare conditions bearing a high risk of cancer development, of normal organogenesis and of cancer cell biology may feed each other and promote innovative approaches. Remarkable, fascinating similar stories can be told for nephroblastoma and normal renal organogenesis. It is hoped that something similar can soon be developed for HB. Despite being exquisitively rare, a series of cancer family syndromes are associated with a higher risk of developing hepatoblastoma, including familial polyposis coli, Beckwith-Wiedemann syndrome, and related overgrowth syndromes. Those rare cancer family syndromes may allow identifyication of the early crucial events which favor cancer development. In this regard it is worth highlighting the fact that when a tumour is finally diagnosed, we usually deal with advanced and - with respect to tumour evolution - ''old'' lesions with massive genomic instability and late molecular changes.

No one can sell any findings with easy enthusiasm. In fact, the evidence seems to indicate that as soon as basic research comes up with new and, what almost always seems to be, definitive insights into cancer cell biology, immediately many other "doors" open unexpectedly. Furthermore, it would not be surprising to discover that the HB family represents quite a heterogeneous group of diseases also in terms of the fundamental underlying transcription pathways involved in their pathogenesis. This is just to anticipate that the path to the development of definitive cure based on biologically-driven innovative approaches is likely to be long.

The other important pipeline, which is expected to bring new insights into the genetic molecular mechanisms sustaining primary childhood hepatic tumor growth and development, is the one represented by modern "genomic medicine." In this context this term refers to all those techniques which are capable of profiling in an increasingly short period of time and at a rapidly decreasing cost, the entire cell genome (including single nucleotide polymorphism), its products and/or other components of the complex genetic machinery such as microRNA. The investigation into the gene profiling of childhood HB has already been initiated; its initial findings have been limited to tumor "*prognostification*" (Cairo et al. 2008). However, more information is forthcoming (Armengol et al. 2009).

If in a purely conceptual way all that has been stated is unquestionably true, special plans should be made for rare tumors, such as primary childhood liver tumors. Large-scale cooperation has, is, and will be the key to the success of clinical research on these rare neoplasms. In fact, it was only by collecting a large critical mass of patients that it has been possible to run meaningful, prospective, and clinical trials with sophisticated clinical designs. This remains important even when planning basic research projects; in fact, a significant amount of biological material must be made available to scientists and possibly linked to clinical information to speed up the investigation process. This is a major challenge for clinical and basic cancer research on rare tumors. The ones who will be involved in designing modern research strategies on HB must keep all this clearly in mind.

Another major problem interferes with the achievement of all the research success one would hope to make available for these children. The difficulty is in allowing children affected by rare tumors – like HB – access to new drugs. Indeed, in many ways children affected by this rare neoplasm suffer from the same problems that patients affected by other rare conditions have, which is the fact that they are "orphan patients": neglected by research, dedicated scientists, innovative drugs, financial drives, which makes industries develop new drugs and finally, denied easy access to new drugs.

Needless to say while we wait for all this to happen we have to continue to try to improve the prognosis for these children using the tools we have in our hands at this time. Clinical research has to continue. As mentioned earlier one of the major results of modern clinical research on HB is having identified an increasing number of different risk groups of patients by clinical, histological, and biological characteristics. Paradoxically, one would conclude that this achievement represents a problem for further clinical research. In fact, the identification of these different risk groups have de facto further fragmented the already small cohorts of children that the different cooperative groups in the world are collecting, thus making it difficult, if not impossible, to collect the critical numbers of patients needed to run meaningful, clinical trials. Of course this should be not a matter of concern but a reason for looking for new ways of clinical research such as overcoming the boundaries within which the different study groups have so far run their own trials. We believe that an increased international cooperation is urgently needed; work should be done to have emerging countries like India and China join in future research cooperative efforts. Telematic communications is allowing to conceive of totally new ways of working together. We must move with determination in these directions as otherwise the children with HB will be deprived of all the benefits that modern basic and clinical research can bring to them.

References

Armengol C, Cairo S, Fabre M et al (2009) Wnt signaling and hepatocarcinogenesis: the hepatoblastoma model. Int J Biochem Cell Biol [Epub ahead of print 10.1016/j.biocel.2009.07.012

Cairo S, Armengol C, De Reyniès A et al (2008) Hepatic stem-like phenotype and interplay of Wnt/beta-catenin and Myc signaling in aggressive childhood liver cancer. Cancer Cell 14(6):471–484

Enguita-Germán M, Schiapparelli P, Rey JA et al (2010) CD133+ cells from medulloblastoma and PNET cell lines are more resistant to cyclopamine inhibition of the sonic hedgehog signaling pathway than CD133- cells. Tumour Biol 2010 May 18 [Epub ahead of print]

Lee EY, Ji H, Ouyang Z et al (2010) Hedgehog pathway-regulated gene networks in cerebellum development and tumorigenesis. Proc Natl Acad Sci U S A 107(21):9736–9741, Epub 2010 May 11

Lo Muzio L (2008) Nevoid basal cell carcinoma syndrome (Gorlin syndrome). Orphanet J Rare Dis 3:32, Review

Pazzaglia S (2006) Ptc1 heterozygous knockout mice as a model of multi-organ tumorigenesis. Cancer Lett 234(2):124–134, Epub 2005 May 31. Review

Perilongo G, Maibach R, Shafford E et al (2009) Cisplatin versus cisplatin plus doxorubicin for standard risk hepatoblastoma. N Engl J Med 361(17):1662–1670

Si-Tayeb K, Lemaigre FP, Duncan SA (2010) Organogenesis and development of the liver. Dev Cell 18:175–189

Wandzioch E, Zaret KS (2009) Dynamic signaling network for the specification of embryonic pancreas and liver progenitors. Science 324:1707–1710

Wong SY, Reiter JF (2008) The primary cilium at the crossroads of mammalian hedgehog signaling. Curr Top Dev Biol 85:225–260

Zimmermann A (2005) The emerging family fo hepatoblastoma from ontogenesis to oncogenesis. Eur J Cancer 41(11):1503–1514, Review

Index

A. Zimmermann et al. (eds.), *Pediatric Liver Tumors*, Pediatric Oncology,
DOI: 10.1007/978-3-642-14504-9, © Springer-Verlag Berlin Heidelberg 2011

MIX
Papier aus verantwortungsvollen Quellen
Paper from responsible sources
FSC® C105338

If you have any concerns about our products,
you can contact us on
ProductSafety@springernature.com

In case Publisher is established outside the EU,
the EU authorized representative is:
Springer Nature Customer Service Center GmbH
Europaplatz 3, 69115 Heidelberg, Germany

Printed by Libri Plureos GmbH
in Hamburg, Germany